ANESTHESIA AND THE LUNG

DEVELOPMENTS IN CRITICAL CARE MEDICINE AND ANESTHESIOLOGY

Prakash, O. (ed.): Applied Physiology in Clinical Respiratory Care. 1982.
ISBN 90-247-2662-X.

McGeown, Mary G.: Clinical Management of Electrolyte Disorders. 1983.
ISBN 0-89838-559-8.

Stanley, T.H., and Petty, W.C. (eds.): New Anesthetic Agents, Devices and Monitoring Techniques. 1983. ISBN 0-89838-566-0.

Scheck, P.A., Sjöstrand, U.H., and Smith, R.B. (eds.): Perspectives in High Frequency Ventilation. 1983. ISBN 0-89838-571-7.

Prakash, O. (ed.): Computing in Anesthesia and Intensive Care. 1983.
ISBN 0-89838-602-0.

Stanley, T.H., and Petty, W.C. (eds.): Anesthesia and the Cardiovascular System. 1984. ISBN 0-89838-626-8.

Van Kleef, J.W., Burm, A.G.L., and Spierdijk, J. (eds.): Current Concepts in Regional Anaesthesia. 1984. ISBN 0-89838-644-6.

Prakash, O. (ed.): Critical Care of the Child. 1984. ISBN 0-89838-661-6.

Stanley, T.H., and Petty, W.C. (eds.): Anesthesiology: Today and Tomorrow.
1985. ISBN 0-89838-705-1.

Rahn, H., and Prakash, O. (eds.): Acid-base Regulation and Body Temperature.
1985. ISBN 0-89838-708-6.

Stanley, T.H., and Petty, W.C. (eds.): Anesthesiology. 1986.
1986. ISBN 0-89838-779-5.

de Lange, S., Hennis, P.J., and Kettler, D. (eds.): Cardiac Anaesthesia: Problems and Innovations. 1986. ISBN 0-89838-794-9.

De Bruijn, N.P., and Clements, F.M.: Transesophageal Echocardiography.
1987. ISBN 0-89838-821-X.

Graybar, G.B., and Bready, L.L. (eds.): Anesthesia for Renal Transplantation.
1987. ISBN 0-89838-837-6.

Stanley, T.H., and Petty, W.C. (eds.): Anesthesia, the Heart and the Vascular System. 1987. ISBN 0-89838-851-1.

Ronai, A.K.: Autologous Blood Transfusions. 1988. ISBN 0-89838-899-6.

Stanley, T.H. (ed.): What's New in Anesthesiology. 1988. ISBN 0-89838-367-6.

Woerlee, G.M.: Common Perioperative Problems and the Anaesthetist. 1988.
ISBN 0-89838-402-8.

Stanley, T.H., and Sperry, R.J. (eds.): Anesthesia and the Lung. 1989.
ISBN 0-7923-0075-0.

ANESTHESIA AND THE LUNG

edited by

T.H. STANLEY and R.J. SPERRY

Department of Anesthesiology,
The University of Utah Medical School,
Salt Lake City, Utah, U.S.A.

KLUWER ACADEMIC PUBLISHERS

DORDRECHT / BOSTON / LONDON

Library of Congress Cataloging in Publication Data

Anesthesia and the lung.

   (Developments in critical care medicine and
anaesthesiology)
   "Refresher course manuscripts of the presentations
of the 34th Annual Postgraduate Course in Anesthesiology
which took place at the Cliff Conference Center in
Snowbird, Utah, February 17-21, 1989"--Pref.
   1. Lungs--Diseases--Complications and sequelae--
Congresses. 2. Anesthetics--Pathophysiology--Congresses.
3. Lungs--Effect of drugs on--Congresses. 4. Lungs--
Pathophysiology--Congresses. I. Stanley, Theodore H.
(Theodore Henry), 1940-   . II. Sperry, R. J.
III. Utah Postgraduate Course in Anesthesiology (34th :
1989 : Snowbird, Utah) IV. Series. [DNLM: 1. Anes-
thesia--congresses. 2. Lung--drug effects--congresses.
3. Lung Diseases--congresses. WF 600 A579 1989]
RD87.3.L85A54 1989   617'.96   88-27362
ISBN 978-94-010-6893-2   ISBN 978-94-009-0899-4 (eBook)
DOI 10.1007/978-94-009-0899-4

Published by Kluwer Academic Publishers,
P.O. Box 17, 3300 AA Dordrecht, The Netherlands.

Kluwer Academic Publishers incorporates
the publishing programmes of
D. Reidel, Martinus Nijhoff, Dr W. Junk and MTP Press.

Sold and distributed in the U.S.A. and Canada
by Kluwer Academic Publishers,
101 Philip Drive, Norwell, MA 02061, U.S.A.

In all other countries, sold and distributed
by Kluwer Academic Publishers Group,
P.O. Box 322, 3300 AH Dordrecht, The Netherlands.

PREFACE

Theodore H. Stanley, M.D.

Anesthesia and the Lung contains the Refresher Course manuscripts
of the presentations of the 34th Annual Postgraduate Course in
Anesthesiology which took place at The Cliff Conference Center in
Snowbird, Utah, February 17-21, 1989. The chapters reflect recent
advances in the diagnosis, pre-, intra-, and postoperative anesthetic
management of patients with lung disease, presenting for pulmonary
and non-pulmonary surgery. They also deal with ventilation-perfusion
issues, the lung as a metabolic organ, the effects of anesthesia on
pulmonary mechanics and pulmonary blood flow. In addition there
are chapters that will focus around hypoxia; regional differences in
the lung; pulmonary surfactant; recent advances in the understanding
of pulmonary edema; high altitude disease; anesthesia and the control
of breathing; recent developments in oximetry; instrumentation
designed to measure pulmonary oxygen tension, PO_2 and PCO_2 trans-
cutaneously; differential lung ventilation; reactive airways; septic
shock; the adult respiratory distress syndrome and numerous aspects
of ventilatory support. The purposes of the textbook are to 1) act
as a reference for the anesthesiologists attending the meeting, and
2) serve as a vehicle to bring many of the latest concepts in
anesthesiology to others within a short time of the formal presentation. Each chapter is a brief but sharply focused glimpse of the
interests in anesthesia expressed at the conference. This book and
its chapters should not be considered complete treatises on the
subjects addressed but rather attempts to summarize the most salient
points. This textbook is the seventh in a continuing series document-
ing the proceedings of the Postgraduate Course in Salt Lake City.

We hope that this and the past and future volumes reflect the rapid and continuing evolution of anesthesiology in the late twentieth century.

TABLE OF CONTENTS

LIST OF CONTRIBUTORS

Allen, S.J.
  Department of Anesthesiology, Center for Microvascular and Lymphatic
  Studies, The University of Texas Medical School at Houston, 6431
  Fannin, Houston, TX 77004, U.S.A.

Benumof, J.L.
  Anesthesia Research Lab, T-001, The University of California San
  Diego, La Jolla, CA 92093, U.S.A.

Bone, R.C.
  Department of Medicine, Rush Presbyterian/St. Luke Medical Center,
  Chicago, IL 60612, U.S.A.

Downs, J.B.
  Department of Anesthesiology, The University of South Florida
  College of Medicine, Tampa, FL 33612, U.S.A.

Hornbein, Th.F.
  Department of Anesthesiology, The University of Washington School of
  Medicine, Seattle, WA 98195, U.S.A.

Marshall, B.E.
  Department of Anesthesia, The University of Pennsylvania School of
  Medicine, Philadelphia, PA 19104, U.S.A.

Milic-Emili, J.
  Meakins-Christie Laboratories, McGill University, Montreal, Quebec,
  H3A 2B4, Canada

Nunn, J.F.
  Division of Anesthesia, Clinical Research Center, Harrow, Middlesex,
  U.K.

Severinghaus, J.W.
  Anesthesia Research Center, The University of California, San
  Francisco, School of Medicine, San Francisco, CA 94102, U.S.A.

Stanley, T.H.
  Department of Anesthesiology, The University of Utah Medical School,
  Salt Lake City, UT 84132, U.S.A.

West, J.B.
  Department of Medicine, The University of California San Diego, La
  Jolla, CA 92093-0623, U.S.A.

Zapol, W.M.
  Department of Anesthesia, Massachusetts General Hospital, Boston, MA
  02114, U.S.A.

Zimmerman, G.A.
  Department of Medicine, The University of Utah Medical School, Salt
  Lake City, UT 84132, U.S.A.

REGIONAL DIFFERENCES IN THE LUNG

JOHN B. WEST

Department of Medicine, University of California San Diego, La Jolla CA 92093-0623

Marked differences of ventilation, blood flow, gas exchange, alveolar size, intrapleural pressures and mechanical stresses exist within the human lung and some of these are of special interest to the anesthesiologist in the context of anesthesia and postoperative care.

The base of the normal upright lung is normally better ventilated than the apex. If a normal subject lies supine, the dependent regions of the lung are usually better ventilated, and in the lateral decubitus position, the down lung is also better ventilated. Exceptions to this may occur during anesthesia because of changes in lung volume and alteration in the action of the diaphragm. With increasing age or the development of chronic obstructive lung disease, the base of the upright lung may become poorly ventilated. The same situation is seen when a young normal subject breathes at low lung volumes. This change is caused by the closure of small airways in the dependent regions.

The cause of the topographical differences of ventilation in the lung is not completely understood. However there is strong evidence that the uneven ventilation is due to the weight of the elastic lung and its resulting distortion within the chest. The result is that the basal alveoli are relatively compressed whereas the apical alveoli are relatively overexpanded. During inspiration, the volume of the basal alveoli increase more because of the nonlinear shape of the pressure-volume curve of the lung. However in the aging lung where the intrapleural pressures are generally less negative, the base of the lung may actually be compressed causing airway closure.

1

T. H. Stanley and R. J. Sperry (eds.), Anesthesia and the Lung, 1–2.
© 1989 by Kluwer Academic Publishers.

The regional differences of alveolar expansion are substantial. In experimental animals, and probably in man, the apical alveoli are as much as four times larger by volume than those at the base. The relatively overexpanded lung at the apex is accompanied by very negative intrapleural pressures in that region. There is evidence that the most apical alveoli are subject to particularly large expanding stresses and are therefore liable to develope structural failure if weakened by disease. It is possible that the predilection of centrilobular emphysema and other diseases for the apex of the lung can be explained in this way.

Blood flow also increases from apex to base of the upright lung and the changes of blood flow are larger than those for ventilation. As a consequence the ventilation-perfusion ratio is high at the apex and low at the base of the upright lung. This ratio determines the gas exchange in any region of the lung and as a result, the PO_2 is substantially higher at the apex than base. The changes in PCO_2 are in the opposite direction. These regional differences of gas exchange probably play a role in the development of some diseases. However the deleterious effect on the overall gas efficiency of the lung is trivial.

REFERENCE

1.West, J.B. (editor) <u>Regional Differences in the Lung</u>, NY, Academic Press, 1977. This monograph contains a full list of references to regional papers.

REGULATION OF THE PULMONARY CIRCULATION

BRYAN E. MARSHALL

Department of Anesthesia, University of Pennsylvania School of Medicine, Philadelphia, Pennsylvania 19104

INTRODUCTION

Individual investigations have shown that a wide variety of factors influence the pulmonary circulation. These factors include mechanical ventilation, hydration, cardiac output, pH, PCO_2, PO_2, age, sex, and many drugs and diseases. In practice, however, the changes are often quite subtle and this paradox between the expected changes and the apparent observed outcome can be understood by the recognition of two basic peculiarities of the pulmonary circuit. The first is the fact that the pulmonary circuit is quite unlike the systemic circulation in almost every way (1), it is a high conductance (low resistance), low pressure, high flow system. Large changes in flows can be accommodated with small changes in pressure and conversely small changes in pressure or vascular conductance can represent large changes in physiological or pathophysiological conditions. A 5 mmHg change in blood pressure, which in the systemic circulation would be trivial, in the pulmonary circulation represents the pressure change that accompanies a two-fold increase in cardiac output. The second peculiarity derives from the first; the low hydrostatic pressure, the thin walled vasculature, the presence of the alveolar gas space and the requirements for ventilation all interact with each other in non-linear and unexpected ways (2). The result has often been that the fundamental actions of a drug, disease or ventilatory technique observed in vivo are difficult to interpret. The purpose of this presentation is to provide a way of thinking about the pulmonary circulation that appears to be helpful for assessing these complex interactions. The discussion will focus on steady state pulmonary hemo-dynamics or the factors that determine the relationships between mean pressure and mean flow in the lung. In this context, pulmonary vascular impedance will not be considered, for it is important for cardiac function

3

T. H. Stanley and R. J. Sperry (eds.), Anesthesia and the Lung, 3–15.

4

and the transfer of energy rather than the characteristic that determines blood flow (9).

PULMONARY VASCULAR CONDUCTANCE

The conductance of a tube is calculated by dividing the flow by the difference in pressure between the inlet and the outlet. Resistance is the reciprocal calculation. In the pulmonary circuit, vascular conductance or resistance can be calculated by the same concept and either value gives the equivalent information. In what follows, the term conductance is preferred because pulmonary artery pressure is the independent variable in the pressure-flow relationship (i.e. it is possible to exert pressure without flow, but not the reverse) and conductance is related to the slope of the curve representing this relationship.

It would be helpful if a single value could be assigned for the normal pulmonary vascular conductances, but a little thought soon reveals some serious problems. The first is evident when it is appreciated that most animals, including man, have a normal mean pulmonary artery pressure of about 15-20 cm H_2O independent of size and, therefore, of cardiac output. The conductance values that may be derived not only vary by several orders of magnitude between species, but also vary with body size, age and physical status even in the same species. A simple way to normalize all data by expressing the blood flow in terms of the normal resting value for that individual is described in a later section and satisfactorily removes this difficulty.

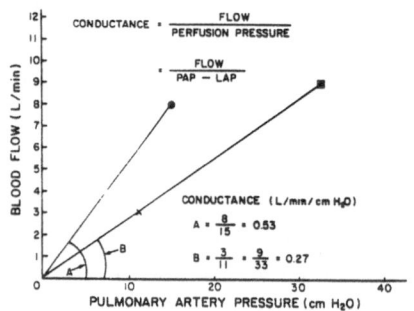

Figure 1.   One relationship for three pressure/flow observations.

The second problem is most easily understood by an example. In Figure
1 are shown three points corresponding to measurements of pulmonary artery
pressure and cardiac output on three different occasions in one
individual. The question is how are the points related? Do they
represent vascular constriction, vascular dilation or the normal pressure-
flow relationship? The most obvious analysis would be the graphical
constriction represented in the figure. Straight lines are drawn
connecting the origin to each of the points and the slope of these lines
is taken to represent the conductance. From this analysis, it would be
assumed that the cross and the filled squares both lie on the same line
and, if the cross is the normal but low flow condition, then the line
might be taken to represent the normal pressure-flow relationship. On
this basis, the increased slope of the line to the filled circle
represents increased conductance resulting from vasodilation. This is
the concept that is used when conductance is calculated clinically by
dividing cardiac output by mean pulmonary artery pressure, but there is a
fallacy underlying this construction because the pressure-flow
relationship is a curve and not a straight line (Figure 2). When a normal

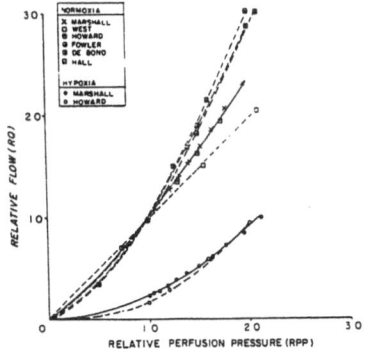

Figure 2.   Pressure-flow curves recalculated for both normoxic and
hypoxic lungs (from references 3-8).

pressure-flow curve is superimposed on the earlier data points, as in
Figure 3, it is apparent that while the cross lies on this curve and,
therefore, represents the normal changes measured under low flow
conditions neither of the other points during high flow conditions are

6

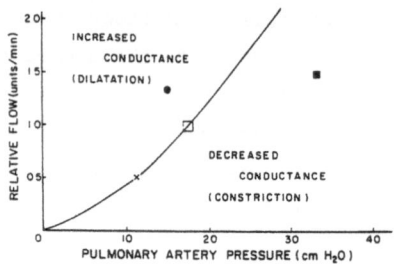

Figure 3. A normal pressure-flow curve is superimposed on the same data as Figure 1.

close to the normal curve. The one to the right represents the values to be expected during vasoconstriction and that to the left during vasodilation.

The implications underlying the curved pressure-flow relationship are illustrated in Figure 4 by considering changes of conductance occurring in simple tubes. As the pulmonary artery pressure increases in the pulmonary circuit the simple rigid tube behavior shown in panel 4a is altered by

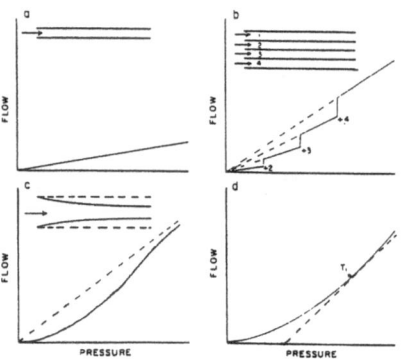

Figure 4   Pressure and Flows in Tubes.

recruitment of new vessels, panel 4b, and/or distension of existing vessels, panel 4c. Both effects undoubtedly occur, but, while in the past the concept of recruitment was preferred, it will become apparent subsequently that distension of the elastic pulmonary vasculature is sufficient to account for the curvature in the practical range of pressure and flow. Either or both mechanisms can lead to the curved pressure-flow relationship shown in panel 4d. The important point about the measurement of conductance at the point T_1 shown in 4d is to understand what it represents. The actual conductance represented by fixed tubes of the same size as existing at the point T_1 would be obtained by the slope of a straight line joining the origin to the point. The slope of the line tangent to the curve at T_1 (shown as a dashed line) combines both the conductance itself and the change of conductance that occurs as the pressure increases, by analogy with muscle mechanics this might be called an incremental conductance. The intercept of the dashed line with the pressure axis has sometimes been given special significance by designating it an opening pressure, but there seems little merit now in this terminology in view of the reduced emphasis on recruitment as the basis for the pressure-flow curve.

The point of this discussion is to emphasize the assumptions that underlie the calculation of conductance in clinical practice. Assuming that vascular conductance is homogenous throughout the lung, the value that is calculated depends only on three parameters; the cardiac output and the mean pressures at the inlet and outlet. For both pressures, it is very important that the anatomic reference for zeroing the pressure transducer be clearly defined, but, while there is little confusion about the measurement of the mean pulmonary artery pressure, there is less certainty about what constitutes the outlet pressure. The outcome of this uncertainty is illustrated in Figure 5 where conductance is calculated with the same values for flow and for pulmonary artery pressure, but with four different choices for the outlet pressure, each of which have

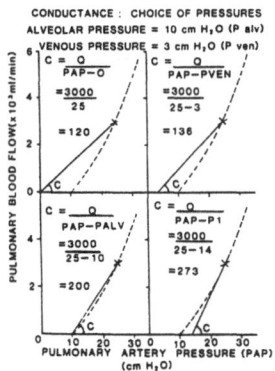

Figure 5.   Calculation of Pulmonary Conductance (or Resistance).

appeared in publication and all of which could be encountered in the same
patient at the same instant. That is to say, values for the conductance
ranging from 120 to 273 units could reasonably be calculated for the same
patient. None of the methods are precisely correct, but the most common
method, that of calculating the perfusion pressure as the difference
between the mean pulmonary artery pressure and the pulmonary artery
occlusion pressure, has the benefit of yielding an intermediate value.

While the calculation of pulmonary conductance (or resistance) may
provide a useful index clinically, to follow gross changes at the bedside,
it should be evident that there are fundamental difficulties in trying to
understand mechanics or interpret data on the basis of this index. The
attempt to represent the interaction of the pulmonary circuit in a single
index results in the loss of much of the information and some other
approach is required if the action of anesthesia is to be adequately
assessed.

A MODEL FOR THE PULMONARY CIRCULATION

The simple diagrams of Figure 4 could be replaced by an accurate
representation of the lung if the number, length, diameter, compliance and
effective viscosity characteristics for each vessel in the lung were
known. This formidable task was systematically approached by Y.C. Fung
and his associates in a series of papers occupying nearly two decades.
This work developed the fundamental equations and the biodynamic data
incorporated into a computer model. The outcome, summarized in a
publication in 1983 (9), was the generation by the computer of a normal
pressure-flow curve for the pulmonary circuit under conditions of normoxia
and the reproduction of experimentally observed changes where the left
atrial, pleural or alveolar pressures were changed.

This model represents a radical change from previous models, all of
which had represented the lungs as rigid tubes or as oversimplified
electrical analogs. The problem with such models is that they are
incapable of providing real insight into mechanics or of realistically
predicting the outcome in conditions other than those for which they were
specifically derived. The model (Figure 6) of Fung and his colleagues is
intellectually much more appealing for the characteristics of the model
are those of the lung vascular components. The model incorporates 11

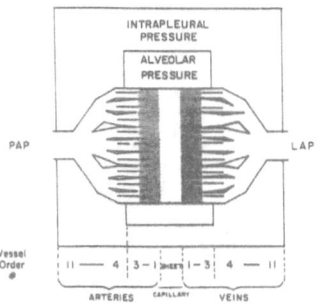

Figure 6. A diagram representing the essential features of the computer model.

orders of arteries and 11 orders of veins and a capillary sheet. The flow through each segment is dependent on the distension of the vessel as determined by its compliance and the transmural pressure. For the larger vessels, the transmural pressure is determined by the difference between the intravascular and the pleural pressure and for the smaller vessels the relevant extravascular pressure is the alveolar pressure. The flow across each tapered segment then determines the perfusion pressure. A single pressure-flow point is calculated by assuming a flow emerging from the pulmonary vein at the outlet pressure. The resting diameter of this vein is increased by the product of the compliance and the transmural pressure at the outlet. The pressure and diameter at the inflow of the first venous segment is then calculated and this intravascular pressure becomes the pressure at the outflow of the next smaller segment. This procedure is continued across the 23 vessel orders until the final pressure, that is the main pulmonary artery is reached.

The entire calculation is then repeated with new values for the cardiac output until a complete pressure-flow curve have been characterized. The variables that need to be stipulated for this procedure include the alveolar and pleural gas pressures and left atrial end diastolic (or outlet) pressure.

GENERALIZATION AND HYPOXIC PULMONARY VASOCONSTRICTION

This model has been modified and adapted in our laboratories as the basis for a model with even greater versatility for analysis of physiologic or pathophysiologic phenomena. The technical details and justification for the modifications have been fully provided elsewhere (10) and are only summarized here. The first modification is to express the flow scale in units relative to the resting value when obtained with the subject breathing oxygen. One effect of this is to generalize the model because the flow ordinate is now independent of size. A flow of 1.0 unit is the normal flow for that individual or group of individuals of any species.

The second modification was to incorporate in the computer model the characteristics of hypoxic pulmonary vasoconstriction. The stimulus for hypoxic pulmonary vasoconstriction (P_{SO2}) has been shown to be a function of the alveolar (P_{AO2}) and mixed venous ($P_{\bar{v}O2}$) oxygen tensions (11). In the computer model, the resting diameter of the smallest six orders of pulmonary arteries were adjusted as a function of the calculated P_{SO2}. The model now required hemoglobin and alveolar and mixed venous oxygen tension. With these modifications, a maximum hypoxic pulmonary vasoconstrictor response corresponding to a P_{SO2} of 30 mmHg produced a shift in the pressure-flow curve to the right in comparison to the curve obtained when the lung was ventilated with oxygen (Figure 7).

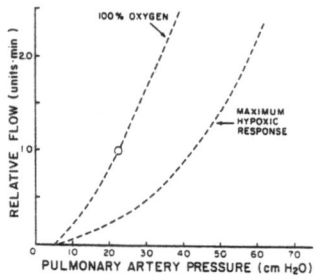

Figure 7. Pressure-flow curves generated by the model for 100% O_2 and a maximum hypoxic response during spontaneous respiration in the awake state.

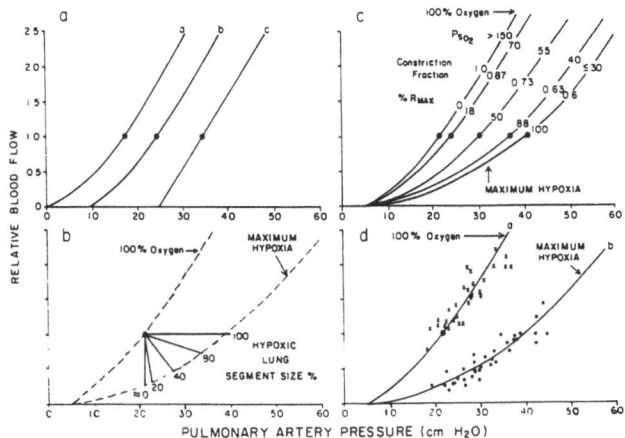

Figure 8   Pulmonary Pressure-Flow Curves.

In Figure 8, the status of the model to this point is summarized.   In panel a are shown three pressure-flow curves that demonstrate the effect that alveolar pressure has on the position of the curve and the even more significant effect that changes in the left atrial or outflow pressure has on both the shape and position of the curve.   Panel 8c demonstrates the graded shift of the pressure-flow curve to the right as the stimulus for HPV increases (i.e. the P_{SO2} is decreased).   While panel 8d shows the good agreement between the pressure-flow curves generated by the computer for 100% oxygen and hypoxic conditions and for data observed under the same conditions.

Panel 8b shows the changes in pressure and flows expected in lung segments of different sizes, but before discussing this, it is necessary to develop further two additional topics.   The real value of utilizing a relative scale for the pulmonary blood flow is demonstrated in Figure 9. The three panels on the left show what happens to pressure and flow when different size segments of the lung are exposed to maximal hypoxic conditions while the rest of the lung (where appropriate) continues to receive 100% oxygen.   When the entire lung is hypoxic, there can be no changes in flow distribution and only the pressure increases.   When smaller segments of the lung are exposed to hypoxia, the constriction in that region results in a reduced blood flow to that region and an increased blood flow to the rest of the lung and obviously an increased

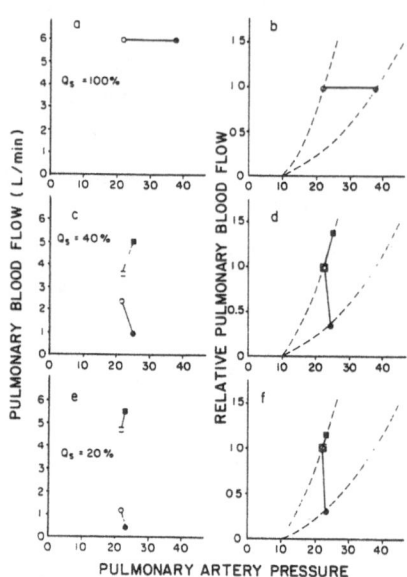

Figure 9   Lung Segment Sizes and the Value of Relative Flow are in absolute units (1/min)

blood pressure that is the same for both segments. When this same data are normalized to relative flow units, as shown on the three panels on the right is Figure 9, the distribution of points is rationalized and easy to understand. The hypoxic lung regions are always on the hypoxic pressure-flow curves, while the hyperoxic rest of the lung remain on the 100% oxygen pressure-flow curve. The position of these points, therefore, provides all the critical information about how effective the hypoxic constriction in diverting blood away from the hypoxic regions as well as showing the increase in pulmonary artery pressure that will result. This is the information that is summarized in panel 8b, with small region of the lung hypoxic flow diversion is very effective and pressure increases are small. This is the most useful homeostatic region where HPV is able to optimize ventilation/perfusion relations and conserve oxygen exchange throughout the lung. When the hypoxic segment becomes large flow diversion is less effective or nonexistent and pressure increases dominate, these are the characteristics of the pathophysiologic outcome of HPV.

In order to utilize these considerations in two lung compartments, with different hypoxic and/or other conditions the model is separated into two with the size of the compartment proportional to the distribution of the blood flow when breathing 100% oxygen. The left lower lobe may receive 25% of the cardiac output normally; such experiments can, therefore, be simulated by initially assigning 25% of the model to the left lower lobe and 75% to the rest of the lung and so on for other models. With these initial conditions, all of the other specific characteristics or conditions of the experiment can be assigned to each compartment. The calculation then proceeds as described before, but now the blood flow distribution is adjusted iteratively until the pulmonary artery pressure derived for each compartment is identical. This procedure defines the pressure and flow distribution between the two compartments.

APPLICATIONS TO PHYSIOLOGY

With these refinements, the predictions of the model can be compared to many experimentally observed results. In Figure 10, the effects of varying the size of the hypoxic segment of the lung or perfusion pressure and flow diversion is illustrated. The close agreement between the computer and the experimental observations is evident and, furthermore,

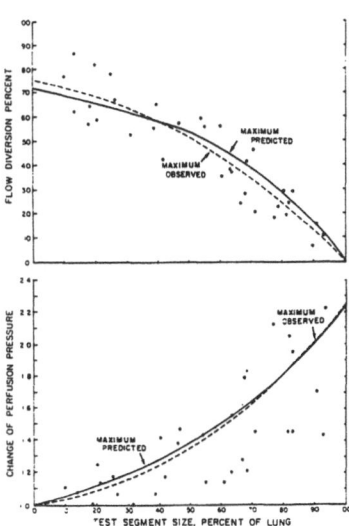

Figure 10. Perfusion pressure and flow diversion responses to hypoxia.

examination of the computer outcome provides an explanation for the
phenomenon that has not been so evident before. First, the reason that
flow diversion is less effective as the segment size is increased, is
attributable to the increased pressure; for, although the same hypoxic
stimulus is assumed to induce the same reduction in the resting diameter
of the smallest six orders of pulmonary arteries, these vessels are
progressively enlarged as the pulmonary artery pressure increases. This
effect is greater on the hypoxic vessels, both because changes in diameter
are magnified the smaller the initial diameter and because the relaxed
vessels soon achieve a maximum diameter limit beyond which they do not
expand.

Another effect that had been observed experimentally, but for which the
physiologic basis had been uncertain, was the observation that the
response to hypoxia was reduced when the pressure in the pulmonary circuit
was raised (12). The data and model simulation shown in Figure 11
demonstrates that the phenomenon is the result primarily of increasing the

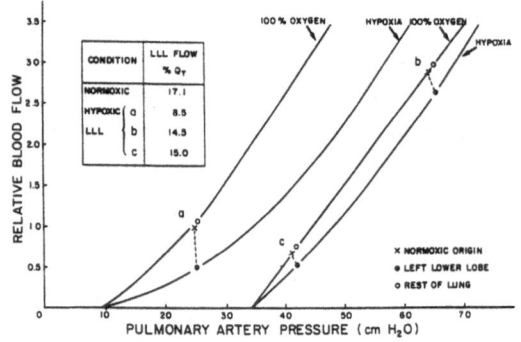

Figure 11. Influence of left atrial pressure on HPV responses.

pressure at the outlet which results in a reduction of the difference in
vascular conductance between the normoxic and hypoxic regions because for
both segments, the vasculature is fully distended.

ACKNOWLEDGEMENT

This work supported in part by grant #GM29628 from the Institute of
General Medical Sciences, NIH.

REFERENCES

1. Harris P. and Heath D. The human pulmonary circulation. Churchill Livingstone, New York, 1986.
2. Fung Y.C. Circulation. Springer-Verlag, New York, 1984.
3. De Bono E.F. and Caro C.G. Am J Physiol 205:1178-1186, 1963.
4. Fowler N.O. Am J Med 47:1-6, 1969.
5. Hall P.W. Circ Res 238-241, 1953.
6. Howard P., Barer G.R., Thompson B., Warren P.M., Abbott C.J. and Mungall I.P.F. Respir Physiol 24:325-345, 1975.
7. Marshall B.E., Marshall C., Benumof J. and Saidman L.J. J Appl Physiol 51:1543-1551, 1981.
8. West J.B. and Dollery C.T. J Appl Physiol 20:175-183, 1965
9. Zhuang F.Y., Fung Y.C. and Yen R.T. J Appl Physiol 55:1341-1348, 1983
10. Marshall B.E. and Marshall C. J Appl Physiol 64:68-77, 1988.
11. Marshall B.E. and Marshall C. J Appl Physiol 55:711-716, 1983.
12. Rehder K. and Marsh M.M. Pulmonary Gas Exchange: Organism and Environment. Academic Press, New York, 1980, pp. 149-185.
13. Marshall B.E. In Anesthesia for Thoracic Procedures (Eds. B.E. Marshall, D.E. Longnecker, H.B. Fairley), Blackwell Scientific, Boston, 1982, pp. 73-118.
14. Marshall B.E. and Marshall C. Effects of Anesthesia. American Physiological Society, Bethesda, 1985, pp. 121-136.

NEW CONCEPTS IN THE REGULATION OF THE PULMONARY VASCULATURE: BIOCHEMICAL ACTIVITIES OF ENDOTHELIAL CELLS THAT INFLUENCE PULMONARY VASCULAR TONE AND BLOOD FLOW

G.A. Zimmerman, MD

Department of Medicine, University of Utah School of Medicine
Salt Lake City, Utah

INTRODUCTION

In contrast to an earlier view that the intima is an inert and passive part of blood vessels, it is now known that it is composed of responsive cells that have the potential to carry out a variety of functions. Biochemical and biologic activities of pulmonary endothelial cells (EC) contribute substantially to the "nonrespiratory" functions of the lung, including several that have clinical significance (1,2). A new concept in vascular cell biology and physiology is that EC of the pulmonary and systemic vascular beds can become "activated" - that is, alter their functional state so that basal, constitutive activities are augmented or new activities are induced - in responses to signals from the local environment (3). Such activation responses may influence the interactions of EC with humoral components of the blood, with blood cells, such as leukocytes or platelets (3), or with smooth muscle cells (4), resulting local or regional changes in vascular function. One type of activation response of EC that is particularly important in cell-cell interactions is the production of autacoids, which are potent biologically-active molecules that act in exquisitely low concentrations over short distances (i.e., in general, they do not circulate in the blood as do hormones) to induce or modulate biochemical or biologic events.

T. H. Stanley and R. J. Sperry (eds.), Anesthesia and the Lung, 17–28.

TABLE 1: AUTACOIDS SYNTHESIZED BY HUMAN ENDOTHELIAL CELLS

1. Prostacyclin (PGI_2) and other eicosanoids
2. Platelet-activating factor (PAF)
3. Endothelium-derived relaxation factors (EDRFs)
4. Endothelium-derived constricting factors (EDCFs)
5. Cytokines (Interleukin-1, platelet-derived growth factor, granulocyte and macrophage colony stimulating factors).

The concept that endothelial products can directly, or indirectly, alter vascular smooth muscle (SMC) tone and activity and thereby regulate local blood flow, hydrostatic pressure, and consequent events (transvascular flux of fluid, delivery of cellular and humoral mediators to areas of inflammation, removal of cellular aggregates or fluid-phase mediators in the flowing blood, etc) has evolved during this decade (5,6) (Table 2); it is changing our views of vascular regulation in physiologic and pathologic conditions, and concepts of pharmacologic manipulation of vascular tone (7).

TABLE 2: CONCEPTS OF VASCULAR REGULATION

1960's   Physical and humoral "signals" are sensed by vascular smooth muscle cells, resulting in changes in tone; EC are inert "bystanders".

1970's   EC metabolize vasoactive mediators (example: conversion of angiotensin I to angiotensin II and degradation of bradykinin by angiotensin converting enzyme in EC plasma membrane), regulating their local and systemic concentrations; "sensing" of signals and primary regulation of vascular tone is at the level of SMC.

1980's   EC generate autacoids that influence SMC activity; EC can "sense" vasoactive signals (changes in pressure or flow; humoral mediators) and "transduce" them into biochemical messages that alter vascular tone. The effect of a mediator or drug that alters vascular tone may involve its direct interaction with EC, SMC, or both. Injury to EC (i.e., pulmonary vascular injury in Adult Respiratory Distress Syndrome, systemic vascular atherosclerosis, etc) alters their influence on SMC activity, potentially turning a vasodilatory signal into one that causes constriction.

The following are capsule summaries of current information on biologically-active mediators that are synthesized by EC that can influence vascular tone and blood flow.

PROSTACYCLIN AND OTHER EICOSANOIDS.

Prostacyclin is one of a remarkable number of biologically-active lipids that are synthesized by human EC (Table 3). It is not produced constitutively or stored by EC, but rather is rapidly synthesized (within seconds) in a regulated fashion from arachidonic acid that is released from membrane phospholipids when the EC are stimulated by an appropriate agonist (8). PGI_2 is released into the fluid phase (i.e., into incubation buffer in vitro or the blood in vivo), where it undergoes rapid non-enzymatic conversion into the biologically-inactive product, $6\text{-}ketoPGF_{1\alpha}$. PGI_2 is a potent inhibitor of platelet adherence and aggregation and a powerful vasodilator (8). The role of PGI_2 in the regulation of systemic and pulmonary vascular tone has been extensively reviewed (1,8,9) and will not be repeated in detail here. In general, the evidence is that PGI_2 is not a circulating hormone that regulates vascular pressure and flow under basal conditions, but that it is released in pathologic states and may have important local vasomotor effects by counteracting vasoconstrictor stimuli, by preventing vasospasm and mechanical obstruction resulting from platelet and/or neutrophil aggregation, and by increasing blood flow in inflammation (1). However, it has also been suggested that continuous generation of PGI_2 contributes to the low basal pulmonary vascular resistance; in addition, it may modulate hypoxic pulmonary vasoconstriction (9,10). Exogenous PGI_2 administered by continuous infusion is evolving as an important adjunct in the management of carefully-selected patients with pulmonary hypertension (11).

TABLE 3: BIOLOGICALLY-ACTIVE LIPIDS PRODUCED BY HUMAN EC*

1. Prostacyclin
2. Prostaglandin E_2 (PGE_2)
3. Platelet-activating factor
4. 15-hydroxyeicosatetraeonic acid (15-HETE)
5. 8,15-dihydroxyeicosatetraenoic acid (8,15-diHETE)
   (*Modified from reference 3.)

Although human EC synthesize certain other eicosanoids (oxygenated products of arachidonic acid) besides PGI_2 (Table 3), there is no evidence that they directly synthesize the important class of eicosanoids termed leukotrienes (LTA_4, LTB_4, LTC_4, LTD_4, LTE_4). However, leukotrienes may influence vascular function. For example, human EC have membrane receptors for LTC_4 and LTD_4 (which can be released from other activated cells, such as mononuclear phagocytes), and cultured human EC synthesize PGI_2 and PAF in response to these sulfidopeptide leukotrienes (3). The synthesis of PGI_2 occurs in a burst that is over in a few minutes, whereas the synthesis of PAF continues for over an hour; furthermore, PGI_2 is released into the fluid phase, whereas PAF is retained by the EC (see below) (3,12). These features provide the basis for differential temporal and spatial effects of the autacoids, PGI_2 and PAF, synthesized by EC in response to LTC_4 or LTD_4. In addition, LTC_4 and LTD_4 induce the endothelial cell-dependent binding of activated neutrophils (PMNs) (3). These observations demonstrate that LTC_4 and LTD_4 can indirectly influence vascular tone by causing the local generation of autacoids (i.e., PAF) or by inducing the recruitment and activation of PMNs, which release vasoactive agents (for example, superoxide anion, H_2O_2, etc). LTC_4 and LTD_4 may also have a direct effect on vascular SMC, causing vasoconstriction. The major response to the infusion of these leukotrienes into the pulmonary vascular circuit of experimental animals is an increase in vascular resistance (9).

While there is no evidence that LTC_4 or LTD_4 is directly synthesized by human EC (apparently EC lack the 5-lipoxygenase required for the initial step in the synthesis of leukotrienes from arachidonate), they may be able to synthesize LTC_4 from LTA_4 supplied by adjacent leukocytes (13). If this conversion occurs in vivo, it provides a mechanism for the local generation of sulfidopeptide leukotrienes by EC. In addition, the release of these eicosanoids from inflammatory cells may influence vascular responses in pathologic conditions such as myocardial infarction (14).

The potential role of leukotrienes and other eicosanoids in the vascular events of shock has been recently reviewed (15).

ENDOTHELIUM-DERIVED RELAXING FACTOR.

A number of physiologically-relevant compounds, in addition to certain pharmacologic agents, relax arterial smooth muscle by an indirect effect that is dependent on an intact, uninjured endothelium (Table 4) (4-6). The original observation by Furchgott (5) resolved a curious discrepancy in vascular pharmacology: acetylcholine (ACH) injected into intact organisms caused vasodilation, whereas it caused vasoconstriction when applied to the surface of isolated vessels. Furchgott showed that the latter effect was due to EC injury, or denudation, and that ACH caused vasodilation of carefully-handled, isolated vessels that had intact endothelium. Furthermore, ACH caused vasoconstriction of the vessls after the endothelium was removed by scraping. Subsequently, many laboratories have confirmed the observaton that in situ and cultured EC release into the fluid phase one or more labile activities that act on vascular smooth muscle (and SMC from certain other sites) to cause relaxation. The activities are termed endothelium-derived relaxation factor(s) (EDRFs). Their effect appears to be greatest in arterial vessels, although they also cause vasodilation in veins (4); in all preparations, the effect of EDRF is most obvious if the vascular segment is preconstricted with an appropriate pharmacologic agent.

TABLE 4: AGENTS THAT CAUSE EDRF SYNTHESIS AND RELEASE BY EC

A. "Physiological" Agonists:

1. Acetylcholine
2. Histamine
3. Vasopressin
4. Epinephrine
5. ADP, ATP
6. Bradykinin
7. Serotonin
8. Thrombin
9. Vasoactive intestinal peptide
10. Shear stress

B. Pharmacologic Agonists:

1. Calcium ionophore A23187
2. Arachidonic acid
3. Hydralazine, others

(From references 6 and 16. There is considerable variation from species to species, and between different vessels from the same species.)

The observations to date indicate that, in EC from an appropriately-responsive vessel, the interaction of one of the physiologic agonists shown in Table 4 with its receptor on the EC surface results in a series of signal transduction events, including the generation of inositol 1,4,5-trisphosphate and the release of Ca++ from intracellular stores, followed by the synthesis and release of EDRF (6). The identity of EDRF was unknown for several years, although its activity could be separated from that of PGI_2 and other eicosanoids. Recently it has been concluded that EDRF is nitric oxide (6,17), synthesized by the activated EC from endogenous L-arginine (18). Both exogenous nitric oxide (NO), and EDRF generated by EC, appear to cause smooth muscle relaxation by inducing activation of soluble guanylate cyclase and an increase in cyclic GMP in the SMC (4,6,16). This is also the apparent mechanism of relaxation induced by pharmacologic agents that act directly on the SMC, such as nitrates (7). There is evidence that EDRF can also cause the disaggregation of platelets and inhibit their adherence to EC by increasing intracellular cyclic GMP levels.

Although there is considerable evidence supporting the identity of EDRF as NO, this conclusion remains controversial. In addition, experimental observations support the possibility that there is more than one molecular species of EDRF that is distinct from PGI_2 and other biologically-active lipids (6).

A major difficulty in judging the clinical relevance of many of the studies of EDRF is that, in addition to the fact that the most compelling experiments have been in in vitro preparations, there is significant interspecies variation (16). However, it has been shown that isolated human vessels undergo endothelial-dependent relaxation (19), and there is evidence for EC-dependent relaxation of coronary arteries of living patients that is lost (causing vasodilators such as ACH to have no effect or to induce vasoconstriction) when the vessels become atherosclerotic (20-22). The latter finding is consistent with observations that low-density lipoprotein inhibits endothelium-dependent relaxation in vitro (23)..

Endothelium-dependent vascular relaxation has been demonstrated in pulmonary vessels from experimental animals (17,24,41). To date, no relevant observations have been reported in humans.

ENDOTHELIN, AN ENDOTHELIUM-DERIVED CONTRACTING FACTOR.

Experiments using protocols similar to those outlined above have indicated that, under certain conditions, EC generate vasoconstrictor activities as well as autacoids that induce vasodilation. Early experiments were done with isolated canine systemic and pulmonary veins; additional observations indicate that rapid stretch can cause EC-dependent constriction of cerebral arteries (4). In general, the EC-dependent constriction is more pronounced in veins than arteries (25). Hypoxia or anoxia potentiates the vasoconstriction (4).

Until recently, the identity of endothelium-dependent contracting factor (EDCF) was unknown. However, a candidate molecule, termed "endothelin", has been identified (26). It is a 21 amino acid peptide that is constitutively synthesized and secreted into the medium of cultured EC. Endothelin has been cloned and sequenced; its primary structure is similar to peptide neurotoxins that act on voltage-dependent ion channels, suggesting that endothelin may be an endogenous agonist of the dihydropyridine-sensitive Ca^{++} channels of SMC (26). Messenger RNA for endothelin is present in both in situ and cultured porcine EC; its level is increased within an hour of adding thrombin or calcium ionophore A23187 to cultured cells (26). This, and the fact that it appears that little endothelin is stored in EC (26), suggest that its release is regulated primarily at the translational level.

The time courses of production and degradaton of EDRF and endothelin are different, even though the release of both may be induced by the same humoral, or hemodynamic, stimulus (4,26). EDRF is produced rapidly and is labile, whereas endothelin is constitutively synthesized, its enhanced production occurs over a longer period, and it is stable (26). Thus endothelin may contribute to long-term regulation of vascular tone and EDRF to rapid, local modulation.

PLATELET-ACTIVATING FACTOR.

Platelet-activating factor (PAF) is the trivial name for 1-O-alkyl-2-acetyl-sn-glycero-3-phosphocholine, a biologically-active phospholipid (27). It has unusual structural features, including an ether bond at the sn-1 position and a short chain acetate group at the sn-2 position, and can activate a variety of human "target" cells - not just platelets - by interacting with putative cell surface receptors (27). The latter property has led to the hypothesis that it acts as a physiologic mediator of cell-cell interactions. However, it is clear from a variety of experiments in animals and humans that it can have pathologic effects if it is produced in an unregulated fashion, in inappropriate locations, or in the absence of molecules that oppose or modify its actions (Table 5).

TABLE 5: IN VIVO BIOLOGIC ACTIVITIES OF PAF.

1. Anaphylaxis (rabbits, baboons)
2. Hypotension (rats, dogs, rabbits)
3. Increased vascular permeability (rabbits, humans)
4. Negative inotropic effects (dogs)
5. Coronary vasoconstriction (swine)
6. Decreased renal blood flow, GFR (dogs)
7. Pulmonary hypertension and edema (rabbits, dogs, sheep)
8. Bronchospasm (guinea pigs, baboons)
9. Leukopenia, thrombocytopenia (rabbits, baboons)
10. Thrombosis (guinea pigs)

PAF has complex cardiovascular effects. In general, injection of high concentrations of PAF into the pulmonary or systemic circulation causes vasconstriction (9,28,29). However, careful studies in intact animals demonstrate biphasic effects on vascular pressure and blood flow (28), and under some conditions PAF may cause vasodilation (30). This suggests that, in appropriately low concentrations, endogenous PAF may act to maintain the low tonic pressure in the pulmonary bed (9). Under some conditions PAF can cause hypotension and shock (14) via direct and indirect effects on systemic vascular tone, on the heart and coronary circulation, and on vascular permeability (14,28,29). Thus, an understanding of its sites of synthesis and the factors that regulate it is important.

PAF is synthesized by a variety of human cell types (27), including EC (3,12,31). PAF has been shown to be synthesized by cultured human EC from umbilical vein, umbilical artery, pulmonary artery, aorta (unpublished observation) and from microvessels (3), and by cultured and in situ endothelium from a variety of bovine vessels (31). No PAF is constitutively produced in EC, nor is it stored in the cells (3,31); rather, it is rapidly (within seconds) synthesized when certain ligands (Table 6) interact with cell surface receptors on the EC, resulting in activation of a guanyl nucleotide-binding regulatory protein ("G protein"), an influx of extracellular calcium, and activation of key synthetic enzymes (phospholipase A_2, and a specific acetyltransferase) (3,32). PAF is raidly degraded by a family of intracellular and extracellular acetylhydrolyses, including one that is found in human plasma (33). Thus, there is a complex series of mechanisms to control its accumulation, again suggesting that its regulated synthesis is a physiologic event. However, some of these regulatory mechanisms may be bypassed under pathologic conditions. For example, hydrogen peroxide, which is an important mediator of oxidant and reperfusion vascular injury, and which does not interact with a cell surface receptor, can induce PAF synthesis by EC (32) (Table 6).

TABLE 6: AGONISTS FOR PAF PRODUCTION BY CULTURED OR IN SITU EC.

A. RECEPTOR-MEDIATED AGONISTS:

Thrombin*
Histamine*
Bradykinin*+
Leukotriene C_4*
Leukotriene D_4*
Angiotensin II+
ATP*+
ADP+

B. AGENTS THAT DO NOT INTERACT WITH RECEPTORS

Hydrogen peroxide*+
Clostridial theta toxin*+
Mellitin (Hymenoptera venom*+
C5b-9 (membrane attack complex of complement)*+

(* = agonist for human EC; + = agonist for bovine EC. This list includes agents that have been studied in our laboratory [3,31,32]. Others have reported that endotoxin, interleukin 1, and tumor necrosis factor a induce PAF synthesis by human EC [3])

PAF is not released into the fluid phase bathing the apical surface of EC activated by receptor-mediated agonists; most, if not all, of the phospholipid remains associated with the cells (3,31). This, and other observations (34), suggest that PAF is not an "EDRF" or "EDCF", although it is possible that PAF is transfered directly to SMC via interdigitations between EC and smooth muscle cells that span the basement membrane of the intima (4). Furthermore, the possibility that PAF is released into the fluid phase at the abluminal surface of the EC has not been completely excluded.

The observation that PAF remains associated with stimulated EC suggests that it has intracellular functions (for example, as a "second messenger"), and/or that it is a cell-associated mediator of cell-cell interactions. The latter hypothesis would require that some, or all, of the newly-synthesized PAF be localized in the plasma membrane of activated EC where it would be in a position to interact with "target" cells. Several pieces of evidence support this possibility, among them the observation that agonists that induce PAF synthesis by EC also induce endothelial cell-dependent neutrophil adhesion (enhanced adhesion of neutrophils that is initiated by activation of the EC, rather than the leukocytes) (43,12,35); the EC-dependent PMN adhesion is tightly coupled to PAF synthesis in terms of the spectrum of agonists and their specificities and concentration-dependencies, the time course of PAF accumulation and the development and reversal of EC-dependent neutrophil adhesion, and other features. Furthermore, the neutrophil adhesion is blocked by specific, competitive PAF receptor antagonists. Thus, the evidence suports the hypothesis that PAF that is synthesized by activated EC can interact with neutrophils, resulting in their adhesion to the EC surface. Some of the PMNs then undergo an activation response, evidenced by alterations in their morphology (12,35); it is likely that these leukocytes release increased quantities of superoxide anion (which can inactivate EDRF; Ref 3), hydrogen peroxide (which can stimulate additional PAF production and have direct vasoactive effects), and other mediators. Thus, this is a potential mechanism by which PAF that is endogenously synthesized by activated EC can indirectly influence vascular tone and blood flow.

Although PAF appears to be retained by EC and most other human cell types, it is released into the fluid phase by human monocytes (36).

Thus the monocyte, particularly monocytes adherent to activated EC, may be the major source of circulating PAF in septic shock. Several recent reports suggest that PAF is a critical mediator of injury to the lung and other tissues in sepsis (37-39), as well as in anaphylaxis (40) and other pathologic conditions (14,27).

REFERENCES

1. Zimmerman, G.A. in <u>Anesthesiology: Today and Tomorrow</u>. (Eds. T.H. Stanley and W.C. Petty). Martinus Nijhoff Publishers, Dordrecht,1985, pp 11-22
2. Ryan, U.S. Annu. Rev. Physiol. 44:223-239, 1982
3. Zimmerman, G.A., Whatley, R.E., McIntyre T.M., and Prescott, S.M. Am. Rev. Resp. Dis. 136:204-207, 1987
4. Vanhoutte, P.M., Rubanyi, G.M., Miller, V.M., and Houston, D.S. Annu. Rev. Physiol. 48:307-320, 1986
5. Furchgott, R.F., and Zawadski, J.V. Nature 288:373-376, 1980
6. Vanhoutte, P.M. Nature 327:459-460, 1987
7. Zelis, R. Am. J. Med 74:3-12, (Supplement) June 27, 1983
8. Majerus, P.W. J. Clin. Invest. 72:1521-1525, 1983
9. Voelkel, N.F., Chang, S.W., McDonnell, T.J., Westcott, J.Y., and Haynes, J. Am. Rev. Resp. Dis. 136:214-127, 1987
10. Meyrick, B., Niedermeyer, M.E., Ogletree, M.L., and Brigham, K.L. J. Appl. Physiol. 59:443-452, 1985
11. Higgenbottam, T. Am. Rev. Res. Dis. 1136:782-784, 1987
12. McIntyre, T.M., Zimmerman, G.A., and Prescott, S.M. Proc. Nat. Acad. Sci. USA 83:2204-2208, 1986
13. Claesson, H., and Haeggstrom, J. in <u>Advances in Prostaglandin, Thromboxane, and Leukotriene Research</u>, Vol 17. (Eds. B. Samuelsson, R. Paoletti, and P.W. Ramwell) Raven Press, New York, 1987, pp 115-119
14. Evers, A.S., Murphee, S., Saffitz, J.E., Jakschik, B.A., and Needleman, P.J. Clin. Invest. 75:992-999, 1985
15. Feuerstein, G., and Hallenbeck, J.M. Annu. Rev. Pharmacol. Toxicol. 27:301-313, 1987
16. Peach, M.J., Loeb, A.L., Singer, H.A., and Saye, T. Hypertension 7 (Suppl I):I-94-I-100, 1985
17. Palmer, R.M.J., Ferridge, A.G., and Moncada, S. Nature 327:524-526,1987
18. Palmer, R.M.J., Ashton, D.S., and Moncada, S. Nature 333:664-667, 1988
19. Bossalier, C., Habib, G.B., Yamamoto H., Williams, C., Wells, S., and Henry, P.D. J. Clin. Invest. 79:170-174, 1987

20. Ludmer, P.L., Selwyn, A.P., Shook, T.L., Wayne, R.R., Mudge, G.H., Alexander, R.W., and Ganz, P. New Eng. J. Med. 315:1046-1051, 1986

21. Harrison, D.G., Armstrong, M.L., Freiman, P.C., and Heistad, D.D. J. Clin. Invest. 80:1808-1811, 1987

22. Fish, R.D., Nabel, E.G., Selwyn, A.P., Ludmer, P.L., Mudge, G.H., Kirschenbaum, J.M., Schoen, F.J., Alexander, R.W., and Ganz, P. J. Clin. Invest. 81:21-31, 1988

23. Andrews, H.E., Bruckdorfer, K.R, Dunn, R.C., and Jacobs, M. Nature 327:237-239, 1987

24. Chand, N., and Altura, B.M. Science 213:1376-1379, 1981

25. DeMay, J.G., and Vanhoutte, P.M. Circ. Res. 51:439-447, 1982

26. Yanagishawa, M., Kurihara, H., Kimura, S., et al. Nature 332:411-415, 1988

27. Hanahan, D.J. Annu. Rev. Biochem. 55:483-509, 1986

28. Kenzura, J.L., Perez, J.E., Bergmann, S.R., and Lange, L.G. J. Clin. Invest. 74:1193-1203, 1984

29. Burhop, K.E., Van Der Zee, H., Bizios, R., Kaplan, J.E., and Malik, A.B. Am. Rev. Resp. Dis. 134:548-554, 1986

30. McMurtry, I., and Morris, K.G. Am. Rev. Resp. Dis. 134:757-762, 1986

31. Whatley, R.E., Zimmerman, G.A., McIntyre, T.M., and Prescott, S.M. Arteriosclerosis 8:321-331, 1988

32. Whatley, R.E., Lewis, M.S., Zimmerman, G.A., McIntyre, T.M., Parker, C.J., Stevens, D.L., and Prescott, S.M. Chest 93 (Suppl):110S-111S, 1988

33. Stafforini, D., McIntyre, T.M., Carter, M.E., and Prescott, S.M. J. Biol. Chem. 262:4215-4222, 1987

34. McIntyre, T.M., Zimmerman, G.A., Satoh, K., and Prescott, S.M. J. Clin. Invest. 76:271-280, 1985

35. Zimmerman, G.A., McIntyre, T.M., and Prescott, S.M. J. Clin. Invest. 76:2235-2246, 1985

36. Elstad, M.R., Prescott, S.M., McIntyre, T.M., and Zimmerman, G.A. J. Immunol. 140:1618-1624, 1988

37. Doebber, T.W., Wu, M.S., Robbins, J.C., Choy, B.M., Chang, M.N., and Shen, T.Y. Biochem. Biophys. Res. Comm. 127:799-808, 1985

38. Chang, S., Feddersen, C.O., Henson, P.M., and Voelkel, N.F. J. Clin. Invest. 79:1498-1509, 1987

39. Sun, X., and Hsueh, W. J. Clin. Invest. 81:1328-1331, 1988

40. Darius, H., Lefer, D.J., Smith, J.B., and Lefer, A. M. Science 232:58-60, 1986

41. Feddersen, C.O., McMurtry, I.F., Henson, P., and Voelkel, N.F. Am. Rev. Resp. Dis. 133:197-204, 1986

PATHOPHYSIOLOGY OF PULMONARY EDEMA: IMPLICATIONS FOR CLINICAL MANAGEMENT

STEVEN J. ALLEN

Department of Anesthesiology, Center for Microvascular and Lymphatic Studies, The University of Texas Medical School at Houston, 6431 Fannin, Houston, Texas

INTRODUCTION

Any understanding of the formation of pulmonary edema requires a familiarity with equations governing lung fluid balance. The one most often discussed is called the Starling equation. A review of the history of this equation makes understanding much easier. Ernest Starling (1866-1927) was a prolific investigator who made major contributions in the areas of cardiovascular, endocrine, gut, nutritional, and microvascular physiology. His work on the formation of lymph was performed early in his career. At the age of 31, he had developed the concept that led to the current form of the Starling equation. Starling's major contribution was the realization that the osmotic pressure exerted by the plasma proteins prevented the formation of edema by counterbalancing the hydrostatic pressure in the vessels. He observed that a decrease in the plasma protein concentration led to the development of edema. Thus, Starling's concept was:

$$Jv = Pc - \pi c \tag{1}$$

where Jv is the rate of fluid flux out of the capillary, Pc is the capillary hydrostatic pressure and πc is the colloid osmotic pressure. Subsequent investigators realized that the interstitial space outside the capillary had its own hydrostatic and colloid pressures as well. Thus, the driving pressures were a result of the differences between the capillary and interstitial pressures as shown in Equation 2.

$$Jv = (Pc-Pt) - (\pi c-\pi t) \tag{2}$$

29

T. H. Stanley and R. J. Sperry (eds.), Anesthesia and the Lung, 29–39.
© 1989 by Kluwer Academic Publishers.

where Pt and πt represent the interstitial (tissue) hydrostatic and colloid osmotic pressures, respectively. Next, the permeability of the capillary membrane to the plasma proteins was recognized as an important factor in fluid exchange. If the membrane became more permeable, then the plasma proteins would exert less of an effect on fluid filtration. The equation was then written:

$$Jv = (Pc-Pt) - \sigma(\pi c - \pi t) \tag{3}$$

where (σ) represents the reflection coefficient. This number represents the fraction of plasma proteins that is "reflected" by the capillary membrane. Finally, an attempt was made to quantitate the amount of fluid that would cross a membrane. In order to determine this, some mechanical properties of the membrane need to be included in the equation. One needs to know the physical ability for water to cross the membrane as well as the surface area of the membrane. The product of these terms is called the filtration coefficient and is represented by Kf. Thus, the current Starling equation is written as:

$$Jv = Kf \, [(Pc-Pt) - \sigma(\pi c - \pi t)] \tag{4}$$

We will discuss each of the components in detail and consider the implications of their manipulation.

COMPONENTS OF STARLING EQUATION

Pulmonary capillary hydrostatic pressure (Pc) represents the major force driving fluid out of the capillary and into the interstitium. The pulmonary capillary wedge pressure (PCWP) is sometimes confused with Pc. In many clinical situations, PCWP represents our best estimate of left atrial pressure (LAP). In order for fluid to flow from the right side of the heart through the lungs and into the left atrium, LAP must be lower than the upstream Pc. In the normal individual, the gradient between the two is so small that they are within a mmHg or two of each other. In congestive heart failure, the pressure rises in the left atrium due to decreased contractility and fluid retention. This pressure elevation is transmitted upstream resulting in an increase in Pc. If the increase is sufficient, fluid enters into the interstitium fast enough to cause pulmonary edema. This mechanism of pulmonary

edema is commonly referred to as "cardiogenic," the implication
being that elevations in Pc are due to, and reflected by, the PCWP.
The degree to which PCWP approaches Pc depends upon the amount
of postcapillary resistance in the pulmonary circulation. In some
cases of pulmonary hypertension, postcapillary resistance may rise
markedly with subsequent widening of the Pc and PCWP difference.
Further, there is evidence that in sepsis, Pc may rise while PCWP
falls. Thus, in some instances, hydrostatic edema may be
accompanied by a normal or low PCWP.

A major problem with lung fluid balance studies is the difficulty in measuring Pc. Pc has been estimated in intact animals
based on data taken from isolated lung preparations. However, the
isolated preparation does not accurately reflect the in vivo
situation. Recently, a technique for estimating Pc has been
reported based on the tracing obtained as a pulmonary artery
balloon is inflated. This technique gives Pc values similar to those
found by direct methods in isolated lungs. Computer analysis may
be necessary to optimize the reproducibility of this method. Normal
Pc is probably around 8 mmHg.

Tissue hydrostatic pressure (Pt) is the hydrostatic force
outside the capillary that opposes Pc. The wider the difference
between these two values, the greater the force to drive fluid out
of the capillary. The lung is one of the few tissues where the Pt is
felt to be negative (probably around -7 mmHg), although there is
much disagreement as to the correct value. Pt changes little (3-5
mmHg) in pulmonary edema.

Capillary colloid osmotic pressure (πc) represents the osmotic
force generated by the plasma proteins that do not easily pass
through the capillary membrane. πc is the major force that opposes
Pc. Thus, simply a drop in πc results in an increase in fluid flux
out of the capillary (Jv) and may enhance the formation of edema.
Guyton and Lindsey studied the effect of πc on the amount of
pulmonary edema formed in dogs with experimentally induced LAP
elevations. In control dogs, πc was 24 mmHg and LAP had to be
raised above 24 mmHg to produce edema. They then lowered the πc
in another group of dogs to 11 mmHg. Pulmonary edema occurred

in these hypoproteinemic dogs with LAP's of only 12 mmHg. Thus, πc is a major determinant of the degree of LAP elevation that results in edema. Direct measurement of πc involves the use of an artificial membrane of arbitrary pore sizes while the capillary membrane consists of pores of various sizes. Thus, the artificial membrane does not exactly reproduce the capillary membrane. Because of this, many investigators measure the protein concentration and calculate the πc from derived equations. Normal πc is 24 mmHg.

Tissue colloid osmotic pressure (πt) is determined by the concentration of osmotically active proteins in the interstitium. πt varies as a result of the reflection coefficient (σ) and the rate at which fluid is entering the interstitium (Jv). Direct measurement of πt is obviously difficult. However, the protein composition of lymph is felt to be similar to the protein composition of the interstitium. Thus, lymph colloid osmotic pressure is used to estimate πt. Normal lung πt is 14 mmHg.

Reflection coefficient (σ) is the fraction of protein that is reflected by the capillary membrane. This is a measure of the relative permeability of the membrane and determines the degree to which the osmotic gradient will oppose the hydrostatic gradient. Some tissues such as the brain are essentially impermeable to proteins and have a σ of 1.0. At the other extreme, liver σ is near 0, that is, the hepatic capillary is completely permeable to plasma proteins and the amount of liver edema and ascites is related almost solely to the hydrostatic pressure. The lung σ lies between these extremes at 0.7. Thus, with normal permeability, the pulmonary capillary membrane may allow a third of the plasma proteins impinging on the pores to leak into the interstitium. Certain compounds and disease states have been demonstrated to decrease σ in the lung (increase permeability).

Filtration coefficient (Kf) represents the physical character- istics of the membrane such as the permeability to water and the total surface area. Similar to Pc, Kf can be measured fairly accurately in isolated lungs but difficult to judge in vivo. Increases in the surface area of the capillary bed or an increase to water permeability will result in more fluid entering the interstitium even if the other factors do not change.

Anti-edema safety factors

Inspection of Equation 4 reveals that increases in Pc or decreases in πc or σ will result in an increase in fluid egress out of the capillary (Jv) and into the interstitium. However, a modest increase in Jv does not necessarily lead to edema formation. All tissues have protective mechanisms that tend to oppose the development of edema when Jv rises above its baseline value. These mechanisms are called the anti-edema safety factors (Table 1).

Increased tissue pressure. When fluid begins to accumulate in the interstitium, the increased fluid volume causes the Pt to rise. This rise tends to oppose Pc and slows Jv. As mentioned above, Pt in the lung can rise only a few mmHg and reaches a plateau (Fig. 1).

Table 1.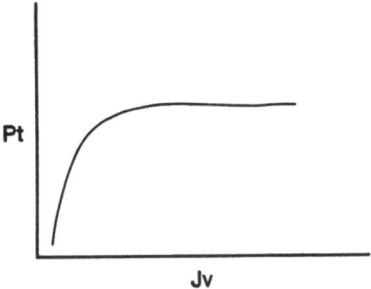

ANTI-EDEMA SAFETY FACTORS

1. increased Pt
2. decreased πt
3. increased rate of
   lymph flow

Fig. 1. Tissue hydrostatic pressure (Pt) vs. fluid flux into the interstitium (Jv). Pt rises quickly to a plateau with initial increases in Jv acting to impede further fluid accumulation.

Decreased tissue osmotic pressure. The capillary membrane acts to sieve protein from the egressing fluid. Thus, the fluid entering the interstitium has a lower protein concentration than plasma. As the amount of fluid entering the interstitium increases, the interstitial proteins are diluted and πt decreases. The effect of a decrease in πt is to increase the osmotic gradient, opposing further fluid flux out of the capillary (Fig. 2).

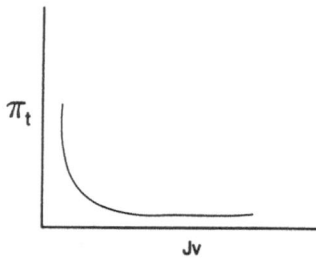

Fig. 2. Tissue colloid osmotic pressure (π_t) vs. fluid flux into the interstitium (Jv). By dropping quickly with initial increases in Jv, π_t acts as an early anti-edema safety factor.

Increased rate of lymph flow. Fluid that enters the interstitium is removed by the lymphatic system. Increases in the rate of fluid entering the interstitium are matched by increases in the rate of lymph flow. This increase in lymph flow rate is produced in the lung by a small increase in tissue driving pressure and a large decrease in lymphatic resistance. However, there is a limit to the increase in lymph flow rate. Thus, once fluid enters the interstitium faster than it can be removed, edema develops.

When the Starling forces are such that the anti-edema safety factors are overwhelmed, edema begins to form. Figure 3 represents the amount of rise in Pc over π_c that an awake sheep will tolerate before developing significant increase in lung water. The control values give a Pc-π_c value of -8 to -10 mmHg. Relative Pc may be elevated 10-15 mmHg before significant increases in lung water develop.

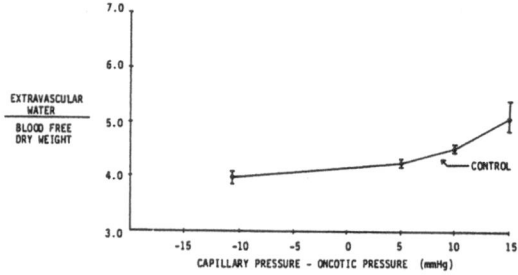

Fig. 3. Extravascular fluid vs. capillary pressure (Pc)-plasma colloid osmotic pressure (π_c) data in unanesthetized sheep. Critical Pc appears to be between +5 and +10 mmHg above π_c. (Reprinted with permission from ref. 9).

EFFECT OF CVP

In the previous section we presented the importance of the increase in lymph flow rate in the prevention of edema. Any factor that results in a decrease in the rate of lymph flow may enhance the development of edema. Lung lymphatic vessels drain into veins in the neck that empty into the superior vena cava. Thus, superior vena caval pressure (SVCP) is the pressure against which lymphatic vessels must pump lymph. At one time, the lymphatics were believed to be capable of generating pressures great enough to overcome any clinically obtainable SVCP. However, recent investigations have focused on the effect of SVCP (outflow pressure) on the actual rate of lymph flow. As shown in Figure 4, lymph flow rate is linearly dependent on outflow pressure.

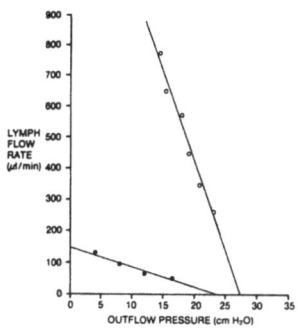

FIG. 4. Lymph flow rate vs. outflow pressure at baseline (filled circle) and after 5 h of increased left atrial pressure (open circle) for a typical experiment. (Reprinted with permission from ref. 13).

Figure 4 also demonstrates that even in the presence of edema, the linear response to outflow pressure is preserved. Thus, elevations in SVCP may impair lymph flow rate sufficiently to reduce removal of interstitial fluid and enhance the development of edema. We performed an experiment to test this hypothesis. The solid line in Figure 5 is the same data from Figure 3. We treated a second group of sheep identically except that we raised the SVCP to 20 mmHg in each sheep. The results of this second group are represented by the dotted line in Figure 5. At control Pc, no increase in lung water was detected in the presence of elevated SVCP. However, at each subsequent Pc elevation, significant increases in lung water were found. Thus, elevations in SVCP may enhance the

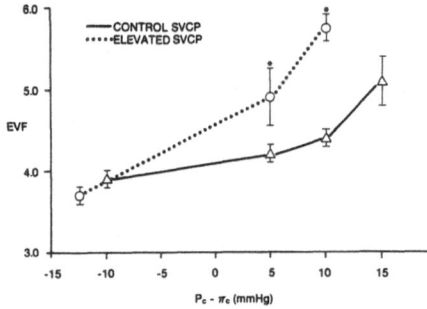

Fig. 5. Extravascular fluid (EVF) vs. capillary pressure (Pc)-colloid osmotic pressure (πc) data for control (solid line) and elevated (dotted line) superior vena cava pressure. Data are plotted as mean $\pm$ SE. (Reprinted with permission from ref. 9).

formation of pulmonary edema by impairing lymph flow. Many therapeutic interventions (positive pressure ventilation, fluid infusions, vasoactive drugs) in critically ill patients result in elevation of SVCP. Thus, routine therapy may actually be creating edema or at least slowing its resolution.

CLINICAL IMPLICATIONS

The development of pulmonary edema may result in a spectrum of clinical findings. An early sign of pulmonary edema is tachypnea although lung compliance is probably not significantly altered by small amounts of edema. Massive pulmonary edema may lead to ventilatory failure and hypoxemia necessitating prolonged intubation and mechanical ventilation.

Congestive heart failure. Pulmonary edema develops when elevations in LAP cause Pc to rise sufficiently to overwhelm the anti-edema safety factors. Treatment of pulmonary edema in this situation is based on reducing the vascular pressures. Typically, a diuretic, such as furosemide, is given to reduce the intravascular volume and, thereby, the intravascular pressures including Pc. The Pc needs to be lowered so that Jv is less than the rate at which the fluid can be removed (lymph flow rate). Furosemide appears to have a venodilatory effect that also results in decreased intravascular pressures. Patients with congestive heart failure often have elevated central venous pressure (CVP). As noted in previous discussion, elevated CVP may not only enhance the formation of pulmonary edema but also impair the lung's ability to clear the excess fluid.

Resuscitation: Crystalloid vs. Colloid. The treatment and prevention of hypovolemia in a patient who has large fluid losses requires a suitable amount of intravascular volume replacement. A major goal of perioperative management is to maintain intravascular volume sufficient to protect the kidneys but insufficient to result in pulmonary edema. In the patient requiring large fluid infusions, the attainment of both goals is often difficult to accomplish. Controversy exists concerning the nature of the optimal replacement fluid. Clinical studies have provided directly opposing conclusions, probably due to the difficulty of measuring the various Starling forces accurately as well as the numerous variables that cannot be controlled in these critically ill patients. From an experimental and theoretical point of view, the use of colloid solutions appears superior to crystalloid. This is because, with the use of colloid solutions, πc may be relatively higher and Pc and central venous pressure may be lower. Thus, the use of colloid solutions, as compared to crystalloid solutions, should result in 1) a smaller decrease in πc, 2) a smaller increase in Pc, and 3) a smaller rise in central venous pressure.

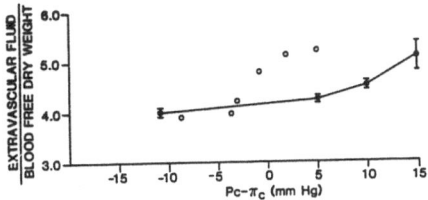

FIG. 6. Extravascular fluid vs. capillary pressure (Pc)-plasma colloid osmotic pressure (πc) data for control (solid line) and endotoxin sheep. Control data are plotted as mean $\pm$ SE. (Reprinted with permission from ref. 9).

ARDS. Much controversy surrounds the question of appropriate fluid management in pulmonary diseases such as ARDS where pulmonary microvascular permeability may be increased. We and others have performed experiments that have examined the impact of E. coli endotoxin induced pulmonary damage on lung fluid balance. The solid line in Figure 6 is the same data presented in Figure 3. The open circles represent sheep subjected to the same protocol except that they were given 1 μg/kg of E. coli endotoxin at the start of the experiment. The data show that endotoxin probably does increase permeability as evidenced by the significant pulmonary edema found at a lower P_c elevation. However, edema did not form even with this increase in permeability unless P_c was elevated above control values. We have performed other experiments with much higher doses of endotoxin in which maintenance of normal P_c prevented the formation of pulmonary edema. Even in situations where permeability has been altered, maintenance of normal P_c and π_c are still important to edema prevention.

SUMMARY

Rational approaches to the prevention and treatment of pulmonary edema begin with a firm understanding of the Starling equation and its components. It is important to remember that the LAP or its estimate (PCWP) may not accurately reflect changes in the true capillary hydrostatic pressure (P_c). Plasma osmotic pressure (π_c) is a major determinant in the amount of fluid that enters the interstitium and maintenance of a normal value is crucial. Finally, elevated central venous pressure may slow the maximal rate of lymph flow from the lungs, impairing a key anti-edema safety factor.

SUGGESTED READING

1. Allen, S.J., Drake, R.E., Williams, J.P., Laine, G.A. and Gabel, J.C. Crit. Care Med. 15:963, 1987.
2. Starling, E.H. J. Physiol. 19:312, 1896.
3. Hakim, T.S., Michel, R.P., Chang, H.K. J. Appl. Physiol. 52:710, 1982.
4. D'Orio, V., Halleux, J., Rodriguez, L.M., et. al. Crit. Care Med. 14:802, 1986.

5. Cope, D.K., Allison, R.C., Parmentier, J.L., et. al. Crit. Care Med. 14:16, 1986.
6. Holloway, H., Perry, M., Downey, J., et. al. J. Appl. Physiol. 54:846, 1983.
7. Bhattacharya, J., Gropper, M.A., Staub, N.C. J. Appl. Physiol. 56:271, 1984.
8. Szabo, G., Magyar, Z. J. Appl. Physiol. 212:1469, 1967.
9. Laine, G.A., Allen, S.J., Katz, J., et. al. J. Appl. Physiol. 61:1634, 1986.
10. Esbenshade, A.M., Newman, J.H., Lams, P.M., et. al. J. Appl. Physiol. 53:967, 1982.
11. Guyton, A.C., Lindsey, A.W. Circ. Res. 7:649, 1959.
12. Allen, S.A., Drake, R.E., Gabel, J.C., et. al. Crit. Care Med. 14:373, 1986..
13. Drake, R.E., Giesler, M., Laine, G., et. al. J. Appl. Physiol. 58:70, 1985.

CONTROL OF BREATHING

THOMAS F. HORNBEIN

Department of Anesthesiology, University of Washington School of Medicine, Seattle, Washington 98195

INTRODUCTION AND GOALS

The primary purpose of this presentation will be to explore the ways in which anesthetics and related drugs - sedatives, tranquilizers, and narcotics - act to produce one of their more notorious side effects, depression of breathing. I will review dose-response relationships, discuss clinical implications, and explore some of the questions of basic ventilatory control revealed by the way in which these drugs modify breathing.

THE NATURE OF DRUG DEPRESSION

Inhalational Anesthetics.

Tidal volume and P_{CO_2}. Ventilatory depression may be perceived clinically as a decrease in minute ventilation, manifest as a rise in arterial or alveolar P_{CO_2}. The dose-response curve differs for different anesthetics, diethyl ether being the least depressant to resting breathing and enflurane the most, with halothane and isoflurane more closely resembling the latter than the former. In spite of these differences, with all these anesthetics tidal volume decreases with increasing anesthetic concentration. The P_{CO_2} below which spontaneous ventilation ceases to occur in the sedated or anesthetized individual was termed by Fink "the apneic threshold." That value lies 5-9 mm Hg below the resting P_{CO_2} and seems to provide the same information regarding ventilatory depression as does the resting P_{CO_2}.

Carbon dioxide response. All inhalation anesthetics, including diethyl ether, produce a dose-proportional decrease in the slope of ventilation-CO_2 response curve.

Hypoxic response. The inhalation anesthetics, halothane, isoflurane, and enflurane, all depress the ventilatory response to hypoxia more than the response to carbon dioxide. For example, halothane at 0.1 MAC

41

T. H. Stanley and R. J. Sperry (eds.), Anesthesia and the Lung, 41–46.
© 1989 by Kluwer Academic Publishers.

depresses hypoxic ventilatory response to approximately 30% of control, while the CO_2 response is virtually unchanged from the awake value; at 1.1 MAC a ventilatory response to hypoxia is absent, while the CO_2 response is decreased to approximately 35% of the awake value. Nitrous oxide behaves similarly. Droperidol selectively increases the ventilatory response to hypoxia. This greater hypoxic depression of inhalation anesthetics appears to result from an effect of these drugs upon the peripheral chemoreceptors.

Response to loading. The ventilatory response to an externally imposed load, an increase in either resistance or capacitance, was originally presumed to be profoundly depressed by even light levels of anesthesia. More recent evidence suggests that mild to moderate loads are well tolerated without resulting in a rise in arterial P_{CO_2}, at least at lower anesthetic concentrations. Little information concerning dose-response relationships is yet available. Increasing anesthetic depth may obtund the ventilatory tolerance to external loads. Response to intrinsic loading (e.g., bronchospasm induced by methacholine in dogs) appears to be unaffected by pentobarbital, which impairs the response to external load-ing; whether humans behave similarly to inhalation anesthetics is not known. Patients with chronic obstructive pulmonary disease exhibiting increased airways resistance when awake may experience a greater rise in P_{CO_2} during anesthesia than that of normal patients if permitted to breathe spontaneously.

Response to stimulation. Noxious stimulation during surgery will result in an increase in ventilation and a decrease in P_{CO_2} of up to 10 mm Hg from the unstimulated state.

Narcotics, Sedatives, and Hypnotics.

These drugs, except ketamine and marijuana, appear to depress ventilation, resulting in a dose-related increase in alveolar or arterial P_{CO_2}. Different classes of drugs appear to affect the pattern of breathing in differing ways: narcotics are associated with a slowing of respiratory frequency but a sustained tidal volume, in contrast to barbiturates and in particular to the inhalation anesthetics, which to varying degrees tend to increase respiratory frequency and decrease tidal volume.

MECHANISMS OF VENTILATORY DEPRESSION

Different drugs depress breathing in different ways. Depression of breathing (signaled by an elevation of P_{CO_2} or a decrease in the ventilatory response to CO_2, hypoxia, or loads) does not necessarily equate with the depression of ventilatory drive when drive is defined as the rate of respiratory motoneuron output during inspiration. Normally this neural output translates to a change in tidal volume so that drive is reflected by the rate of change of lung volume during inspiration

$$drive = \underline{K} \times V_T/T_I$$

where $\underline{K}$ is a proportionality constant, V_T is tidal volume, and T_I is time for inspiration. Minute ventilation ($\dot{V}_E$) = $V_T \times f$, where f is frequency of breaths.

Thus

$$\dot{V}_E = V_T \times f = V_T/T_I \times T_I \times 1/T_T$$

where T_T is duration of the total respiratory cycle or $1/f$.

A decrease in minute ventilation may result from 1) a decrease in drive (V_T/T_I); 2) a shortened time for inspiration (T_I); or 3) a decrease in ventilatory frequency (increase in T_T). Thus anesthetics and sedatives may depress breathing by decreasing drive or by altering timing.

One more caution for the use of tidal volume to measure drive is necessary. The linkage between the respiratory controller's output and the movement of air includes a series of connections that begins with a dorsal horn synapse, proceeds to the neuromuscular junction, includes the behavior of the respiratory muscles themselves, and finally involves the mechanical properties of the chest wall, the diaphragm, and the lungs. Anesthetics can affect lung and chest wall compliance as well as functional residual capacity. In addition, factors such as age, position, and site of surgery may also alter this linkage.

Studies in humans of how anesthetics and other depressant drugs influence the drive-timing relationships are sparse but the information that is available reveals different actions of rather similar drugs. For example, halothane results in a much greater increase in ventilatory frequency than either enflurane or isoflurane, associated with a lesser tidal volume but also a lower P_{CO_2} for a given MAC equivalent.

44

While logically the hypercapnia associated with drug depression might increase ventilatory frequency to limit the rise in P_{CO_2}, in fact most evidence suggests that at least the inhalation anesthetics affect frequency or timing independently of the P_{CO_2}. Changes in P_{CO_2} above or below the resting P_{CO_2} do not appear to influence breathing frequency at any given anesthetic depth. The same behavior may not be true for narcotics, sedatives, or tranquilizers, but little information is yet available.

CONCLUSIONS

Most of the anesthetics and anesthetic adjuvants that we use depress breathing in a dose-related manner. This ventilatory depression may result from a decrease in the rate of inflow during inspiration (drive), a shortened time for inspiration, or a decreased frequency of breathing. Inhalational anesthetics cause a greater depression of the ventilatory response to hypoxia than to CO_2, even at sub-anesthetic concentrations. These effects are of relevance to spontaneous ventilation during anesthesia but perhaps more importantly to breathing in the immediate postoperative period.

GENERAL REFERENCES

1. Hickey, R.F., and Severinghaus, J.W. Regulation of breathing: drug effects. In: Lung Biology in Health and Disease. Regulation of Breathing (Ed. T.F. Hornbein), Dekker, New York, 1978, pp. 1251-1312.
2. Hornbein, T.F. Anesthetics and ventilatory control, In: Effects of Anesthesia, Americal Physiological Society, Clinical Physiology Series, 1985, pp. 75-90.
3. Pavlin, E.G. and Hornbein, T.F. Organ and tissue disturbances produced by acid-base abnormalities. In: Lung Biology in Health and Disease. Extrapulmonary Manifestation of Respiratory Disease (Ed. E.D. Robin), Dekker, New York, 1978, pp. 363-405.

REFERENCES

1. Bainton, C.R. and Mitchell, R.A. Posthyperventilation apnea in awake man. J. Appl. Physiol. 21:411-415, 1966.
2. Biscoe, T.J. and Millar, R.A. Effects of inhalation anaesthetics on carotid body chemoreceptor activity. Br. J. Anaesth. 40:2-12, 1968.
3. Bromage, P.R., Camporesi, E., and Leslie, J. Epidural narcotics in volunteers: sensitivity to pain and to carbon dioxide. Pain 9:145-160,1980.
4. Byrick, R.J. and Janssen, E.G. Respiratory waveform and rebreathing in T-piece circuits: a comparison of enflurane and halothane waveforms. Anesthesiology 53:371-378, 1980.
5. Christensen, V. Respiratory depression after extradural morphine (Letter). Br. J. Anaesth. 52:841, 1980.

6. Clark, F.J. and Von Euler, C. On the regulation of depth and rate of breathing. J. Physiol. Lond. 222:267-295, 1972.
7. Davies, R.O., Edwards, M.W., and Lahiri, S. Halothane depresses the response of carotid body chemoreceptors to hypoxia and hypercapnia in the cat. Anesthesiology 57:153-159, 1982.
8. Doblar, D.D., Muldoon, S.M., Abbrecht, P.H., Baskoff, J., and Watson, R.L. Epidural morphine following epidural local anesthesia: effect on ventilatory and airway occlusion pressure responses to CO_2. Anesthesiology 55:423-428, 1981.
9. Eger, E.I., II, Dolan, W.M., Stevens, W.C., Miller, R.D., and Way, W.L. Surgical stimulation antagonizes the respiratory depression produced by Forane. Anesthesiology 36:544-549, 1972.
10. Foldes, F.F., Duncalf, D., and Kuwahara, S. The respiratory, circulatory, and narcotic antagonistic effects of nalorphine, levallorphan and naloxone in anaesthetized subjects. Can. Anaesth. Soc. J. 16:151-161, 1969.
11. Glynn, C.J., Mather, L.E., Cousins, M.J., Wilson, P.R., and Graham, J.R. Spinal narcotics and respiratory depression. Lancet 2:356-357, 1979.
12. Hanks, E.C., Ngai, S.H., and Fink, B.R. The respiratory threshold during halothane anesthesia. Anesthesiology 22:393-397, 1961.
13. Hickey, R.F., Fourcade, H.E., Eger, E.I., II, Larson, C.P., Bahlman, S.H., Stevens, W.M., Gregory, G.A., and Smith, T.C. The effects of ether, halothane and Forane on apneic thresholds in man. Anesthesiology 35:32-37, 1971.
14. Isaza, G.D., Posner, J.D., Altose, M.D., Kelsen, S.G., and Cherniack, N.S. Airway occlusion pressures in awake and anesthetized goats. Respir. Physiol. 27:87-98, 1976.
15. Knill, R.L., Bright, S., and Manninen, P.H. Hypoxic ventilatory responses during thiopentone sedation and anaesthesia in man. Can. Anaesth. Soc. J. 25:366-372, 1978.
16. Knill, R.L. and Clement, J.L. Site of selective action of halothane on the peripheral chemoreflex pathway in humans. Anesthesiology 61:121-126, 1984.
17. Knill, R.L. and Clement, J.L. Ventilatory responses to acute metabolic acidemia in humans awake, sedated, and anesthetized with halothane. Anesthesiology 62:745-753, 1985.
18. Knill, R.L., Clement, J.L., and Thompson, W.R. Epidural morphine causes delayed and prolonged ventilatory depression. Can. Anaesth. Soc. J. 28:537-543, 1981.
19. Knill, R.L. and Gelb, A.W. Ventilatory response to hypoxia and hypercapnia during halothane sedation and anesthesia in man. Anesthesiology 49:244-251, 1978.
20. Knill, R.L., Kieraszewicz, H., Dodgson, G.G., and Clement, J.L. Chemical regulation of ventilation during isoflurane sedation and anaesthesia in humans. Can. Anaesth. Soc. J. 30:607-614, 1983.
21. Kryger, M.H., Yacoub, O., Dosman, J., Macklem, P.T., and Anthonisen, N.R. Effect of meperidine on occlusion pressure responses to hypercapnia and hypoxia with and without external inspiratory resistance. Am. Rev. Respir. Dis. 114:333-340, 1976.
22. Mitchell, R.A. and Herbert, D.A. Potencies of doxapram and hypoxia in stimulating carotid-body chemoreceptors and ventilation in anesthetized cats. Anesthesiology 42:559-566, 1975.

23. Moote, C.A., Knill, R.L., and Clement, J. Ventilatory compensation for continuous inspiratory resistive and elastic loads during halothane anesthesia in humans. Anesthesiology 64:582-589, 1986.
24. Munson, E.S., Larson, C.P., Jr., Babad, A.A., Regan, M.J., Buechel, D.R., and Eger, E.I., II. The effects of halothane, fluroxene and cyclopropane on ventilation: a comparative study in man. Anesthesiology 27:716-728, 1966.
25. Nunn, J.F. and Ezi-Ashi, T.I. The respiratory effects of resistance to breathing in anesthetized man. Anesthesiology 22:174-178, 1966.
26. Pietak, S., Weenig, C.S., Hickey, R.F., and Fairley, H.B. Anesthetic effects on ventilation in patients with chronic obstructive pulmonary disease. Anesthesiology 42:160-166, 1975.
27. Pokorski, M., Barnard, P., McGregor, K., and Lahiri, S. Dependence of ventilatory stimulation by naloxone on anesthesia and surgery in the cat (abstr.) Federation Proc. 42:741, 1983.
28. Polacheck, J., Strong, R., Arens, J., Davies, C., Metcalf, I., and Younes, M. Phasic vagal influence on inspiratory motor output in anesthetized human subjects. J. Appl. Physiol.: Respirat. Environ. Exercise Physiol. 49:609-619, 1980.
29. Santiago, T.V., Remolina, C., Scoles, V., and Edelman, N.H. Endorphins and the control of breathing. N. Engl. J. Med. 304:1190-1195, 1981.
30. Savoy, J., Arnup, M.-E., and Anthonisen, N.R. Response to external inspiratory resistive loading and bronchospasm in anesthetized dogs. J. Appl. Physiol.: Respirat. Environ. Exercise Physiol. 53:355-360, 1982.
31. Slee, T., Sharar, S., Pavlin, E.G., and Macintyre, P.E.: The effect of airway impedance on work of breathing during halothane anesthesia. Anesth. Analg., in press.
32. Tusiewicz, K., Bryan, A.C., and Froese, A.B. Contributions of changing rib cage-diaphragm interactions to the ventilatory depression of halothane anesthesia. Anesthesiology 47:327-337, 1977.
33. Ward, D.S. Stimulation of hypoxic ventilatory drive by droperidol. Anesth. Analg. Cleveland 63:106-110, 1984.
34. Weiskopf, R.B., Raymond, L.W., and Severinghaus, J.W. Effects of halothane on canine respiratory responses to hypoxia with and without hypercarbia. Anesthesiology 41:350-360, 1974.
35. Wheeler, M.E. and Farber, J.P. Naloxone administration and ventilation in awake cats. Brain Res. 258:343-346, 1983.

PULMONARY SURFACTANT: AN ENDOGENOUS MEDIATOR OF ALVEOLAR STABILITY AND A THERAPEUTIC AGENT

G.A. Zimmerman, MD
Department of Medicine, University of Utah School of Medicine
Salt Lake City, Utah

INTRODUCTION

Physiologic lung function depends on surfactant, a complex lipoprotein that is a major component of the alveolar lining fluid and that dynamically regulates alveolar surface tension, decreasing it at end expiration (preventing closure of the alveoli) and allowing it to increase at end inspiration (contributing to elastic recoil). The discovery that surfactant deficiency is the primary defect in Infant Respiratory Distress Syndrome, and that surfactant is synthesized by the alveolar Type II cells, ushered in the modern era of lung cell biology. Basic observations on the nature and metabolism of surfactant and the regulation of Type II cell function have, particularly in the last 5 years, contributed clinically-relevant information (1-10). The initiation of controlled trials of administration of surfactant preparations for the treatment of Infant Respiratory Distress Syndrome, and consideration of similar trials to determine the role of surfactant in the therapy of other conditions such as the Adult Respiratory Distress Syndrome (ARDS), have resulted directly from these basic investigations.

The alveolar Type II cell is the most numerous and metabolically-active of the alveolar lining cells (2,9,11). Its major functions are thought to be the synthesis and secretion of components of surfactant, and proliferation and differentiation in response to lung injury. Other potential functions include: 1) antioxidant defenses; 2) secretion of enzymes and other components of the alveolar lining material, in addition to surfactant, which may be important in alveolar defense; and 3) control of the electrolyte composition of the alveolar subphase (11,12). The most well-studied of these processes

47

T. H. Stanley and R. J. Sperry (eds.), Anesthesia and the Lung, 47–53.
© 1989 by Kluwer Academic Publishers.

is surfactant production. The pulmonary surface-active material, or "surfactant," is found at the air-liquid interface of the lung and is responsible for regulating the surface tension at this interface (9,13). If unopposed, the increase in surface tension that occurs at low lung volumes promotes alveolar collapse at the end of expiration, resulting in atelectasis and regional inequality of alveolar volumes. Both of these cause disordered gas exchange (12,13). Thus surfactant contributes to the ability of the lung to mantain a stable functional residual capacity, a requirement for normal gas exchange. In addition, surfactant influences perimicrovascular pressure and therefore transcapillary fluid exchange (19), acts as an alveolar integumentary barrier, facilitates the clearance of inhaled particles, and enhances the bactericidal capacity of alveolar macrophages (13) (Table 1).

TABLE 1: FUNCTIONS OF SURFACTANT

1. Lowers and dynamically alters surface tension in direct proportion to surface area. This has several beneficial consequences:

   A. Contributes to the maintenance of a stable functional residual capacity.
   B. Minimizes differences in alveolar volume.
   C. Prevents atelectasis.
   D. Minimizes the work of breathing.
   E. Retards the development of pulmonary edema.

2. Lung defense against certain bacteria (staphylococci, pneumococci).

The consequences of a surfactant deficit are well-known in neonates with the Infant Respiratory Distress Syndrome, the only human disease clearly attributable to surfactant lack. Abnormalities of surfactant composition and biophysical function also occur in the Adult Respiratory Distress Syndrome (19). Quantitative and/or qualitative defects in surfactant may play a role in other pathologic conditions as well (Table 2).

TABLE 2: CLINICAL CONDITIONS THAT MAY BE ASSOCIATED WITH A DECREASE IN SURFACTANT

CONDITION	SURFACTANT ABNORMALITY
INFANT RESPIRATORY DISTRESS SYNDROME	Quantitative Deficiency
ADULT RESPIRATORY DISTRESS SYNDROME	Altered Composition; Functionally Inactive
PULMONARY EDEMA	? - Quantitative Decrease
CONSTANT TIDAL VOLUME VENTILATION	
A. "Post-op" (abdominal, chest)	? - Functionally inactive
B. Restrictive lung/chest wall disorders	"
C. Inspiratory muscle fatigue	"
D. Mechanical ventilation	"
E. General anesthesia	"
PULMONARY EMBOLUS	? - Quantitative Deficiency

Surfactant is a phospholipid-protein complex that is rich in phosphatidylcholine (PC) (70-80% of total lipid) and phosphitidylglycerol (5-10%), and is unusual because of the high proportion of saturated fatty acids in the phosphatidylcholine molecules (9,20). The major saturated fatty acid is palmitic acid, with approximately 60% of the phosphatidylcholine (PC) being dipalmitoyl PC (9,12). In addition to phospholipids, proteins are essential for the functions of surfactant. Surfactant-associated proteins appear to be found only in the lung, to be highly conserved in nature, and have been demonstrated in subcellular organelles in Type II cells and Clara cells. Two groups of surfactant apoproteins have been identified. One group, consisting of proteins of 26-36 KDa molecular weight, is variably glycosylated, and has a segment of primary sequence that is similar to collagen (1). It also has lipid binding sites and binds to mannose and other carbohydrates in a Ca++-dependent fashion, indicating that it has lectin-like properties (8). It will associate with synthetic lipids to form a complex that spreads to form an interfacial film, and reduces surface tension in vitro (1,3). The gene for a 32 KDa human surfactant apoprotein has been cloned (1) and expressed in mammalian cell lines (8). The apoproteins of the second group are smaller, with molecular weights of 5-18 KDa, and are extremely hydrophobic - so hydrophobic that they are soluble in organic solvents but not water (1,4,5,6,10). This property facilitates their interaction with lipids. Recent studies suggest that the low molecular weight apoproteins may be required for maximal reduction of surface tension (6). As with the high molecular weight proteins, the 5-18 KDa class can combine with synthetic phospholipids to form a synthetic surfactant that lowers surface tension in vitro (4,10). A human cDNA for a precursor protein of a 6 KDa apoprotein, and a cDNA for an 18 KDa protein, have been cloned (6,10).

The exact molecular basis for the synthesis and release of surfactant is unknown, but production and organization of the components occurs in the endoplasmic reticulum of the Type II cell and the surfactant is stored in organelles known as lamellar bodies (9,11-13). These are secreted by exocytosis onto the alveolar surface and the surfactant is arranged as "tubular myelin", a unique physical form that appears as a lattice structure on electron micrographs (14). The tubular myelin then adsorbs to the air-fluid interface and assumes a different physical conformation with a typical linear appearance (9,11-13). This conformation appears to be required for the normal ability of the material to lower surface tension. The synthesis and secretion of surfactant by Type II cells are regulated processes (2,9); a protein kinase C and a cyclic AMP-dependent protein kinase influence secretion (2). Type II cell activity is affected by certain hormones, by autacoids such as platelet-activating factor (27), and by the pattern of ventilation (7,9,11-13). There is also evidence that alveolar Type II cells take up surfactant from the alveolar surface and reprocess it, perhaps for later secretion (9,24). Both the low- and high-molecular weight apoproteins enhance the uptake of surfactant by alveolar Type II cells (21).

Investigation of the effects of the pattern of ventilation on surfactant activity has suggested extraordinary qualities of the material that may be of clinical importance. While studying the mechanism for decreased lung compliance during constant tidal volume ventilation with low or normal tidal breaths, Thet, Massaro and co-workers found that this pattern of breathing resulted in increased amounts of surfactant in the aggregated form, of which tubular myelin is one physical configuration (14,15). In the aggregated form the <u>chemical</u> composition of surfactant is the same, but the <u>physical</u> state prevents the surfactant from rapidly diminishing surface tension (17). The development of an increased fraction of aggregated surfactant results in increased alveolar surface tension in normal, excised animal lungs (14,15,17). These findings suggest that an alteration in the physical and biologic properties of surfactant can be caused by the pattern of ventilation, a concept developed earlier by Clements (13). Such alterations may explain the atelectatic, liver-like lungs that were observed in animals subjected to constant volume ventilation by Drinker and other early investigators of physiologic alterations caused by mechanical ventilation (16). Under experimental conditions the amount of aggregated surfactant can be returned to normal by a single deep breath (approximately 3 times normal tidal volume), and its formation appears to be prevented by a) a periodic sign during constant ventilation with normal tidal volumes, b) continuous ventilation at two or three times the normal tidal volume, or c) by the addition of positive end expiratory pressure to continuous normal volume ventilation (14,15,17).

Considering these observations, it is possible that alteration in surfactant function caused by an abnormal pattern of breathing may explain the propensity for atelectasis in postoperative abdominal and thoracic surgery patients, whose pattern of ventilation is routinely one of low constant tidal volumes without sighs. Since increased surface tension appears to favor alveolar fluid accumulaton (18), the amount of aggregated surfactant may also be important in the genesis of pulmonary edema in some circumstances. Alteration in the amount of aggregated surfactant has been proposed as a mechanism for ventilation-perfusion abnormalities in pulmonary embolism, oxygen toxicity, and the adult respiratory distress syndrome (17).

If the studies that indicate improvement in surfactant function by alteration in the ventilatory pattern (discussed above) are applicable to humans, they may provide a cellular, biochemical, and biophysical basis for common respiratory therapy practices in the operating room and intensive care unit. These include the use of larger than normal tidal volumes during mechanical ventilation, use of the sustained maximum inspiration ("incentive spirometry") in postoperative care, and the use of positive end expiratory pressure in some circumstances.

Synthetic and partially-purified natural surfactants have been administered to humans for the treatment of lung disease (21-24). Logically, the first condition in which these agents have been tested is the Infant Respiratory Distress Syndrome, where remarkable success has been reported in some trials of prophylactic and/or therapeutic use of surfactant preparations (21-23). Trials for other conditions, such as ARDS, are being considered (24), although the role of surfactant deficiency in the pathophysiology of this syndrome is not clearly defined and surfactant deficiency is a secondary, rather than primary, event. Current efforts are also focused on using basic information on the nature of the surfactant phospholipids and apoproteins to define the characteristics that are requried for an effective and safe synthetic preparation, and on using basic observations of alveolar Type II cell biology to devise strategies to therapeutically influence the synthesis and secretion of surfactant in vivo (24,25).

In addition to their use as therapeutic agents, surfactant preparations appear to be valuable tools for sorting out specific defects that contribute to disordered lung function in humans and in experimental animals (23,26). Experiments of this sort have suggested that increased epithelial or microvascular permeability add to the physiologic consequences of surfactant deficiency in Infant Respiratory Distress Syndrome.

REFERENCES

1. White, R.T., Damm, D., Miller, J., et al. Nature 317:361-363, 1985
2. Sano, K., Voelker, D., and Mason, R.J. J. Biol. Chem. 260:12725-12729, 1985.
3. Revak, S.D., Merritt, T.A., Hallman, M., and Cochrane, C.G. Am. Rev. Resp. Dis. 134:1258-1261, 1986.
4. Phelps, D., Smith, L.M., and Tausch, H.W. Am. Rev. Resp. Dis. 135:1112-1117, 1987.
5. Glasser, S.W., Korfhagen, T.R., Weaver, T., et al. Proc. Nat. Acad. Sci USA 84:4007-4011, 1987.

6. Jacobs, K.A., Phelps, D.S., Steinbrink, R., et al. J. Biol. Chem. 262:9808-9811, 1987.

7. Whitsett, J.A., Weaver, T.E., Clark, J.C., et al. J. Biol. Chem. 262:15618-15623, 1987.

8. Haagsman, H.P., Hawgood, S., Sargeant, T., et al. J. Biol. Chem. 262:13877-13880, 1987.

9. Wright, J.R., and Clements, J.A. Am. Rev. Resp. Dis. 135:426-444, 1987.

10. Revak, S.D., Merritt, T.A., Degryse, E., et al. J. Clin. Invest. 81:826-833, 1988.

11. Mason, R.J., Williams, M.C. Am. Rev. Resp. Dis. 115:81-91, 1977 (Suppl).

12. Mason, R.J., et al. Fed. Proc. 36:2697-2702, 1977.

13. Clements, T. Am. Rev. Resp. Dis. 115:67-71, 1977 (suppl).

14. Thet, L.A., et al. J. Clin. Invest. 64:600-608, 1979.

15. Thet, L.A., et al. Clin. Res. 27:494, 1979 (Abstract).

16. Drinker, C.K., Hardenbergh, E. Surgery 24:113-118, 1948.

17. Massaro, D., et al. Am. J. Med. 69:113-115, 1980.

18. Albert, R.K., Lakshminaryan, S., Hildebrandt, J., et al. J. Clin. Invest. 63:1015-1018, 1979.

19. Hallman, M., Spragg, R., Harrell, J.H., et al. J. Clin. Invest. 70:673-683, 1982.

20. Roony, S.A. Am. Rev. Resp. Dis. 131:439-460, 1985.

21. Taeusch, H.W., Clements, J., and Benson, B. Am. Rev. Resp. Dis. 128:791-794, 1983.

22. Merritt, T.A., Hallman, M., Bloom, B.T., et al. N. Eng. J. Med. 315:785-790, 1986.

23. Jobe, A., and Ikegami, M. Am. Rev. Resp. Dis. 136:1256-1275, 1987.

24. Jobe, A.H., Young, S.L. Am. Rev. Resp. Dis. 136:1032-1033, 1987.

25. Whitsett, J.A., Pilot, T., Clark, J.C., and Weaver, T.E. J. Biol. Chem. 262:5256-5261, 1987.

26. Ikegami, M., Berry, D., Elkady, T., et al. J. Clin. Invest. 79:1371-1378, 1987.

27. Kumar, R., King, R.J., Martin, H.H., and Hanahan, D.J. Biochim. Biophys. Acta 917:33-41, 1987

HIGH ALTITUDE DISEASES

JOHN B. WEST

Department of Medicine, University of California San Diego, La Jolla CA
92093-0623

This is a brief review of several high altitude diseases. They
range from the benign acute mountain sickness to the potentially fatal
high altitude cerebral edema.

Acute Mountain Sickness

Newcomers to high altitude frequently complain of headache, fatigue,
dizziness, palpitations, nausea, loss of appetite, and insomnia. This
constellation is know as acute mountain sickness and is presumably caused
by a combination of hypoxemia and respiratory alkalosis. Some physicians
believe that the underlying pathology may be mild cerebral edema. It is
known that hypoxemia is a cerebral vasodilator and measurements of
retinal blood flow show that this can double in lowlanders moved to an
altitude of 5,300 m (17,500 ft.). Although the hypoxemia causes cerebral
vasodilatation, the reduced arterial PCO_2 and increased pH as a result of
the hyperventilation cause cerebral vasoconstriction. The interaction
between these two competing factors at high altitude is not well
understood.

Acute mountain sickness is often most apparent at night when
ventilation tends to be somewhat depressed and hypoxemia most severe.
The hypoxemia can be exaggerated by periodic breathing which is very
common. However the symptoms of acute mountain sickness generally
subside over a period of one to two days, though interestingly some
people are not able to tolerate altitudes as low as 2,400 m (8,000 ft.).

Acute mountain sickness usually needs little treatment although
aspirin may be useful for the headache. The incidence of acute mountain
sickness can be reduced by taking acetazolamide (Diamox) 250 mg two or
three times a day before ascending to high altitude.

T. H. Stanley and R. J. Sperry (eds.), Anesthesia and the Lung, 55–58.

Chronic Mountain Sickness

Long term residents of high altitude sometimes develope an ill-defined syndrome characterized by fatigue, reduced exercise tolerance, severe hypoxemia and excessive polycythemia. This is called chronic mountain sickness or Monge's Disease. Extremely high levels of hematocrit are sometimes seen. During a recent visit to La Paz, Bolivia I was shown data on several patients with hematocrits in the low to mid 70's.

It appears that some of these patients have lost part of their hypoxic ventilatory response with the result that their ventilation falls, they develop severe hypoxemia, and the resulting tissue hypoxia stimulates the development of the high hematocrit levels. Presumably the fatigue and reduced exercise tolerance come about as a result of the high viscosity of the blood. The condition often responds well to removal to lower altitudes.

Recent work suggests that even more moderate degrees of polycythemia at high altitude may be counterproductive. The erythropoietin mechanism controlling the production of red blood cells was developed at sea level over thousands of years where it performs a useful role in maintaining a normal hemoglobin level in the face of blood loss through trauma, parasites and malnutrition. However at high altitude where the tissue hypoxia is caused by an entirely different mechanism, the polycythemia may be an inappropriate response. Winslow has shown that a reduction of hematocrit in high altitude permanent dwellers may result in an improvement of exercise tolerance.

High altitude pulmonary edema

Occasionally skiers, trekkers and climbers at high altitude develop pulmonary edema. The incidence varies from about 0.5 to 2% in different series. A typical history is that a subject ascends rapidly to altitude and is very active getting there or on arrival. He often has symptoms of acute mountain sickness though they may not be very severe. He then become more short of breath and lethargic. There may be chest pain. Physical signs include tachycardia, tachypnea, and crackles at the lung bases. He develops a dry cough which later progresses to one productive cough of frothy white sputum, and eventually blood-tinged sputum. The condition may progress over a few hours with increasing respiratory distress, cyanosis, bubbling respirations, coma and death.

The mechanism of the condition is not yet understood. The wedge pressure is normal so left ventricular failure is not the cause. There is an associated pulmonary hypertension due to hypoxic pulmonary vasoconstriction. One hypothesis proposed by Hultgren is that the hypoxic pulmonary vasoconstriction is uneven and those capillaries not protected from the high pressures leak. However recent measurements indicate that the alveolar fluid has a high protein content so that the condition is not simply caused by an increased hydrostatic pressure. It is possible that the regions of the lung that have very high flows develop damage to the capillaries increasing their permeability.

The treatment of the condition is descent to a lower altitude. If oxygen is available this should also be given. Diuretics such as furosemide should be used with great caution because the patients are often dehydrated.

High altitude cerebral edema

Fortunately this condition is uncommon though in one series of 278 trekkers to an altitude of 4,243 m, the incidence was 1.8% A typical history is that the patient develops symptoms of acute mountain sickness with headache, photophobia and perhaps irritability. This then progresses with the appearance of ataxia, irrationality, hallucinations and clouding of consciousness. Coma may supervene and death follow in a matter of a few hours or a day or so.

The most likely mechanism is cerebral edema related to the high cerebral blood flow consequent upon the cerebral vasodilatation produced by the hypoxemia. There is papilledema and blurring of vision. Sometimes pulmonary edema occurs as well.

The treatment is to remove the patient to a lower altitude as quickly as possible. Oxygen should be given if this is available, though the efficacy of this appears to be less than a reduction in barometric pressure. Patients with high altitude cerebral edema who are rapidly evacuated to lower altitudes often improve with dramatic suddenness.

High altitude retinal hemorrhages

These are common in climbers above altitudes of about 5,000 m. The condition is almost always symptomless and self-limiting. However if the hemorrhage is very near the optic disc there may be some blurring of vision. The hemorrhage is often flame-shaped and adjacent to a vessel. They generally disappear completely soon after descent. Presumably the etiology is the high cerebral blood flow caused by the hypoxemia.

REFERENCE

1.   Ward, M.P., J.S. Milledge and J.B. West High Altitude Medicine and Physiology. London, Chapman and Hall, 1989.

Preparing the Patient With COPD for Surgery

Roger C. Bone, M.D.

Obstructive lung disease is not really a disease but a
physiologic impairment which occurs as a result of
varying combinations of diseases such as chronic bronchitis, obstructive emphysema, asthma, bronchiectasis,
mucoviscidosis (cystic fibrosis), and central airway
obstruction. Chronic bronchitis is defined clinically
as sputum production on most days of the week for at
least three months of the year in two or more consecutive years. Pathologically, it is defined in terms of
mucous and serous gland and goblet cell hyperplasia in
the bronchial walls. In the strictest sense, emphysema
is defined as "a condition of the lung characterized by
increase beyond the normal in the size of air spaces
distal to the terminal bronchioles, with destructive
changes in their walls. However, the term is often used
more loosely in referring to chronic cigarette smokers
who develop hyperinflation of the lungs by physical
examination and chest roentgenogram and/or airflow
obstruction and loss of elastic recoil of the lung
detected in the pulmonary function laboratory. Chronic
bronchitis and emphysema usually occur in varying
combinations in the same patient. In 90 percent of

T. H. Stanley and R. J. Sperry (eds.), Anesthesia and the Lung, 59–68.
© 1989 by Kluwer Academic Publishers.

cases, chronic cigarette smoking can be implicated as
the causative factor, although there appear to be
genetic predispositions. Because of the confusion of
terms, more nonspecific diagnoses such as chronic
obstructive pulmonary disease (COPD), chronic obstructive airways disease (COAD), chronic nonspecific lung
disease (CNSLD), and chronic airflow obstruction (CAO)
have been applied. Although these terms are still in
common use, it is preferable to use the more specific
terms, chronic bronchitis and emphysema. In this condition the airflow obstruction is due to combinations of
airway narrowing or obstruction due to smooth muscle
spasm, excessive, thick mucus, and airway mucosal edema
(chronic bronchitis), decreased driving pressure for
expiratory airflow due to the loss of elastic recoil of
the lung (emphysema), and airway collapse during
expiration.

TREATMENT

The treatment of ARF is described as conservative
if the patient is managed without an artificial airway
and mechanical ventilation. About 75 percent or more of
patients can usually be managed conservatively. Certainly, the additional complications of an artificial
airway and mechanical ventilation should be a warning to
use this mode of therapy only as a last resort. The
patient's presenting blood gas values while breathing
room air can provide some indication as to the patient's
likely course. Bone et al. found that the initial PaO_2

and pH together could be used in a quadrant diagram to predict roughly the course. Their diagram basically shows that patients with PaO_2 less than 35 mm Hg, especially if acidotic, are very likely to require mechanical ventilation. A small review of 25 consecutive patients at the Atlanta Veterans Administration Medical Center similarly showed that 12 patients presenting with PaO_2 less than 36 mm Hg incurred a 50 percent incidence of intubation and mechanical ventilation whereas, of 13 patients with PaO_2 equal to or greater than 36 mm Hg, only one required mechanical ventilation.

Conservative therapy is directed at correcting life-threatening hypoxemia, improving airflow, treating primary or secondary infection and avoiding complications. If at all possible, patients should be managed in intensive care units. Rogers et al. found the mortality rate fell from 55 percent on the general wards to 19 percent in an intensive care unit. O'Donohue et al. also showed a mortality rate of 47 percent on general medical wards and 7.1 percent in a respiratory intensive care unit. Conservative management should be the initial approach in all patients who are sufficiently alert to cooperate with therapy.

The administration of oxygen is, in the mind of laymen, the panacea for shortness of breath. In ARF, the potentially lethal effects of severe hypoxemia are reason enough to make this the first priority. Because hypoxemia and oxygen delivery are discussed in a separate article, they will not be presented in detail here. Administering oxygen-enriched air to these patients sufficient to increase the PaO_2 to 50 to 60 mm Hg decreases hypoxic pulmonary arterial vasoconstriction and pulmonary arterial pressure, improves the handling of a water load by the renal tubules, decreases hypoxia-related bronchoconstriction, and improves oxygen transport to the tissues. In these patients, very small increases in inspired oxygen concentration often result in significant improvement in the PaO_2. The effects of oxygen administration are not all beneficial. Relief of hypoxic pulmonary vasoconstriction may result in increased perfusion of poorly ventilated areas of lung and decreased perfusion of well-ventilated areas. Elimination of the hypoxic ventilatory drive may cause a decrease in alveolar ventilation. Finally, the increase in the ratio of oxyhemoglobin to deoxyhemoglobin decreases the binding of carbon dioxide by hemoglobin (the Haldane effect). All these mechanisms tend to elevate the $PaCO_2$, primarily in the patient with pre-existing hypercapnia. This may result in increased respiratory acidosis and depressed sensorium.

From a practical standpoint, patients who are not chronically hypercapneic may be given oxygen with little concern for hypercapnia, and up to 40 to 50 percent oxygen may be given if necessary to maintain the PaO_2 at 50 to 60 mm Hg. In the patient who is chronically hypercapneic, more judicious oxygen administration is necessary. The most commonly used methods of administering small "doses" of oxygen are the Venturi masks and low-flow oxygen by nasal prongs. Venturi face masks provide 24 or 28 percent (or higher, if necessary) oxygen; however, for long-term use, they must be removed for the patient to eat, drink, or receive a medication aerosol. Nasal prongs with a flow of 1 to 2 liters per min are a suitable alternative, which, although the specific oxygen percentage is variable, do not have to be removed intermittently. At times, special flowmeters to deliver less than 1 liter per min may adequately treat hypoxemia when higher flowrates and 24 percent Venturi masks have produced serious ventilatory depression. It is important not to become alarmed with the almost expected rise in $PaCO_2$ with oxygen administration. As long as the patient remains coherent, easily arousable, and does not develop profound acidemia (pH < 7.25), conservative treatment with the low-flow oxygen should continue.

Improving airflow involves bronchodilator therapy, corticosteroids to reduce airway edema and inflammation, and the mechanical removal of tracheobronchial secretions.

Inhaled sympathomimetic drugs are extremely effective with a minimum of side effects. Parenteral or oral sympathomimetics may also be helpful; however, the major thrust in ARF should be administering aerosol drugs. Older nonselective bronchodilators such as epinephrine and isoproterenol have given way to newer drugs with longer duration of action and more selective action on the bronchial tree (beta-2 adrenergic activity) and less action on the cardiovascular system (beta-1 activity). Since patients with chronic bronchitis and emphysema are older, avoiding excessive cardiac stimulation is theoretically valuable. In ARF, I prefer to use medication aerosols generated by compressed air, although some physicians use metered-dose inhalers. Metaproterenol (Alupent, Metaprel) is marketed in a 5 percent solution for inhalation. Doses of 0.3 to 0.5 ml (15 to 25 mg) diluted in 2.5 ml normal saline may be given hourly for 3 to 4 doses, then every 3 to 4 hours thereafter. Isoetharine (Bronkosol) in a 1 percent solution, although less beta-2 selective, may be administered in doses of 0.5 to 1.0 ml (5 to 10 mg) diluted in 1 to 2 ml normal saline at similar or even slightly more frequent intervals. Terbutaline (Brethine, Bricanyl), although marketed in a solution for injection, has been used as an aerosol in doses of 1 to 2 mg at similar intervals. Although effective and without apparent problems, the injectable form of terbutaline has not been officially approved by the Food and Drug Administration for inhalation.

Intravenous aminophylline, which is 85 percent anhydrous theophylline, is also an effective bronchodilator in chronic bronchitis and emphysema. Besides specific effects on the airways, it has been shown to improve right and left ventricular performance, improve the ventilatory response to hypoxia, increase mucociliary clearance, and improve respiratory muscle contractility. Its bronchodilator effect appears to be additive with sympathomimetic drugs, and it should be used in combination with them. The therapeutic range of serum theophylline is 10 to 20 mg per liter. Recent data suggest that a greater improvement in airflow is associated with maintaining the serum concentration near 20 mg per liter rather than at 10 mg per liter. Close monitoring of the serum theophylline concentration is essential since clearance in critically ill patients may fluctuate. Adverse effects of serum concentrations above 25 mg per liter include cardiac arrhythmias and seizures. Since theophylline pharmacokinetics are affected by cigarrete smoking, congestive heart failure, pneumonia, and severe airways obstruction, some modification of the maintenance dose is necessary in patients with these conditions. The recommendations of Powell et al. provide an initial dosage which can then be modified depending on the serum concentrations achieved.

Loading dose = Desired serum concentration/ 1.6 mg per kg

Maintenance infusion = Desired serum concentration X 0.05 mg per kg per hr

The maintenance infusion is multiplied by the following factors in the presence of these respective conditions:

current smoking, 1.6; congestive heart failure, 0.4;
pneumonia, 0.4; and severe airways obstruction, 0.8. It
is important to restate that these calculations are used
to arrive at a beginning dosage, and the infusion rate
may require adjustment if the serum concentration is too
high or too low.

A third method of bronchodilatation is the use of
an aerosolized parasympatholytic such as atropine
sulfate. This drug has been shown to be effective in
chronic bronchitis and mucoviscidosis. The optimum dose
for patients with chronic bronchitis and emphysema
appears to be 0.025 mg per kg. Aerosolized atropine may
be administered every 4 hours in an alternating manner
with inhaled sympathomimetics so that the patient
receives one or the other every 2 hours. Recent data
from Lefcoe et al. support the use of parasympatholy-
tics in combination with sympathomimetics and theophylline. Side effects of atropine at this dose are minimal, but if the dose is increased, dry mouth, tachycardia, and urinary retention may become problems. Con-
trary to medical folklore, no data exist to support the
contention that parasympatholytic drugs cause adverse
effects related to the theoretical drying and inspissa-
tion of mucus in the airways.

The value of corticosteroids in the treatment of
acute asthma has been known for many years; however,
their use in chronic bronchitis and emphysema has
been controversial. Data are now available that

corticosteroids are useful in ARF from chronic
bronchitis and emphysema and in stable patients as well.
Although many physicians advocate extremely large doses
(250 to 500 mg methylprednisolone or its equivalent),
there appears to be no advantage over much smaller
doses. Intravenous methylprednisolone 0.5 mg per kg or
hydrocortisone 2.5 mg per kg given every 6 hours should
provide optimum patient benefit.

Antibiotic and Adjunctive Therapy

Antibiotic treatment of ARF from chronic bronchitis
and emphysema is controversial in the literature but
seldom omitted in clinical practice. If acute bacterial
pneumonia is present, sputum Gram's stain and sputum and
blood cultures should be obtained. If the Gram's stain
shows a total predominance of one organism, initial
therapy may be directed specifically at that organism.
If there are multiple organisms, then antibiotic cover-
age should include treatment both for gram-positive and
gram-negative organisms until culture results are available. Penicillin, ampicillin, or a cephalosporin combined with an aminoglycoside are usually adequate. If
the ARF is associated with acute bronchitis, ampicillin
500 mg orally every 6 hr or tetracycline 500 mg orally
every 6 hr may be administered. However,a recent controlled trial of tetracycline versus a placebo showed no
differences in subjective or objective parameters in
exacerbations of chronic bronchitis. The use of an
antibiotic in this situation is probably optimal and is

left to the clinical judgment of the physician.

Adjunctive therapy such as hydration, suctioning of secretions, postural drainage and vibration, and bland aerosol therapy is often administered, although few data exist to document effectiveness. The term "vigorous pulmonary toilet" has been applied to adjunctive therapy; however, it is somewhat misleading, since the term implies therapeutic value. Dehydration can thicken bronchopulmonary secretions, but the value of forcing intravenous or oral fluids into well-hydrated patients is doubtful. There are also no data to support the use of postural drainage and chest percussion or vibration in patients with acute exacerbations of chronic bronchitis and emphysema. Bland aerosol therapy (saline mist) is empirical and probably of little or no benefit. Properly performed nasotracheal suction in patients who are unable to clear copius secretions effectively may be beneficial.

ANESTHETIC INFLUENCES ON THE PULMONARY CIRCULATION

BRYAN E. MARSHALL

Department of Anesthesia, University of Pennsylvania School of Medicine,
Philadelphia, Pennsylvania 19104

INTRODUCTION

Most current textbooks (1,2) conclude that general anesthetic agents,
whether injectable or inhalational, have relatively little apparent effect
on the pulmonary circulation. This conclusion is primarily based on
measurements of pulmonary artery pressure or calculations of the overall
pulmonary vascular conductance (or resistance), both of which are
functions of so many variables that only gross changes are detectable.
The available data concerning anesthesia has rapidly expanded in both
quantity and sophistication and the work has established that general
anesthetic agents alter lung mechanics, blood volume distribution, cardiac
output, myocardial contractility, vascular tone, blood pH and carbon
dioxide tension, pulmonary blood flow distribution and the effectiveness
of the major active regulator of pulmonary blood flow, hypoxic pulmonary
vasoconstriction (HPV). All of these factors influence the pulmonary
circulation and, therefore, anesthesia could be expected to be accompanied
by more or less profound changes. In the previous lecture concerning the
regulation of the pulmonary circulation, some of these factors were
discussed and a model was introduced that provides quantitative insight as
to the outcome and mechanisms of multiple influences on the pulmonary
circulation and gas exchange (3,4). With such an approach, it is possible
to suggest which of the many changes introduced during general anesthesia
have predominant effects.

OUTCOME

There are two principal ways by which the outcome of anesthetic
influences on the pulmonary circulation become manifest. The first is by
a change in pulmonary vascular conductance; for example, stimulation of
pulmonary vasoconstriction or application of increased positive end-

T. H. Stanley and R. J. Sperry (eds.), Anesthesia and the Lung, 69–77.

expiratory pressure will reduce conductance, while increased cardiac output or administration of drugs that inhibit vascular smooth muscle constriction (i.e. nitroprusside or nitroglycerin) will increase conductance. The result of changing pulmonary vascular conductance is a concomitant change in pulmonary artery pressure and/or cardiac output. The second manifestation is an alteration of regional blood flow so as to change the distribution of ventilation/perfusion ratios. The result is a change in gas exchange that particularly influence oxygenation.

Most general anesthetics have influences that both reduce and enhance these manifestations and considerable confusion has been introduced, particularly from studies of intact humans by attempts to identify quantitative effects of anesthetics from fragmentary data (5).

THE CENTRAL ROLE OF HYPOXIC VASOCONSTRICTION

As has been emphasized already, pulmonary vascular tone is influenced by passive mechanical factors and by numerous vasoactive drugs. Furthermore, a large number of circulating humoral or neurogenic mediators can influence the final responsiveness of the pulmonary vasculature. Yet, the principal regulator of pulmonary vascular tone that has so far been established is hypoxic pulmonary vasoconstriction. It is, therefore, important to understand the strength of and the stimulus for this response and its influence on both physiology and pathophysiology during anesthesia.

That the response is a powerful one is reflected in the two to three fold decrease in conductance that may accompany breathing hypoxic gas mixtures. The response has an almost immediate onset when hypoxia is introduced and lasts as long as observations have been recorded. The profound effect on arterial oxygenation is illustrated in Figure 1 by comparison of the arterial oxygen tension expected with increasing fraction of atelectatic lung both with and in the absence of an active HPV response.

Even the influence of pH and PCO_2 appears to be secondary to the HPV response. Because the vasoconstriction associated with acidosis is progressively reduced with increasing oxygen tension and is abolished when both alveolar and mixed venous oxygen tension approach 700 mmHg.

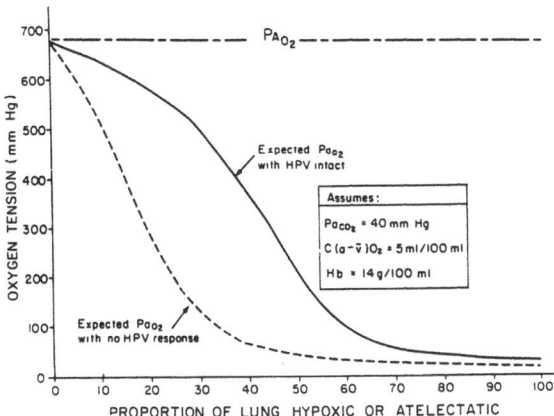

Figure 1. Role of HPV in preserving arterial oxygen tension.

The stimulus for HPV is a resultant of both alveolar and mixed venous oxygen tension. The latter becomes increasingly significant as alveolar oxygen tension is reduced (Figure 2) and, of course, in atelectasis the "alveolar" oxygen tension is the mixed venous oxygen tension. It is

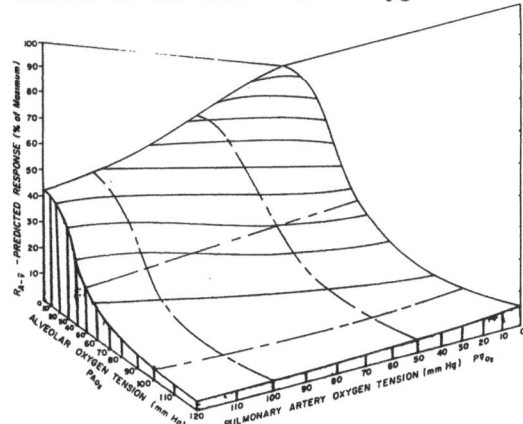

Figure 2. The alveolar and mixed venous oxygen tension stimulation of HPV.

readily appreciated that HPV may serve to improve ventilation/perfusion ratios or to reduce the perfusion of atelectatic lung and both of these effects result in a predominantly beneficial improvement in oxygenation. But these same influences are also the cause of pathophysiologic increases in pulmonary vascular tone. Thus, patients with limited cardiac reserve following cardiac surgery may demonstrate right heart failure if the mixed

venous oxygen tension is low enough (<30 mmHg) to cause a generalized HPV
response. In this latter context, the HPV cannot be regarded as
homeostatic and the rationale for the empirical therapeutic use of
nitroprusside in this situation is evident. A somewhat similar pattern
appear to account for some types of persistent fetal hypertension where
HPV increases the pulmonary vascular tone sufficiently so as to prevent
closure of the ductus arteriosus. The realization that HPV is markedly
inhibited by alkalosis is, therefore, particularly interesting because one
of the few therapies with considerable success in these infants is to
induce alkalosis by hyperventilation and/or administration of bicarbonate.

APPLICATIONS TO ANESTHESIA

All that remains is to add the specific influence of anesthetic drugs
on the hypoxic vasoconstrictor response. The apparent inconsistencies
between the observed effects of a variety of in vivo studies (see, for
example, Table 2 in reference number 2) can be largely resolved by the
considerations summarized in Figure 3. This figure shows that while most
inhalational anesthetics in the usual clinical doses inhibit the HPV

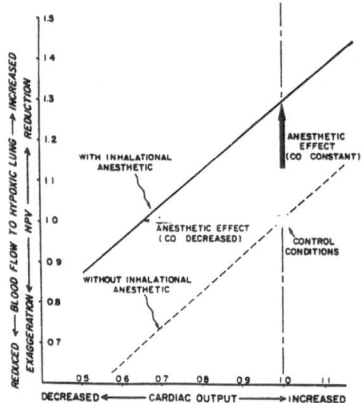

Figure 3. Influence of inhalational anesthetics on observed response to
HPV. Abscissa shows relative cardiac output and ordinate shows apparent
HPV effect. In absence of inhalational anesthetics, dashed line indicates
changes in blood flow to an hypoxic lung region that occurs as total
cardiac output changes. Solid line parallel to this shows same
relationship in presence of inhalational anesthetics. Vertical arrow
demonstrates the true reduction of HPV response associated with
inhalational anesthetics when cardiac output is not changed. Horizontal
arrow illustrates how action of anesthetic agent simultaneously depresses
HPV directly and enhances HPV through cardiac depression and leads to an
apparently unchanged response to HPV.

response by 20-50%, this may not be observed if the cardiac output changes simultaneously. The explanation for this result is that decreasing the cardiac output decreases the mixed venous oxygen tension ($P_{\bar{v}O2}$) and potentiates the hypoxic constriction stimulation (Figure 4). The actions

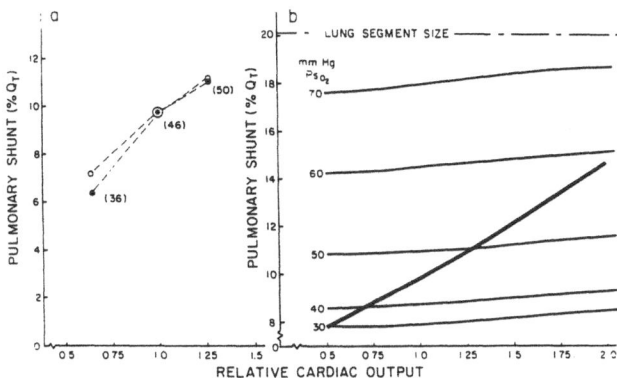

Figure 4. Pulmonary shunt increases with cardiac output because the $P\bar{v}O_2$ increases and reduces the HPV effect.

of the anesthetic, the one a direct inhibition and the other an indirect potentiation may offset each other, sometimes completely. A precise derivation from additional data suggests the following form of the relationship (Figure 5) (3).

$$\text{\%Depression HPV} = \frac{100\ (\text{Anesthetic:MAC})^{2.92}}{4.9 + (\text{Anesthetic:MAC})^{2.92}}$$

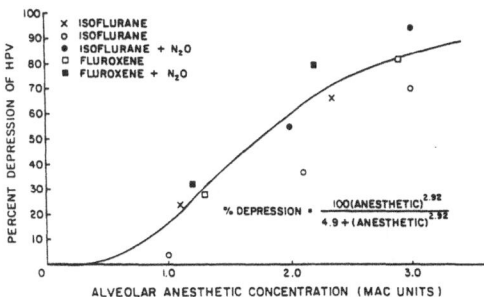

Figure 5. Depression of HPV by inhalational anesthetics in vivo.

74

This result is incorporated into the computer model by modifying the amount of the constriction induced by hypoxia according to the alveolar anesthetic concentration in MAC units.

This model now allows the pressure and flow distribution to be predicted for two compartments of any size and with any combination of the defined variables. The individual quantities representing ventilation or PEEP, pleural pressure, alveolar oxygen or inhalational anesthetics and so forth can be selected independently for each compartment and thus the influence of an anesthetic can be examined overall and by each of the contributing components.

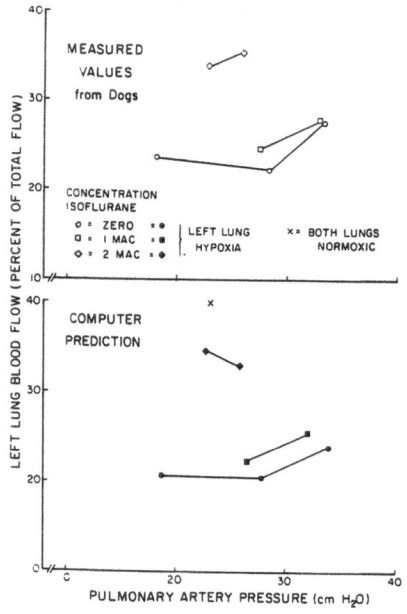

Figure 6. The influence of isoflurane on the left lung blood flow when ventilated with an hypoxic gas mixture. The upper panel shows the mean values for experimental data from six dogs. The cross represents the values for left lung pressure and flow when ventilated with 100% oxygen without isoflurane. The open circles connect the values for pressure and flow to the left lung when ventilated with an hypoxic gas mixture in the absence of isoflurane, but with three levels of cardiac output. The addition of 1 and 2 MAC isoflurane increases the left lung blood flow by inhibition of the hypoxic constriction. The lower panel shows the output from the computer model in the same circumstances. The cross, circles, square and diamonds have the same meaning as the upper panel and it is evident that the data are similar in both.

In one experiment in dogs (6), isoflurane in 1.0 or 2 MAC concentrations was administered to the left lung that was alternately ventilated with oxygen or an hypoxic gas mixture. The procedure was repeated at various levels of cardiac output. The experimental results are depicted in the upper half of Figure 6 and in the lower half are shown the computer model simulation of this experiment. It is evident that the changes are comparable both quantitatively and qualitatively.

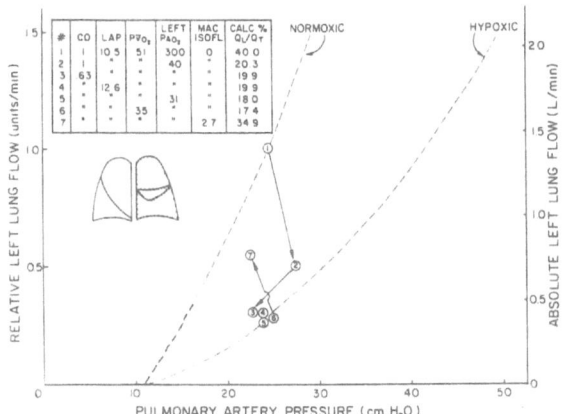

Figure 7. Analysis of factors influencing response to HPV during isoflurane anesthesia in intact dogs.

The basis for these effects are analyzed for the 2.0 MAC concentrations of isoflurane in Figure 7. The initial conditions during 100% oxygen breathing with no isoflurane are shown at position 1. The left lung flow is 1.0 relation unit and the pulmonary artery pressure is 25 cm H_2O. In the presence of 2 MAC isoflurane and hypoxia, the left lung is located at position 7. The points numbered 2-6 in between demonstrate prediction of the computer model of how each change associated with the anesthesia and hypoxia contributed to the final outcome. The analysis demonstrates that the principal effects in this experiment were: 1-2, the reduction of flow to the left lung and increase of pulmonary artery pressure due to HPV; 2-3, the decrease in cardiac output associated with the introduction of isoflurane _in vivo_; and 6-7, the specific inhibition of hypoxic pulmonary vasoconstriction by isoflurane. The smaller contributions by the changes in left atrial pressure and mixed venous oxygen tension are also identified. The graphical representation of the pathway as a discrete series of steps allows the complex interaction of all of the changes on the pulmonary circulation that accompany anesthesia to be readily assessed.

SUMMARY

This discussion has argued that the complexity and subtleness of the interactions exhibited by the pulmonary circulation have made it difficult to identify any but the most gross of effects of anesthesia on the pulmonary circulation and, in particular, the calculation of an index such as pulmonary vascular conductance (or resistance) has come to be recognized of little value for detailed analysis.

Instead, the value of displaying data graphically as pressure and flow ordinates is presented and the importance of the pressure-flow curve has been emphasized. A generalized computer model of the pulmonary circulation is presented which is based on the real morphologic and biodynamic properties of the pulmonary circulation. The model incorporates all of the usual factors that influence the pulmonary circulation, including the alveolar, pleural and left atrial pressure, the cardiac output and pulmonary artery pressure, the hemoglobin concentration and the influence of alveolar and mixed venous oxygen tension on hypoxic pulmonary vasoconstriction. This model is used to demonstrate and explore the effects of pressure change, anesthetic agent and one-lung anesthesia on pulmonary function.

It is evident that anesthetic agents and techniques can have profound effects on the pulmonary circuit and it appears that the necessary tools to identify and investigate these effects are just now coming to hand.

ACKNOWLEDGEMENT

This work supported in part by grant #GM29628 from the Institute of General Medical Sciences, NIH.

REFERENCES

1. Bergman N.A. General Anesthesia. Butterworths, Boston, 1980.
2. Pavlin E.G. Anesthesia. Churchill Livingstone, New York, 1986.
3. Marshall B.E., Longnecker D.E., Fairley H.B. Anesthesia for thoracic procedures. Blackwell Scientific, Boston, 1982.
4. Marshall B.E. and Marshall C. J Appl Physiol 64:68-77, 1988.
5. Marshall B.E. and Marshall C. Effects of anesthesia. American Physiological Society, Bethesda, 1985.

6. Domino K.B., Borowec L., Alexander C.M., Williams J.J., Chen L., Marshall C. and Marshall B.E. Anesthesiology <u>64</u>:423-429, 1986.

VENTILATION-PERFUSION MISMATCHING DURING ANESTHESIA

J. F. NUNN.
Division of Anaesthesia, Clinical Research Centre, Harrow, U.K.

THE THREE-COMPARTMENT MODEL OF GAS EXCHANGE

This model is useful, not because it has any pretensions to be a
correct representation of affairs, but because it is practical,
capable of precise definition and of direct relevance to therapy. It
presents the lung as though it comprises three compartments - ideally
perfused and ventilated alveoli, alveolar dead space and shunt (Figure
1). Physiological dead space is easily quantified by the Bohr
equation, and shunt by the shunt equation.

It has long been known that anaesthesia (with or without paralysis)
results in an increase in the alveolar component of the physiological
dead space so that the VD/VT ratio from carina downwards approximates
to 0.3 (Figure 2); this is increased to 0.5 if the volume of the
endo-tracheal tube is included.

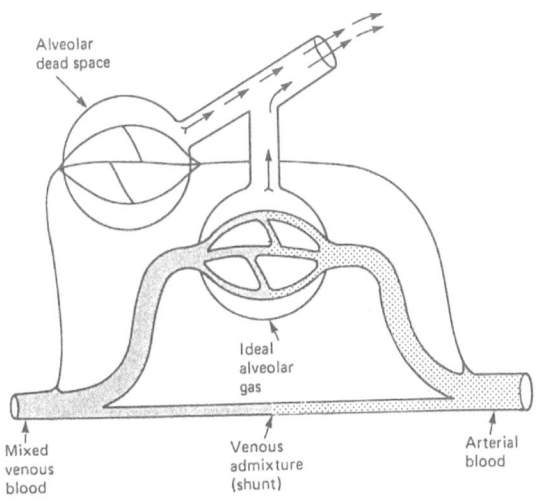

Figure 1

T. H. Stanley and R. J. Sperry (eds.), Anesthesia and the Lung, 79–84.
© 1989 by Kluwer Academic Publishers.

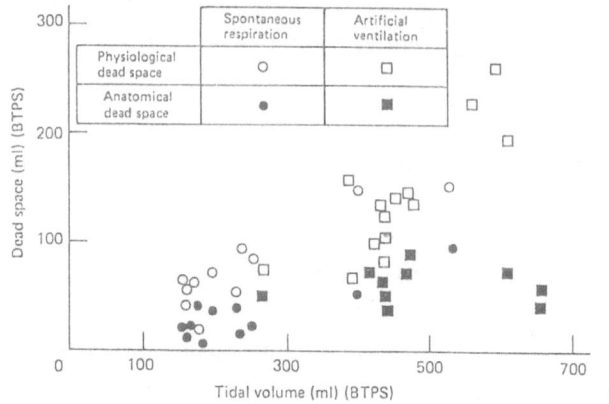

Figure 2

The shunt is also increased during anaesthesia (with or without paralysis) and is usually within the range 5 - 15 % of cardiac output. Figure 3 shows mean values for shunt for 8 individual studies, cited in reference 1.

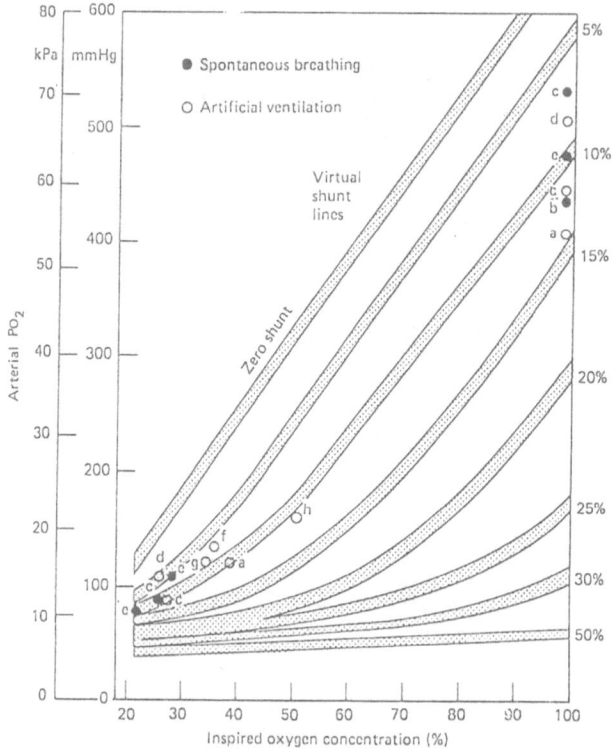

Figure 3

VERTICAL STRATIFICATION OF $\dot{V}/\dot{Q}$ RATIOS

Hulands et al. (2) investigated normal tidal breathing in the
supine anesthetized patient and found only slight preferential
ventilation of the posterior slices of the lungs compared with the
anterior slices with the dependent parts receiving approximately
double the perfusion of the uppermost parts at FRC. $\dot{V}/\dot{Q}$ ratios at the
top of the lung averaged about 1.5 times the ratios at the bottom. It
was not possible to demonstrate an area without perfusion (Zone 1).

Huland's group found no change in the distribution of ventilation
following the induction of anaesthesia with paralysis and artificial
ventilation. There was, however, a slight increase in the
maldistribution of perfusion and therefore the $\dot{V}/\dot{Q}$ ratios. The
changes were of minimal clinical significance.

DISTRIBUTION OF VENTILATION AND PERFUSION IN TERMS OF $\dot{V}/\dot{Q}$ RATIOS

Analysis of the distribution of pulmonary ventilation and perfusion
in terms of $\dot{V}/\dot{Q}$ ratios is a particularly complex and challenging
technique, particularly under the conditions of anaesthesia.

Rehder et al (3) studied young healthy volunteers, and both
ventilation and perfusion were found to be distributed to a wider
range of $\dot{V}/\dot{Q}$ ratios after induction of anaesthesia and paralysis
(Figure 4). The true intrapulmonary shunt had a mean value of less

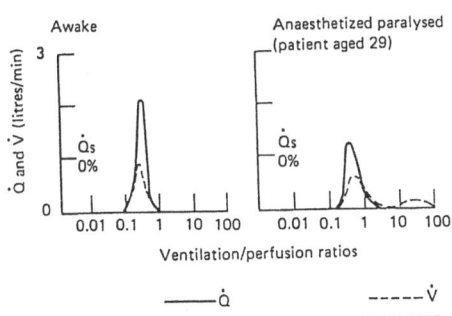

Mean values		
$\dot{Q}s/\dot{Q}t$	0%	0.9%
V_D/V_T	35%	26%
PaO_2	143 mmHg	117 mmHg

F_{IO_2} 30%
Age range 24-33

Figure 4

than 1 per cent during anaesthesia but the alveolar/arterial Po_2 gradient was slightly increased and this was attributed to the increased spread of the distribution of perfusion to areas of poorer ventilation (lower $\dot{V}/\dot{Q}$ ratio). Alveolar dead space was increased, partly due to increased spread of distribution of ventilation to areas of higher ventilation/perfusion ratio. In a group of surgical patients of similar age range to Rehder's volunteers, Prutow et al. (4) found an average increase in shunt of 8 per cent during anaesthesia. Pulmonary blood flow to areas of zero and low $\dot{V}/\dot{Q}$ correlated with the reduction in FRC.

Bindslev et al (5) studied typical surgical patients, aged 37 to 64. They were studied awake, anaesthetized and breathing spontaneously, anaesthetized paralysed and ventilated artificially and finally with PEEP. In this group of older patients, they found that the true intrapulmonary shunt was increased during anaesthesia (Figure 5). However, the shunt calculated from the alveolar/arterial Po_2 gradient according to the three-compartment lung model would be larger still and the difference would be due to perfusion of areas of low $\dot{V}/\dot{Q}$ ratio. The dead space/tidal volume ratio was increased during anaesthesia in spite of the tracheal tube bypassing the upper airway. PEEP reduced the shunt but also reduced the cardiac output and therefore the mixed venous oxygen content. The decreased admixture of more desaturated blood resulted in virtually no change in arterial Po_2.

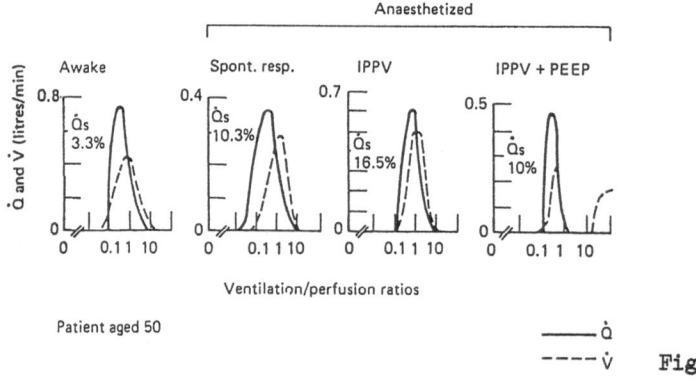

Figure 5

Dueck et al (6) studied elderly patients (mean age 60), who all had some deterioration in pulmonary function. His results can most easily be appreciated by considering the patients in three groups (Figure 6).

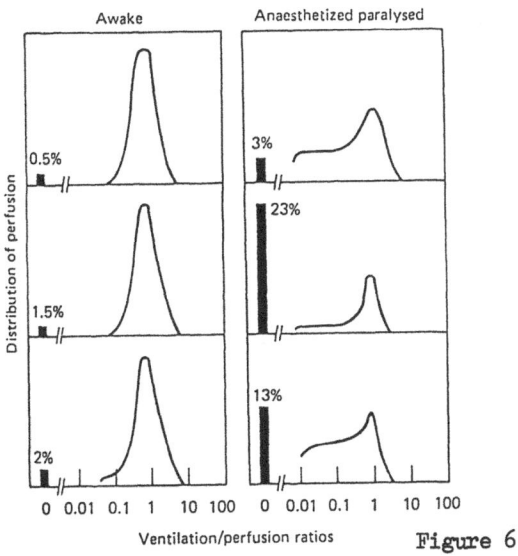

Figure 6

In the first, there was only a small increase in the true shunt following the induction of anaesthesia, but there appeared a "shelf" of perfusion of regions of very low $\dot{V}/\dot{Q}$ ratios in the range 0.01 - 0.1. In the second group, this "shelf" was less prominent but there was a substantial increase in true shunt. Finally, in the third group, there was both a "shelf" and an increase in true shunt. All of these changes are compatible with a decrease in FRC below closing capacity.

These three studies of ventilation/perfusion relationships during anaesthesia complement one another and give us greatly increased insight into the effect of anaesthesia on gas exchange.

CONCLUSIONS

The effects of anaesthesia on alveolar/arterial Po_2 gradient may be summarized as follows:

1. Changes in alveolar/arterial Po_2 gradient are markedly affected by age, being minimal in the young.

2. The increase in alveolar/arterial Po_2 gradient is due partly to an increase in true intrapulmonary shunt and partly to increased distribution of perfusion to areas of low (but not zero) $\dot{V}/\dot{Q}$ ratios.

3. The increase in alveolar dead space appears to be due to increased distribution of ventilation to areas of high (but not usually infinite) $\dot{V}/\dot{Q}$ ratios.

4. The major differences are between the awake and the anaesthetized states. Paralysis and artificial ventilation do not greatly alter the parameters of gas exchange, in spite of the quite different spatial distribution of ventilation.

5. PEEP reduces the shunt but the beneficial effect on arterial Po_2 is offset by the decrease in cardiac output which reduces the mixed venous oxygen content.

REFERENCES.

1. Nunn,J.F. (1987) Applied Respiratory Physiology, 3rd edition. London: Butterworths.
2. Hulands,G.H., Green,R., Iliff,L.D. and Nunn,J.F. Clin. Sci. 38 451-460, 1970.
3. Rehder,K., Knopp,T.J. Sessler,A.D. and Didier,E.P. J. appl. Physiol. 47 745-753, 1979.
4. Prutow,R.J., Dueck,R., Davies,N.J.H. and Clausen,J. Anesthesiol. 57 A477 1982.
5. Bindlsev,L., Hedenstierna,G., Santesson,J., Gottlieb,I. and Carvallhas,A. Acta Anaesthesiol. Scand. 25 360-371, 1981.
6. Dueck,R., Young,I., Clausen,J. and Wagner,P.D. Anesthesiol. 52 113-125, 1980.

ANESTHESIA AND CHANGES IN LUNG VOLUME.

J. F. NUNN.
Division of Anaesthesia, Clinical Research Centre, Harrow, UK.

Perhaps the most fundamental effect of anesthesia on the respiratory system is the decrease of the functional residual capacity. The cause of this change probably lies in the effect of anesthesia on the respiratory muscles. During normal breathing by the conscious subject in the supine position, the diaphragm retains considerable tone at the end of expiration. This holds the lung volume above that which it would attain if determined solely by the equilibration of elastic forces. This may well be a special mechanism to prevent the weight of the viscera pushing the diaphragm too far into the chest in the supine position. Muller and his colleagues (1) have used diaphragmatic electromyography to demonstrate that this residual end-expiratory tone is lost during anesthesia with halothane. Under these circumstances, the end-expiratory position of the diaphragm is the same as in the paralysed patient.

Freund, Roos and Dodd (3) first demonstrated that general anesthesia caused phasic activity of the expiratory abdominal muscles which are normally silent in the conscious supine subject. This activation of expiratory muscles seems to serve no useful purpose and it does not appear to have any significant effect on the change in functional residual capacity.

Bergman (3) was the first to report a decrease of functional residual capacity (FRC) during anesthesia. This was followed by many studies which have established the following characteristics of the change.

1. FRC is reduced during anesthesia with all anesthetic drugs which have been investigated, by a mean value of about 16 - 20 per cent of the FRC (in the supine position). However, there is

T. H. Stanley and R. J. Sperry (eds.), Anesthesia and the Lung, 85–91.

considerable individual variation and changes range from about +19 per cent to -50 per cent.

2. FRC does not seem to fall progressively during anesthesia and appears to reach its final value within the first few minutes of anesthesia. It does not return to normal until some hours after the end of anesthesia.

3. Inhalation of high concentrations of oxygen does not appear to be a factor in the change and does not usually result in progressive changes.

4. FRC is reduced to the same extent during anesthesia whether the patient is paralysed or not.

5. Expiratory muscle activity has no significant effect on the change in FRC.

6. The reduction in FRC has a weak but significant correlation with the age of the patient.

7. Artificial ventilation of the conscious subject causes only a small reduction in FRC.

8. Anaesthesia does not change FRC in the sitting position.

(see references 4, 5 and 6)

Froese and Bryan (7) in a classic study of lateral chest radiographs during anesthesia clearly showed that the diaphragm ascended into the chest by about 2 cm during anesthesia with or without paralysis and this change accorded roughly with the decrease in FRC (Figure 1).

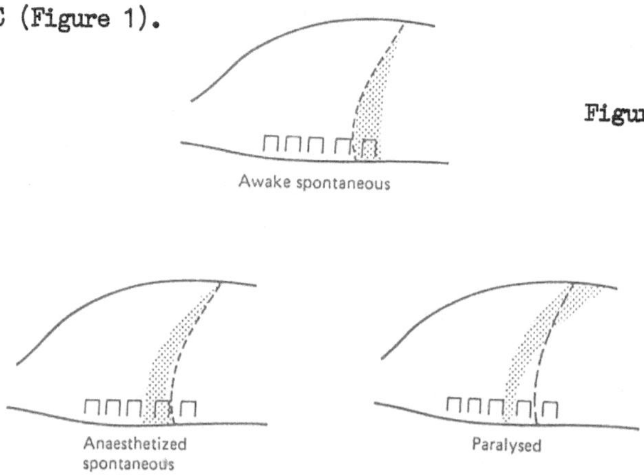

Figure 1

Awake spontaneous

Anaesthetized spontaneous

Paralysed

The next generation of studies used new imaging techniques to make more precise measurements of geometric changes and to relate these to observed changes in FRC and central blood volume. Hedenstierna and his colleagues (8) used computerized tomography to indicate the changes following anesthesia and paralysis which are summarized in Figure 2. The ascent of the diaphragm was found to correspond to

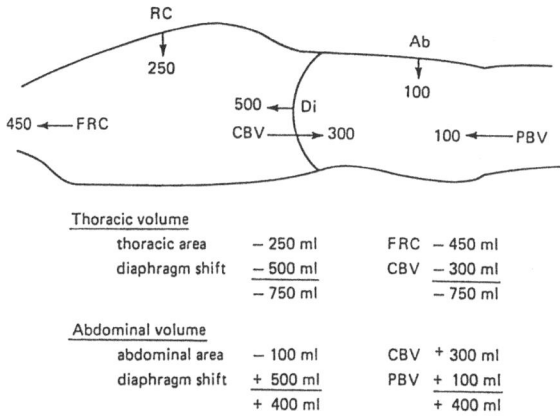

Thoracic volume

thoracic area	− 250 ml	FRC − 450 ml
diaphragm shift	− 500 ml	CBV − 300 ml
	− 750 ml	− 750 ml

Abdominal volume

abdominal area	− 100 ml	CBV + 300 ml
diaphragm shift	+ 500 ml	PBV + 100 ml
	+ 400 ml	+ 400 ml

Figure 2

slightly more than the observed decrease in FRC (450 ml). However, there was also a decrease in the volume of the rib cage of 250 ml which was more than offset by a shift of blood volume from thorax to abdomen. The decrease in diameter of the rib cage corresponding to a volume change of 250 ml would be only about 2 mm and it is not surprising that this had been missed by earlier investigators. Abdominal blood volume increased by a total of 400 ml which almost entirely offset the ascent of the diaphragm. The resultant decrease in abdominal volume was only 100 ml which would be very difficult to measure by conventional methods.

CONSEQUENCES OF THE CHANGE IN FUNCTIONAL RESIDUAL CAPACITY

In the supine position, the expiratory reserve has a mean value of only 1 litre in males and 660 ml in females. Therefore, the reduction in FRC following the induction of anesthesia will bring the lung

volume close to residual volume. This has major effects on lung
function, particularly in respect to airway closure, airway calibre,
compliance and gas exchange.

Airway closure

A reduction of FRC, such as follows the induction of anesthesia,
might be expected to reduce the end-expiratory lung volume below the
closing capacity (CC), at least in older patients, and so result in
airway closure, absorption collapse of lung and shunting.

Pulmonary collapse can easily be demonstrated in conscious subjects
who voluntarily breathe oxygen close to residual volume (9). Figure 3
shows the effect on arterial Po_2 of breathing air at different lung
volumes in the author at the age of 45. "Miliary atelectasis" was put
forward by Bendixen, Hedley-Whyte and Laver (10) as an explanation of
the increased alveolar/arterial Po_2 difference during anesthesia.
Computerized tomography has now shown "compression collapse" in
dependent zones of the lung following the induction of anesthesia

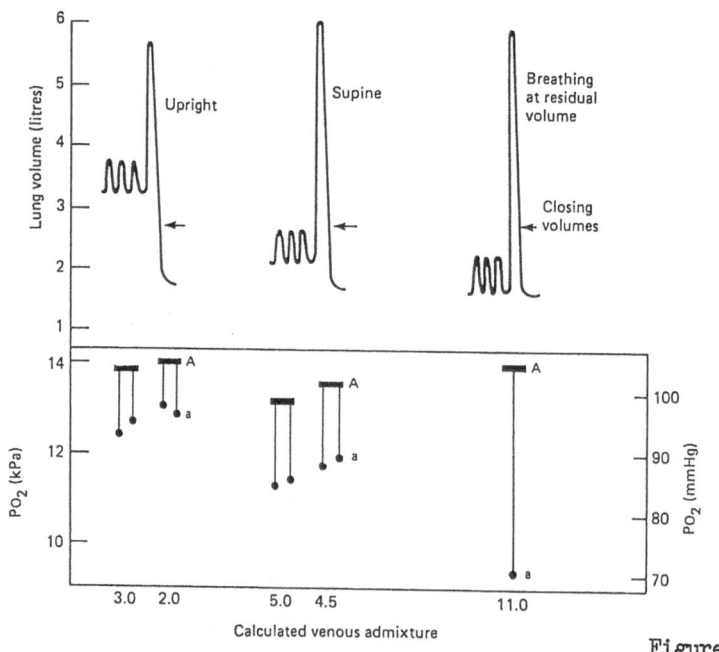

Figure 3

(11). For technical reasons, it would be extremely difficult to define these areas with conventional radiography.

Airway calibre

Figure 4 shows the hyperbolic relationship between lung volume and airway resistance. This is due to the fact that the airways participate in the overall change in lung volume and, other things being equal, as the lung volume decreases, the airway calibre is reduced and the airway resistance increased. Figure 4 clearly shows that the curve is steep in the region of FRC in the supine position and therefore the reduction in FRC which occurs during anesthesia should result in a marked increase in airway resistance. However, the effect of decreased lung volume is to a large extent offset by the bronchodilator effect which seems to be shared by most of the inhalational anesthetics.

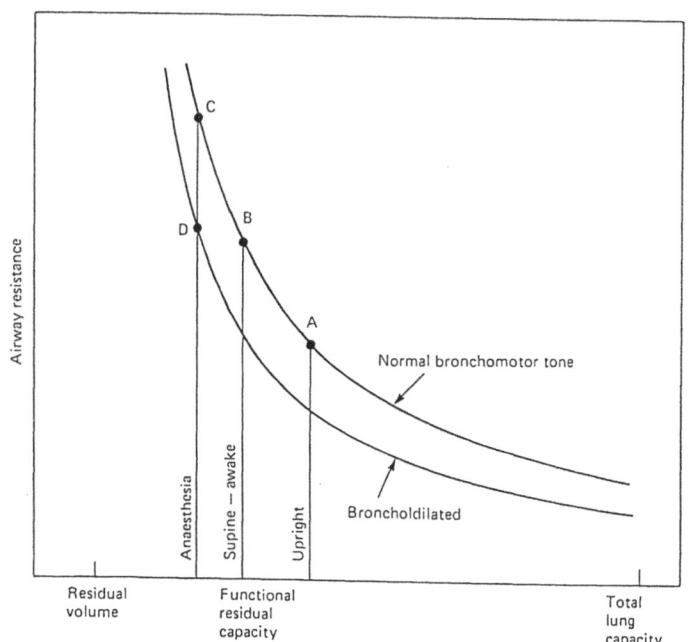

Figure 4

Compliance

Figure 5, based on the work of Westbrook et al. (12) and Butler and
Smith (13), summarizes the effect of anesthesia on the
pressure/volume relationships of the lung and chest wall. The diagram
shows the major differences between the conscious state and
anesthesia. There are, however, only minor differences between
anesthesia with and without paralysis.

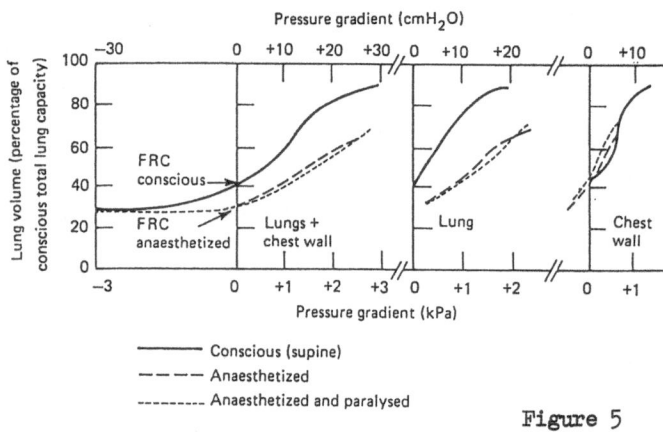

Conscious (supine)
Anaesthetized
Anaesthetized and paralysed

Figure 5

The left-hand section shows the relationship for the whole
respiratory system comprising lungs plus chest wall. The curves
obtained during anesthesia clearly show the reduction in FRC (lung
volume with zero pressure gradient from alveoli to ambient). The
subatmospheric section of the curve also shows the very small volume
change which can be achieved by application of a subatmospheric
pressure to the airway of an anesthetized patient. This implies a
very low expiratory reserve volume. Application of a positive
pressure as high as 3 kPa (30 cm H_2O) to the airways expands the lungs
to barely 70 per cent of the pre-operative total lung capacity, which
implies a reduced overall compliance. The two sections of Figure 5 on
the right show that the major changes are in the lung rather than the
chest wall.

REFERENCES

1. Muller, N., Volgyesi, G., Becker, L., Bryan, M.H. and Bryan, A.C. J. Appl. Physiol. 47: 279-284, 1979.
2. Freund, F., Roos, A. and Dodd, R.B. J. Appl. Physiol. 19: 693-697, 1964.
3. Bergman, N.A. J. Appl. Physiol. 18: 1085-1089, 1963.
4. Hewlett, A.M., Hulands, G.H., Nunn, J.F. and Heath, J.R. Br. J. Anaesth. 46: 486-494, 1974.
5. Hewlett, A.M., Hulands, G.H., Nunn, J.F. and Milledge, J.S. Br. J. Anaesth. 46: 495-503, 1974.
6. Rehder, K. and Marsh, H.M. Handbook of Physiology, Section 3: 737-752, 1987.
7. Froese, A.B. and Bryan, A.C. Anesthesiology 41: 242-255, 1974.
8. Hedenstierna, G., Standberg, A., Brismar, B., Lundquist, H., Svenson, L. and Tokics, L. Anesthesiology 62: 247-254, 1985.
9. Nunn, J.F., Coleman, A.J., Sachithanandan, T., Bergman, N.A. and Laws, J.W. Br. J. Anaesth. 37: 3-11, 1965.
10. Bendixen, H.H., Hedley-Whyte, J. and Laver, M.B. New Engl. J. Med. 269: 991-996, 1963.
11. Brismar, B., Hedenstierna, G., Lundquist, H., Standberg, A., Svenson, L. and Tokics, L. Anesthesiology 62: 422-428, 1985.
12. Westbrook, P.R., Stubbs, S.E., Sessler, A.D., Rehder, K. and Hyatt, R.E. J. Appl. Physiol. 34: 81-86, 1973.
13. Butler, J. and Smith, B.H. Clin. Sci. 16: 125-146, 1956.

OXIMETRY I: NOMENCLATURE, HISTORY, ACCURACY and USES

John W. Severinghaus, MD

University of California Medical School, San Francisco

NOMENCLATURE [1]:

Pulse oximeter reading is designated S_pO_2. Arterial and venous saturation, S_aO_2 and S_vO_2, are $100[O_2 \text{ content}]/[O_2 \text{ capacity}]$. O_2 capacity is determined by exposing the blood to a bubble of O_2, measuring the O_2 content by a physical or electrochemical method, and subtracting the dissolved O_2 determined by measuring Po_2 after bubble equilibration. O_2 capacity is not determined by 1.35 times hemoglobin concentration. HbCO and HbMet reduce O_2 content and capacity but do not reduce S_aO_2 at high Po_2. The value computed from Po_2 and pH with a blood gas apparatus approximates S_aO_2 but may differ if P50 is abnormal. A bench oximeter (IL, Corning or Radiometer OSM3) reads $HbO_2\%$ (not S_aO_2) as a percentage of total Hb (including HbCO and HbMet). S_aO_2 may be calculated as $100HbO_2/(Hb+HbO_2)$. S_aO_2 is sometimes called functional saturation, and HbO_2 fractional saturation.

HISTORICAL ASPECTS OF OXIMETRY [2]

Oximetry depends on the color change in blood. Hemoglobin was named by Felix Hoppe-Seyler in 1862, and shown by George Gabriel Stokes to be the carrier of oxygen, which changed its color. The spectroscope also dates from 1860 in Bunsen and Kirchhoff's laboratory in Heidelberg. By 1874, Karl von Vierordt had spectroscopically measured the change in the red light penetrating his hand when he tourniqueted his arm, the first oximeter. No one pursued von Vierordt's discovery for almost 60 years, nor applied it to routine monitoring of the adequacy of oxygenation in patients for over 100 years.

In 1929, an American physiologist, Glen Millikan, went to Cambridge for graduate work in Barcroft's laboratory, where FJW Roughton put him to the task of optically measuring the speed of combination of oxygen with hemoglobin after mixing in a flowing stream. Millikan's 1932 PhD thesis described a light source shining through a flowing stream of blood into photocells covered with purple and yellow filters to measure the solution saturation at varying points (times) downstream.

In 1932 in Göttingen, Germany, a physiologist, Ludwig Nicolai, resurrected von Vierordt's work, using a light "chopper" and an AC electronic light detector, to study oxygen consumption in his own hand. His student Kurt Kramer recorded saturation in-vivo by transilluminating the arteries of animals, and introduced the new barrier layer photocells. Karl Matthes in Leipzig about 1936 developed the first ear saturation meter, and was the first to use two wavelengths in vivo to compensate for variations in light intensity and for tissue thickness.

At the outset of the war, because of military aviation hypoxia problems, Millikan and John Pappenheimer developed a light-weight ear "oximeter" which used ideas of both German workers, Kramer's copper oxide barrier photocells and Matthes' two colored filters. Despite the discovery (later) that the ear doesn't transmit green light, it worked, because Millikan's green filter and its photo-cell happened to transmit and detect infrared light.

93

T. H. Stanley and R. J. Sperry (eds.), Anesthesia and the Lung, 93–97.
© *1989 by Kluwer Academic Publishers.*

Millikan's oximeter was useful to show changes in saturation, but one had to set it at the outset to read an assumed 97% while breathing air or 100% breathing O_2. It drifted and was sensitive to skin pigment and thickness. In England, also working on the aviation hypoxic problem during the war, JR Squire concluded that one should set a zero for tissue density by squeezing blood out pneumatically, and then record the increased density as blood was let back in, comparing the *fall* of light produced by the blood at two wavelengths, one sensitive to oxygen and one insensitive. The method anticipates the concept inherent in pulse oximetry, except that it detects all the blood, not just arterial.

In the 1950's, Earl Wood at the Mayo Clinic modified Millikan's ear piece, adding a pneumatic cuff like that of Squire, and constructed cuvette oximeters and densitometers for use in cardiac catheterization laboratories. In Groningen, Netherlands, Brinkman and Zijlstra developed surface (forehead) oximetry, a device called the Cyclops, which was used for many years in physiology and even in anesthesia. Their work also led to invasive reflectance oximetry, developed by M. Polanyi at the American Optical Company, used for both cuvette and catheter oximetry, and later used by Oximetrix as part of a central venous or arterial catheter oximeter.

In 1964, Robert Shaw, a surgeon and inventor in San Francisco, began design and construction of a self-calibrating, 8 wavelength ear oximeter to identify the separate Hb species. This was marketed about 1970 by Hewlett Packard. Because of its large earpiece and great expense, this HP oximeter was seldom used for clinical monitoring, but was widely used in physiology and in cardiac catheterization laboratories.

Origin of pulse oximetry

In 1972 in Tokyo, Takuo Aoyagi was developing cardiac output measurement by dye dilution using an ear-piece densitometer. Pulsatile variations made it impossible to extrapolate and obtain accuracy. Dr. Yoshimura had shown a way to normalize the signal using the AC to DC ratio at one wavelength. Aoyagi conceived the idea of minimizing the pulses by electrically balancing the red light signal with an infrared light signal where the dye had no absorption. He found that this compensation varied with oxygen saturation. He decided to use this ratio to measure saturation as an added . advantage in his dye densitometer. He realized that the pulsatile *changes* in light transmission through living tissues would be due solely to pulsatile alteration of the arterial blood volume in the tissue. Thus the variable absorption of light by tissue, bone, skin, pigments etc. would be eliminated from analysis. It was this key idea which permitted development of instrumentation which required no calibration after its initial factory setting, since all human blood has essentially identical optical characteristics in the red and infrared bands chosen for oximetry. The first commercial instrument, the OLV-5100, was made available in 1975 as an ear oximeter by Aoyagi and his associates.

Meanwhile, Akio Yamanishi and M. Konishi, engineers working for Minolta, were improving photo-plethysmographic methods by introducing LED light sources and silicon photo diodes. They used both tissue transillumination and reflection, the latter with fiberoptic light pipes. Yamanishi wrote that he learned in January, 1974 of Weinman's method for determining the effective blood thickness in a finger from the logarithms of the AC and DC components of light transmission, caused by arterial pulsation. Yamanishi had been reading Millikan and Wood to find other uses for light technology, and proposed using Weinman's method for oximetry in a patent application prepared in February, 1974, less than 2 months before learning of Aoyagi's proposed ear pulse oximeter presentation. Minolta proceeded to market their invention as the Oximet MET-1471 in June, 1977 with a finger tip probe and fiberoptic cables from the instrument.

Scott Wilbur in Boulder, Colorado, also appears to have independently invented pulse oximetry about 1976-8 while working on an exercise heart rate counter with finger plethysmographic methods.

He also realized that the logarithm of the AC to DC ratios of the red and infrared light transmissions would be oxygen dependent, and obtained a patent on this process. His company, Biox, now Ohmeda, originally considered the probable market to be pulmonary and cardiac function laboratories, which had been the prime users of the Hewlett Packard ear oximeter.

Credit for the revolution in patient monitoring with pulse oximetry belongs to anesthesiologist William New of Stanford University Medical School who recognized the great need it could fulfill in clinical medicine, and with an engineer, Jack Lloyd, founded the Nellcor Company [3].

ACCURACY OF PULSE OXIMETERS

In the design and calibration of pulse oximeters, manufacturers have generally only been able to obtain data in normals at oxygen saturations above 70%. The lower response cannot be extrapolated because it is neither linear nor logarithmic. We developed a new method to test pulse oximeter response to very severe hypoxia in normal subjects [4].

Oxygen saturation, $S_{p}O_2\%$, was recorded during rapidly induced 42.5 ± 7.2 sec plateaus of profound hypoxia at 40-90% saturation by 1 or 2 pulse oximeters from each manufacturer. Usually, one probe of each pair was mounted on the ear, the other on a finger. Semi-recumbent healthy normotensive non-smoking caucasian or asian volunteers (age range 18-64) performed the test six times each. After insertion of a radial artery catheter, subjects hyperventilated 3% CO_2, 0-5% O_2, balance N_2. Saturation S_cO_2, computed on-line from mass spectrometer end tidal Po_2 and Pco_2, was used to manually adjust F_1O_2 breath by breath to obtain a rapid fall to one or two hypoxic plateaus lasting 30-45 sec, followed by rapid resaturation. Arterial $HbO_2\%$, measured in blood using a Radiometer OSM-3$^\bullet$) sampled near the end of the plateau, averaged $55.5 \pm 7.5\%$. In studies done in 1988 (the 10 regression data), triplicate comparisons were obtained in each subject at 4 levels of S_aO_2, about 86%, 74%, 62% and 50%. $S_cO_2\%$ calculated from the mass spectrometer and $S_aO_2\%$ from pH and Po_2 by Corning 178$^\bullet$ differed from $HbO_2\%$ by $+0.2 \pm 3.6\%$ and $0.4 \pm 2.8\%$ resp.

Table 1: Responses of 13 finger pulse oximeters in normal adults. Ten were studied over the range from 40% to 100%. Mean error (bias) and s.d. (precision) of S_pO_2-$S_aO_2\%$ are at S_aO_2 <72% ($55.5 \pm 7.5\%$).

Mfg*	N	Slope	Int	$S_{y.x}$	R	Mean	SD	N
			REGRESSION				ERROR @55%	
CSI	214	1.01	-0.82	3.56	0.952	-0.63	3.45	334
CTK						0.22	5.84	120
DTX	119	0.97	6.7	4.77	0.933	1.63	5.11	114
INV						-5.55	6.62	60
KON	96	0.99	1.5	2.53	0.976	0.81	2.93	60
MAR						-2.9	5.4	36
NEL	108	1.23	-17.7	4.60	0.948	-3.48	5.29	179
NOV	75	1.15	-17.3	7.36	0.82	-2.06	6.93	120
OHM	120	1.42	-35.1	5.15	0.953	-10.65	6.49	59
PHY	120	1.19	-14.1	2.39	0.985	-0.26	3.64	60
PUR	240	1.02	-3.84	2.46	0.979	-1.92	3.23	120
RAD	120	1.41	-34.7	5.70	0.942	-9.76	7.79	72
SIM	240	1.065	-7.05	4.29	0.943	-3.45	5.08	144

*Criticare, Critikon, Datex, InVivo, Kontron (Roche), Marquest, Nellcor (with ECG synchronization), Novametrix, Ohmeda, PhysioControl, Puritan Bennett, Radiometer, and SiMed. (Other instruments tested included Biochem Int, Sensor Medics and Sentinel, but results suggested these were not yet ready for marketing).

When our testing began in 1986, most instruments read significantly too low with finger probes at 55% mean S_aO_2. Several early models of the instruments occasionally defaulted to zero saturation during rapid desaturation. Bias and precision differed widely between instruments, being as erroneous as $-12\% \pm 15\%$. By September, 1987, these problems had been largely corrected by program alterations by the manufacturers, as suggested by the latest data shown in table 1.

USES OF PULSE OXIMETRY

MONITORING OF OXYGENATION
> Anesthesia, recovery, ICU, NMR, CAT
> Reduce need for ICU, low risk groups
> Central nursing station with telemetry
> Office procedures: Dentistry, Endoscopy
> Monitoring spinal or epidural narcotics.
> Home or hospital monitoring of SIDS
> Critical Care Transport

MONITORING OF CIRCULATION
> Monitor during microvascular reimplantation
> Measure blood pressure (cuff occlusion)
> Determine ductus patency
> Test circulatory obstruction from cervical rib.
> Test patency of arterial grafts
> Indicate carotid artery compression during neck surgery
> Assess circulatory adequacy in unusual positions
> Monitor viability of transplant graft.

CLINICAL TESTS
> Assess hypoxic ventilatory response.
> Quantitate sleep apnea, adults and infants, SIDS.
> Measure circulation time with single breath of N_2.
> Improved Allen's test for radial and ulnar artery patency.

TEACHING
> Physiology during anesthesia.
> Effectiveness of CPR
> Bio-feedback for peripheral vasodilation.
> Relationship of CPAP and PEEP to atelectasis.

USES OF PULSE WAVEFORMS
> Diagnosis of irregularities
> Absolute amplitude as monitor of circulation.
> Substitute for arterial line
> Monitor circulatory obstruction

RESEARCH ASPECTS

Regulation of respiration studies
Exercise physiology.
Cardio-pulmonary tests.
Mountaineering studies.
Animal research.

THERAPY CONTROL

Maintain deliberate hypoxia in premature infants.
Servo-controlled saturation, prematures.
Conserve O_2 in home O_2 therapy
Determine optimal PEEP and CPAP
Monitor apneic oxygenation during bronchoscopy etc.
Trial of extubation or ending O_2 therapy

REFERENCES:

1) Payne J P and J W Severinghaus: *Pulse Oximetry*, Springer Verlag, London, 1-197, 1986.

2) Severinghaus J W, P Astrup: The history of blood gas analysis. Int. Anesth. Clinics 25, No. 4, 1987, Little Brown and Co, Boston, 224 pp.

3) Yelderman M, W New, Jr: Evaluation of pulse oximetry. Anesthesiology 59: 349-362, 1983.

4) Severinghaus J W, K H Naifeh: Accuracy of response of six pulse oximeters to profound hypoxia. Anesthesiology 67:551-558, 1987.

WHAT IS THE REQUIRED INSPIRED OXYGEN CONSUMPTION DURING ANESTHESIA?

J. F. NUNN.

Division of Anaesthesia, Clinical Research Centre, Harrow, UK.

THE OXYGEN CASCADE

Oxygen moves down a partial pressure gradient from inspired gas, through alveolar gas, arterial blood, systemic capillaries and cells, to reach its lowest level within the mitochondria where it is consumed (Figure 1). The steps by which the Po_2 decreases from inspired gas to the mitochondria are known as the oxygen cascade and are of great

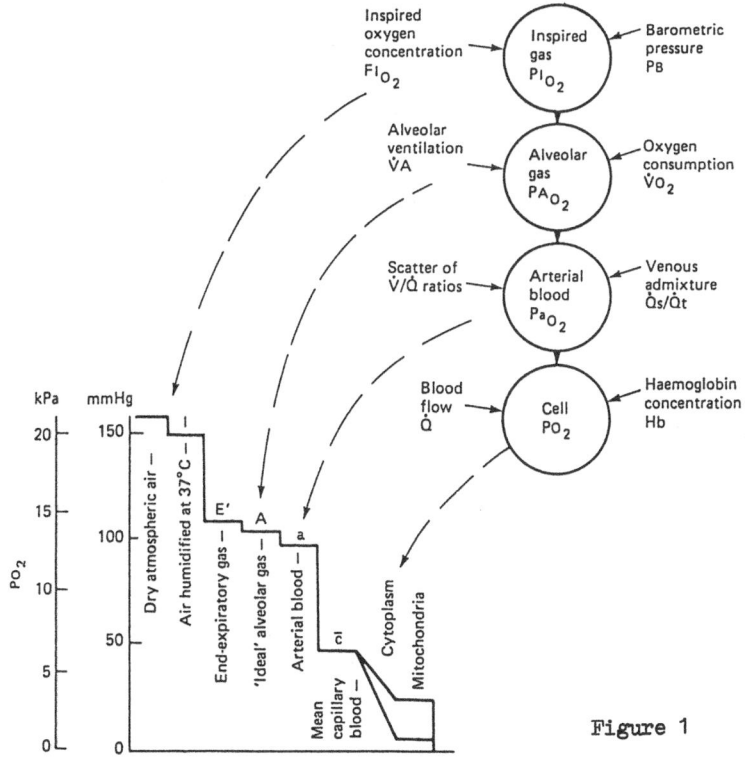

Figure 1

T. H. Stanley and R. J. Sperry (eds.), Anesthesia and the Lung, 99–105.

practical importance. Any one step in the cascade may be increased
under pathological circumstances and this may result in hypoxia.
Within limits, the effect of certain increased steps in the cascade
can be offset by raising the concentration of oxygen in the inspired
gas. However, the quantitative relationships are totally different
depending on which step in the cascade is abnormal.

The above considerations apply to the steady state. It is also
necessary to consider the effect of certain unsteady states,
particularly apnea. The oxygen stores of the body are normally small
but may be improved by elevation of the inspired oxygen concentration
in anticipation of apnea.

Factors influencing alveolar oxygen tension

The equation for the calculation of the alveolar Po_2 is as follows:

$$\text{alveolar } Po_2 \doteq \genfrac{}{}{0pt}{}{\text{dry}}{\substack{\text{barometric}\\\text{pressure}}} \left(\genfrac{}{}{0pt}{}{\text{inspired}}{\substack{\text{oxygen}\\\text{concentration}}} - \frac{\text{oxygen uptake}}{\text{alveolar ventilation}} \right)$$

This equation is only approximate and does not include the effect of
exchange of a soluble gas such as nitrous oxide, as in so-called
"diffusion anoxia" or the "third gas effect".

Dry barometric pressure. Other factors remaining constant, the
alveolar Po_2 will be directly proportional to the dry barometric
pressure which falls with increasing altitude. Alveolar Po_2 is
reduced by approximately 20 mm Hg at 5,000 ft (Denver).

Inspired oxygen concentration. The alveolar Po_2 will be raised or
lowered by an amount equal to the change in the inspired gas Po_2,
provided that other factors remain constant (Figure 2).

Oxygen consumption. The role of oxygen consumption has received
insufficient attention. An increased oxygen consumption will decrease
the alveolar Po_2 (sometimes very markedly) if the alveolar ventilation
is not increased by the appropriate amount.

Alveolar ventilation There is a hyperbolic relationship between

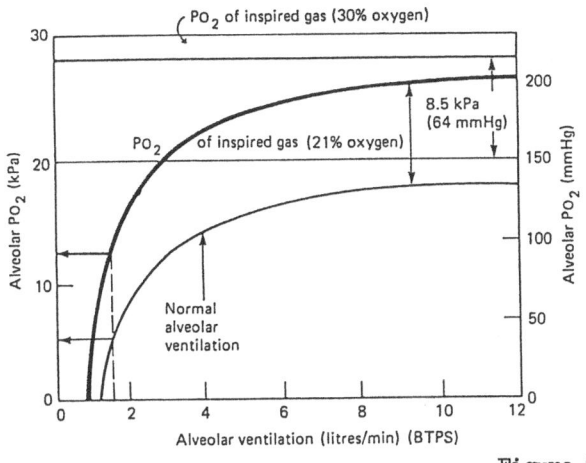

Figure 2

alveolar Po₂ and alveolar ventilation. As ventilation is increased, the alveolar Po₂ rises asymptomatically towards (but never reaches) the Po₂ of the inspired gas (Figure 2). It will be seen from the shape of the curves that changes in ventilation <u>above</u> normal level have comparatively little effect upon alveolar Po₂. In contrast, changes in ventilation <u>below</u> the normal level may have a very marked effect on alveolar Po₂. At very low levels of ventilation, the alveolar ventilation is critical and small changes may precipitate gross hypoxia.

The alveolar/arterial Po₂ difference

The next step in the oxygen cascade is of great clinical relevance. In the healthy young adult breathing air, the alveolar/arterial Po₂ difference does not exceed 15 mm Hg but may rise to above 35 mm Hg in aged but healthy subjects. These values are usually increased during anesthesia and in the presence of any lung disease which causes shunting or mismatching of ventilation and perfusion.

Unlike the alveolar Po₂, the alveolar/arterial Po₂ difference cannot be predicted from other more easily measured quantities, and there is no simple means of knowing the magnitude of the alveolar/arterial Po₂ difference in a particular patient without measuring the arterial blood gas tensions. It is important to understand the factors which influence the difference and the principles of restoration of arterial Po_2 by increasing the inspired oxygen concentration.

During anesthesia the increased alveolar/arterial Po_2 gradient depends on the alveolar Po_2 but is, on average, that which would be caused by a 10 % shunt (Figure 3).

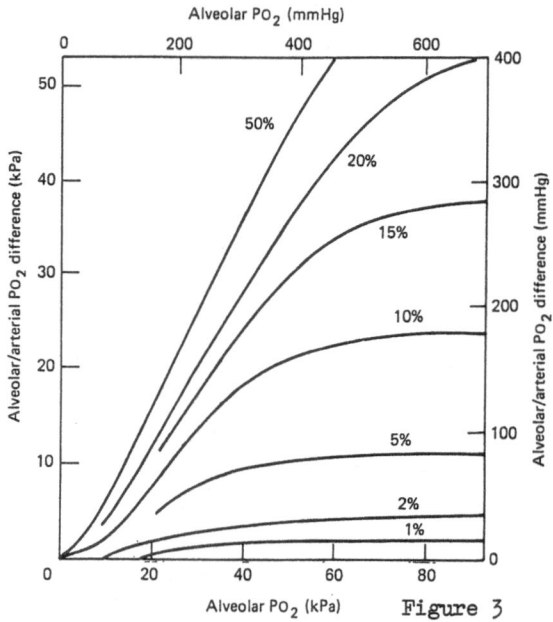

Figure 3

COMPENSATION FOR ABNORMAL RESPIRATORY FUNCTION DURING ANESTHESIA BY RAISING THE INSPIRED OXYGEN CONCENTRATION

If patients are allowed to breathe spontaneously, the alveolar ventilation is usually decreased to a greater extent than is appropriate to the diminished oxygen consumption. Figure 4 shows the relationship between alveolar Pco_2 and alveolar ventilation. Along the curve is shown the inspired oxygen concentrations required to maintain a normal alveolar Po_2, as derived from the alveolar air equation above (for basal oxygen consumption). It will be clear that, if more than about 30 % oxygen is required to restore normal alveolar (not arterial) Po_2, then attention should be directed to the Pco_2.

The situation is quantitatively quite different when preventing hypoxaemia due to an increased alveolar/arterial Po_2 gradient due to

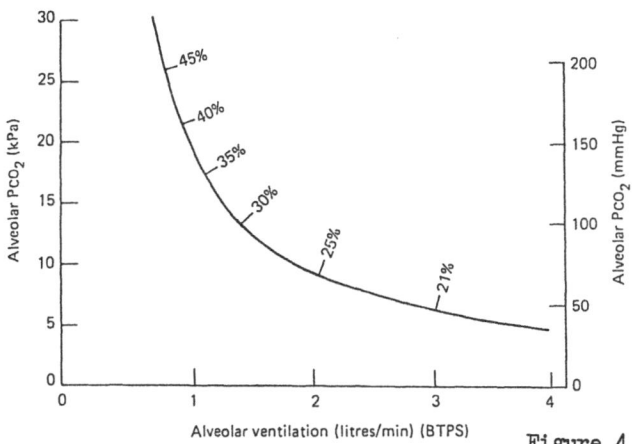

Figure 4

Alveolar ventilation (litres/min) (BTPS)

venous admixture. It is greatly complicated by the fact that the
magnitude of the gradient is itself influenced by the absolute value
of the alveolar Po_2. Thus increasing the alveolar Po_2 by raising the
concentration of oxygen in the inspired gas will actually increase the
gradient (Figure 3) and the effect on arterial Po_2 is not simply
additive (as it is for the alveolar Po_2).

INSPIRED OXYGEN CONCENTRATION REQUIRED DURING ANESTHESIA

Uncomplicated anesthesia

The overall relationship between inspired oxygen concentration and
arterial Po_2 for different values of shunt is shown in figure 5. The
circles show the mean values for 8 studies conducted during
anaesthesia (individually cited in 1).

Greater detail for lower inspired oxygen concentrations with
artificial ventilation is shown in Figure 6 (from 2). The alveolar
Po_2 is a highly predictable function of the inspired oxygen
concentration and 20 % oxygen ensures a normal value. However, due to
the unpredictable alveolar/arterial Po_2 gradient, an inspired oxygen
concentration of less than 30 % will not guarantee a normal arterial
Po_2 under these circumstances.

During spontaneous breathing (Figure 7, also from 2), the alveolar
Po_2 is decreased by an amount which is not easily predictable. Taken
in conjunction with the alveolar/arterial Po_2 gradient (also

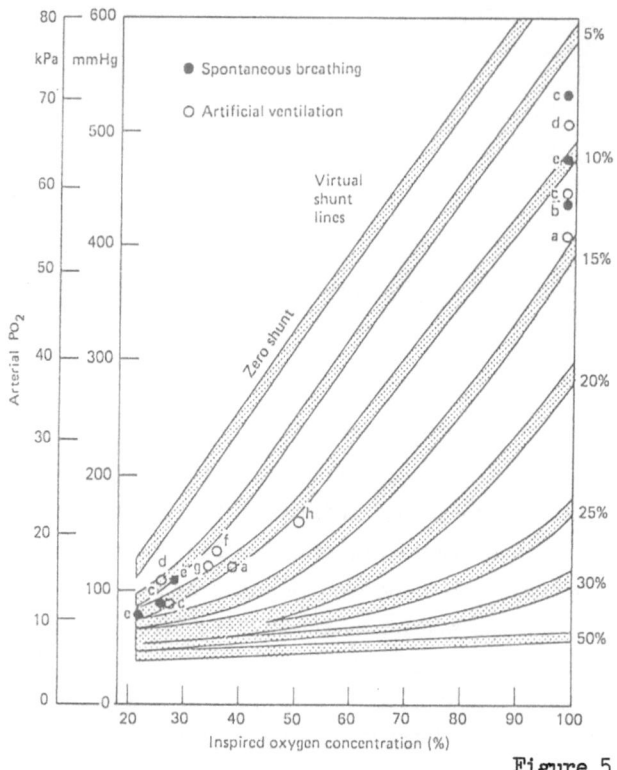

Figure 5

unpredictable), this requires an inspired oxygen concentration in excess of 35 % to ensure a normal arterial Po₂.

During one-lung anesthesia, there is a variable and largely unpredictable shunt through the uninflated lung. This requires an increased inspired oxygen concentration. A typical value would be 50 % (3) but monitoring with a pulse oximeter is the best approach.

Prior to apnea (eg before tracheal intubation) safety is enhanced by breathing 50 - 100 % to increase the oxygen stores (Table 1).

Principal stores of body oxygen

	While breathing air	While breathing 100% oxygen	
In the lungs (FRC)	450 ml		3 000 ml
In the blood	850 ml		950 ml
Dissolved in tissue fluids	50 ml	?	100 ml
In combination with myoglobin	? 200 ml	?	200 ml
Total	1 550 ml		4 250 ml

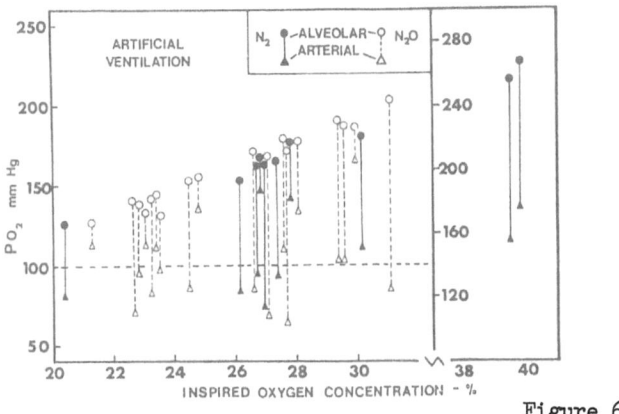

Figure 6

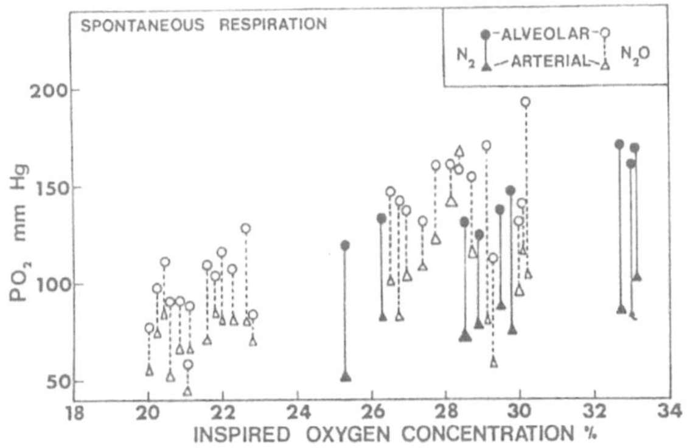

Figure 7

REFERENCES

1. Nunn, J.F. Appplied Respiratory Physiology, 3rd Edition.
    London: Butterworths. 1987.
2. Webb, S.J.S. and Nunn, J.F. Anaesthesia 22: 69-81, 1967.
3. Khanam, T. and Branthwaite, M.A. Anaesthesia 28: 280-290, 1973.

POSTOPERATIVE HYPOXIA

THOMAS F. HORNBEIN

Department of Anesthesiology, University of Washington School of Medicine, Seattle, Washington 98195

INTRODUCTION

Emergence from anesthesia is akin to birth: passage from a phase where all is controlled through the first faltering breaths toward a state of autonomous function. This transition (which begins as anesthesia is discontinued and ends, usually, with discharge from the postanesthesia recovery area) is the target for this exploration of the causes, consequences, prevention, and treatment of postoperative ventilatory failure, i.e. arterial hypoxemia and/or hypercapnia.

Patients may bring to this time three pieces of baggage:

- their state of health, particularly cardiopulmonary, prior to surgery;
- what the surgery may have done to make things worse;
- the residua of the anesthetic experience, most notably of the drugs used to effect anesthesia and facilitate surgery.

The environment into which the patient emerges is one that by custom and cost possesses less intense observation and modulation than that received during surgery. As the individual is nurtured to fly on his or her own, hypoxia is a risk that encompasses more than the effect on the arterial PO_2; oxygenation of vital tissues, particularly heart and brain, are at stake. The objectives of this presentation will be:

- to review the pharmacological contributors to ventilatory depression after surgery and anesthesia;
- to identify interactions between drug depression, the state of the patient's presurgical health, and the nature of the surgical intervention that may render certain patients more susceptible to ventilatory failure after surgery;
- to underscore the role of sleep as a factor in postoperative ventilatory failure, to identify its interaction with postoperative pain relief, and to establish duration for the period of susceptibility.

107

T. H. Stanley and R. J. Sperry (eds.), Anesthesia and the Lung, 107–110.
© 1989 by Kluwer Academic Publishers.

CONDITIONING FACTORS FOR POSTOPERATIVE VENTILATORY FAILURE

<u>Preoperative factors</u> include the patient's general health and underlying pathology, the presence and severity of pulmonary and circulatory disease, state of nutrition, age, obesity, smoking history, and the extent to which the patient can and has been tuned for surgery.

<u>Intraoperative surgical influences</u> include the nature of the operation and its anatomical location (e.g., proximity to the diaphragm, the patient's position, duration of surgery, fluid losses, translocations and replacements, and nociceptive potential of the surgical violation).

<u>Intraoperative anesthetic influences</u>. While some may on occasion be of a mechanical nature, akin to those of surgery, most are a function of the pharmacological effects and side effects of drugs used for anesthesia and to facilitate surgery:

- Anesthetics conventionally depress ventilation, with aftereffects that may be long-lasting. Most of the anesthetics and adjuvants that we use - narcotics, sedatives, and tranquilizers - depress the ventilatory response to carbon dioxide in a dose-dependent manner; some exert an even more profoundly depressant effect upon the ventilatory response to hypoxia, doing so even at concentrations much less than those required to produce anesthesia. With our ability to determine mechanically the state of gas exchange during anesthesia, these pharmacological side effects of the tools of our trade often become relevant only upon emergence when the patient is being asked to do his own breathing. Residual neuromuscular blockade is yet one more potential contributor to this polypharmaceutic trespass.

- This pharmacology interacts with whatever deficits the patient may have brought to the postanesthesia period from his preanesthetic and surgical state and from the surgical experience itself. For example, the individual with chronic pulmonary disease may tolerate less well a given level of anesthetic or analgesic drug presence than will the healthy individual. Similarly, pain resulting from the surgical intervention may modify the capacity for effective gas exchange, e.g. after upper abdominal surgery.

- The patient awakening from anesthesia may shiver, sometimes intensely. The increase in metabolic demands is well-tolerated in most patients but may result in further impairment of arterial blood oxygenation or increased cardiovascular stress in less healthy patients.

- Compared with the awake state, sleep decreases ventilatory drives. Superimposed upon age or obesity, sleep may result in breathing dysrhythmias including hypoventilation and central, obstructive, or combined apneas. Residual anesthetic drugs may enhance these tendencies in the early postoperative period, while the medications conventionally used for relief of pain may contribute to disruption of sleep patterns and a tendency to impaired gas exchange for O_2 and CO_2 for several days following surgery. The choice of postoperative pain therapy may influence the frequency of sleep-related ventilatory failure for several days into the postoperative period.

APPROACH TO MANAGEMENT

Hypoxemia during recovery from anesthesia might relate to: 1) depression of the output of the bellows or 2) impaired gas exchange for oxygen, namely shunt and ventilation-perfusion inequalities.

Monitoring for hypoxia. In addition to the usual blood pressure and heart rate measurements, electrocardiogram, and assessment of the patient's sensorium, for some awakening patients there is the potential for continuous noninvasive assessment of blood oxygen saturation by pulse oximetry.

Prevention of postoperative hypoxia depends in part on what has gone before in regard to preoperative preparation of the patient, the tailoring of anesthesia to the potential for problems of gas exchange, and selection and judicious application of postoperative pain relief. The delaying of extubation until control of the airway by the individual is ensured may avert the potential problem of obstruction. The use of oxygen by mask or prongs in the extubated patient presumably provides a margin of safety conventional to the recovery area, albeit less used in transport from operating room to recovery area.

Treatment. 1) increased F_{IO_2}; 2) pharmacological antagonists of ventilatory depression: narcotic antagonists, cholinesterase inhibitors, respiratory stimulants; 3) airway protection; 4) mechanical ventilation.

REFERENCES

Reviews.
1. Pavlin, E.G. and Hornbein, T.F. Anesthesia and the Control of Ventilation. Chapter 25 in: Handbook of Physiology, Part 2, pp. 793-813. Baltimore, The Williams & Wilkins Co., 1986.
2. Bishop, M.J. and Cheney, F.W. Respiratory complications of anesthesia and surgery, Seminars in Anesthesia 2:91-99, 1983.

Selected Articles.

1. Alexander, J.I., Spence, A.A., Parikh, R.K., and Stuart, B. The role of airway closure in postoperative hypoxaemia, Brit. J. Anaesth. 45:34-40, 1973.
2. Bay, J., Nunn, J.F., and Prys-Roberts, C. Factors influencing arterial PO_2 during recovery from anaesthesia. Brit. J. Anaesth. 40:398-407, 1968.
3. Becker, L.D., Paulson, B.A., Miller, R.D., Severinghaus, J.W., and Eger, E.I., II. Biphasic respiratory depression after fentanyl droperidol or fentanyl alone used to supplement nitrous oxide anesthesia. Anesthesiology 44:291-296, 1976.
4. Catley, D.M., Thornton, C., Jordan, C., Lehane, J.R., Royston, D., and Jones, J.G. Pronounced, episodic oxygen desaturation in the postoperative period: its association with ventilatory pattern and analgesic regimen, Anesthesiology 63:20-28, 1985.
5. Cherniack, N.A. The clinical assessment of the chemical regulation of ventilation. Chest 70:274-281, 1976.
6. Garibaldi, R.A., Britt, M.R., Coleman, M.L., Reading, J.C., and Pace, N.L. Risk factors for postoperative pneumonia, Am. J. Med. 70:677-680, 1981.
7. Jones, H.D. and McLaren, C.A.B. Postoperative shivering and hypoxaemia after halothane, nitrous oxide and oxygen anaesthesia, Brit. J. Anaesth. 37:35-41, 1965.
8. Knill, R.L., Moote, C.A., Rose, E.A., and Skinner, M.I. Marked hypoxemia after gastroplasty due to disorders of breathing in REM sleep. Anesthesiology 67:A552, 1987.
9. Knill, R.L., Moote, C.A., Skinner, M.I., Rose, E.A., and Lok, P.Y.K. Morphine-induced ventilatory depression is potentiated by non-REM sleep. Canad. J. Anaesth. 34:S101-S102, 1987.
10. Knill, R.L., Rose, E.A., Skinner, M.I., Moote, C.A., and Lok, P.Y.K. Episodic hypoxaemia during REM sleep after anaesthesia and gastroplasty. ACTA Anaesth. Scand. Suppl. 86, 31:No. 102, 1987.
11. Macintyre, P.E., Pavlin, E.G., and Dwersteg, J.F. Effect of meperidine on oxygen consumption, carbon dioxide production, and respiratory gas exchange in postanesthesia shivering. Anesth. Analg. 66:751-755, 1987.
12. Mankikian, B., Cantineau, J.P., Bertrand, M., Kieffer, E., Sartene, R., and Viars, P. Improvement of diaphragmatic function by a thoracic extradural block after upper abdominal surgery. Anesthesiology 68:379-386, 1988.
13. Moote, C.A., Knill, R.L., Skinner, M.I., Rose, E.A., and Lok, P.Y.K. Morphine produced a profound disruption of nocturnal sleep in humans. Canad. J. Anaesth. 34:S100-S101, 1987.
14. Pavlin, E.G., Holle, R., and Schoene, R. Recovery of airway protection in humans after paralysis with curare. Anesthesiology (in press).
15. Remmers, J.E. Obstructive sleep apnea: A common disorder exacerbated by alcohol. Am. Rev. Respir. Dis. 130:153-155, 1984.
16. Rigg, J.R.A. Pulmonary atelectasis after anaesthesia: Pathophysiology and management. Canad. Anaesth. Soc. J. 28:305-313, 1981.
17. Simonneau, G., Vivien, A., Sartene, R., Kunstlinger, F., Samii, K., Noviant, Y., and Duroux, P. Diaphragm dysfunction induced by upper abdominal surgery: Role of postoperative pain. Am. Rev. Respir. Dis. 128:899-903, 1983.

THE 1981 AMERICAN MEDICAL RESEARCH EXPEDITION TO MT. EVEREST

JOHN B. WEST

Department of Medicine, University of California San Diego, La Jolla CA 92093-0623

In recent years, much has been learned about the body's responses to severe hypoxia by making measurements at extreme altitudes. Exceptional opportunities for new knowledge were generated by the American Medical Research Expedition to Everest which took place in 1981. Laboratories were set up at altitudes of 17,700 ft.(5400 m), 20,700 ft.(6300 m) and 26,400 ft.(8050 m) while a few measurements were even obtained on the summit, the highest point on earth at 29,028 ft.(8848 m).

When normal man goes to high altitude, pulmonary ventilation increases because of stimulation of the peripheral chemoreceptor by hypoxemia, much as occurs in some patients with severe lung disease. We were interested to find that the extent to which ventilation increased when hypoxic mixtures were inhaled at sea level (hypoxic ventilatory response) was a good predictor of tolerance to extreme altitude. The reason is probably that a climber at great altitudes needs to hyperventilate to a very dramatic extent to maintain an adequate alveolar PO_2 so as to avoid lethal arterial hypoxemia. This was an interesting finding because it suggests that measurements made at sea level prior to an expedition can identify climbers who are likely to do poorly at extreme altitudes.

Another interesting finding in the area of control of ventilation was that all the American members of the expedition showed striking periodic breathing during the night. This Cheyne-Stokes breathing produced marked fluctuations in the arterial oxygen saturation as measured by an oximeter, and profound degrees of arterial hypoxemia following the apneic periods. It was fascinating to find that the Sherpas developed no periodic breathing at the same altitude. The explanation may be that the Sherpas are born with a reduced ("blunted") ventilatory response to hypoxia. This means whereas the Westerners have

T. H. Stanley and R. J. Sperry (eds.), Anesthesia and the Lung, 111–116.
© 1989 by Kluwer Academic Publishers.

an unstable control system because of the very high gain (hypoxic ventilatory response) the Sherpas have a stable ventilatory control system.

Polycythemia always occurs in lowlanders when they go to high altitudes, and on Mt. Everest hematocrits can easily increase from the normal value of 45% to the low 60's. Although this degree of polycythemia has often been seen as a useful response because it increases the oxygen carrying capacity of the blood, some physicians have pointed out that polycythemia of this magnitude increases the viscosity of the blood and therefore cardiac work, and tends to produce uneven blood flow in peripheral capillaries. As a result of these untoward effects, it has been suggested that hemodilution might reduce the tendency for frostbite at high altitude and improve exercise tolerance.

We decided to test this by taking four of the climbers with the highest hematocrits at the end of the expedition, and comparing their exercise tolerance and mental function before and after hemodilution. Blood was removed and replaced with human albumin solution in order to return the hematocrit to more normal levels. We found that there were very small differences as a result of the hemodilution, and in particular, exercise tolerance as measured on the bicycle ergometer was not improved. This suggests that hemodilution is not justified. A more interesting conclusion is that the polycythemia of high altitude may be an inappropriate response. The control system that determines the hematocrit level has probably been developed over many thousands of years at sea level were the polycythemic response to tissue hypoxia is valuable in the case of a reduced hemoglobin concentration caused by trauma, malnutrition, or intestinal parasites. However at high altitude where the tissue hypoxia is caused by an entirely different mechanism, namely the reduced inspired PO_2, the polycythemic response may be inappropriate.

Some of the most interesting data were obtained at extreme altitudes including a few measurements on the summit itself. Two of the three Americans who reached the summit were physicians, Dr. Christopher Pizzo, and Dr. Peter Hackett. Pizzo made the first direct measurement of barometric pressure on the summit obtaining the value of 253 mm Hg. It is interesting that this value and many others that we obtained at slightly lower altitudes all considerably exceed the barometric pressures predicted from the standard altitude-pressure tables used by aviation physicians. The reason is that the barometric pressure at altitudes like the summit of Mt. Everest are latitude-dependent. They are higher near the equator than the poles because of the very large mass of very cold air in the stratosphere above the equator. Paradoxically the coldest air in the atmosphere is above the equator. This results from radiation and convection phenomena and the large mass of cold air causes the barometric pressure at altitudes of 25,000 to 30,000 feet to be much higher than would be the case if the mountain were near the poles. It turns out that this increase in barometric pressure just makes it possible for man to reach the highest point on earth without supplementary oxygen, a remarkable coincidence indeed.

Dr. Pizzo took a number of alveolar gas samples at extreme altitudes including several on the summit itself. As a result of these measurements, it is clear that alveolar PCO_2 falls steadily as a climber goes to higher and higher altitudes, and that on the summit the alveolar PCO_2 is only about 7.5 mm Hg in well-acclimatized subjects. This indicates the astonishing high level of alveolar hyperventilation.

When the alveolar gas measurements are plotted on an oxygen-carbon dioxide diagram, an interesting point emerges. It turns out that both the alveolar PO_2 and PCO_2 fall as the climber goes to higher and higher altitudes. The PO_2 falls because the inspired value is decreasing, while the alveolar PCO_2 falls because of increasing hyperventilation. It transpires that when a well-acclimatized climber is above an altitude of about 23,000 ft.(7,000 m), the alveolar PO_2 is maintained constant at a value of about 35 mm Hg. This is accomplished by extreme levels of hyperventilation. This appears to be one of the most important features of acclimatization to extreme altitude because it defends the alveolar PO_2 against the very low values in the air around the climber.

We were not able to take samples of arterial blood on the summit. However it is possible to get a good estimate of the arterial PO_2 by calculating the change in PO_2 along the capillary using the alveolar gas and blood data that we were able to collect. The results showed that the arterial PO_2 on the summit is less than 30 mm Hg, the difference between the arterial and alveolar values being explained by diffusion-limitation of oxygen transfer under these extreme conditions. It turns out that predicted from the standard altitude-pressure tables used by aviation physicians. The reason is that the barometric pressure at altitudes like the summit of Mt. Everest are latitude-dependent. They are higher near the equator than the poles because of the very large mass of very cold air in the stratosphere able the equator. Paradoxically the coldest air in the atmosphere is above the equator. This results from radiation and convection phenomena and the large mass of cold air causes the barometric pressure at altitudes of 25,000 to 30,000 feet to be much higher than would be the case if the mountain were near the poles. It turns out that this increase in barometric pressure just makes it possible for man to reach the highest point on earth without supplementary oxygen, a remarkable coincidence indeed.

Dr. Pizzo took a number of alveolar gas samples at extreme altitudes including several on the summit itself. As a result of these measurements, it is clear that alveolar PCO_2 falls steadily as a climber goes to higher and higher altitudes, and that on the summit the alveolar PCO_2 is only about 7.5 mm Hg in well-acclimatized subjects. This indicates the astonishing high level of alveolar hyperventilation.

When the alveolar gas measurements are plotted on an oxygen-carbon dioxide diagram, an interesting point emerges. It turns out that both the alveolar PO_2 and PCO_2 fall as the climber goes to higher and higher altitudes. The PO_2 falls because the inspired value is decreasing, while the alveolar PCO_2 falls because of increasing hyperventilation. It transpires that when a well-acclimatized climber is above an altitude of about 23,000 ft.(7,000 m), the alveolar PO_2 is maintained constant at a value of about 35 mm Hg. This is accomplished by extreme levels of hyperventilation. This appears to be one of the most important features of acclimatization to extreme altitude because it defends the alveolar PO_2 against the very low values in the air around the climber.

We were not able to take samples of arterial blood on the summit. However it is possible to get a good estimate of the arterial PO_2 by calculating the change in PO_2 along the capillary using the alveolar gas and blood data that we were able to collect. The results showed that the arterial PO_2 on the summit is less than 30 mm Hg, the difference between the arterial and alveolar values being explained by diffusion-limitation of oxygen transfer under these extreme conditions. It turns out that the PO_2 in the arterial blood rises very slowly along the pulmonary capillary because the lung is working so low on the oxygen dissociation curve. Such diffusion-limitation of oxygen transfer is almost never seen in the normal lung at sea level but occurs to a striking degree at extreme altitudes, particularly on exercise.

It was possible to get some information about the acid-base status of the climber because both Drs. Pizzo and Hackett took samples of venous blood from each other on the morning after their successful summit climbs. These samples allowed us to calculate the base excess of the blood and when the measured value for the alveolar PCO_2 on the summit was taken into account, the arterial pH comes out to exceed 7.7. This extraordinary degree of respiratory alkalosis is partly explained by the fact that renal excretion of bicarbonate is apparently very slow at extreme altitude. We do not fully understand the reasons for this but one clue may be that climbers living at an altitude of 21,700 ft.(6,300 m) were apparently chronically dehydrated. We know that in the presence of volume depletion, the kidney is reluctant to excrete cations which would be necessary to compensate for the respiratory alkalosis, because in doing so the kidney tends to exaggerate the dehydration.

A series of psychometric tests were made on the climbers before, during and after the expedition. Since it is well known that the central nervous system (CNS) is exquisitely sensitive to hypoxia, it was not surprising to find that aspects of mental function were impaired at extreme altitudes. However it was surprising to find that two of the tests remained abnormal when the expedition members returned to sea level. Both short term memory and a test of manipulative skill (finger-tapping test) were abnormal in the majority of expedition members immediately upon return. Furthermore, in 13 out of 16 expedition members, the test of manipulative skills remained abnormal for up to a year after the expedition and for a longer period of time in some members. Thus it appears that it is not possible to spend periods at these great altitudes with the inevitable severe hypoxemia and have the CNS escape completely unscathed.

Measurements of maximal oxygen consumption were made at an altitude of 21,700 ft.(6,300 m) using the bicycle ergometer. Several measurements were made with expedition members inhaling low oxygen concentrations to simulate conditions at even higher altitudes. We found that when climbers were breathing 14 percent oxygen at an altitude of 21,700 ft. (6,300 m) which gave an inspired PO_2 of only 43 mm Hg, equal to that on the summit of Mt. Everest, the maximal oxygen consumption was reduced to just over 1 liter/minute. This is an extremely low value equivalent to that seen when a person walks slowly on the level. However this very small maximal oxygen uptake apparently explains how it is possible for man to reach the summit of Mt. Everest without supplementary oxygen, a feat first accomplished by the European climbers Reinhold Messner and Peter Habeler in 1978.

The American Medical Research Expedition to Everest clarified a number of the responses that occur in patients with profound hypoxemia caused by severe lung and heart disease. However the profound physiological changes which occur should not blind us to the fact that one of the most important factors in the success of a man on a high mountain is his attitude, that is, his energy, motivation and enthusiasm.

REFERENCES

1. West J.B. Human physiology at extreme altitude on Mount Everest. Science 223:784-788, 1984.

2. West, J.B. Everest - The Testing Place. New York: McGraw-Hill, 1985. (This is a general account of the expedition including the major scientific findings.).

EFFECTS OF ANESTHETICS ON PULMONARY GAS EXCHANGE

BRYAN E. MARSHALL

Department of Anesthesia, University of Pennsylvania School of Medicine, Philadelphia, Pennsylvania 19104

INTRODUCTION

While much has been written about problems of gas exchange during anesthesia, not all the questions have been resolved. This complexity is well illustrated in the current controversy concerning the use of inhalational agents for the maintenance of anesthesia during one-lung ventilation and thoracic surgery. Most authors have suggested caution in the use of inhalational agents in these circumstances because inhibition of hypoxic pulmonary vasoconstriction (HPV) may contribute to hypoxemia (6,21,29); others have concluded that the inhibition does not occur or is unimportant in practice (5,13). The data on which these contrasting conclusions are based will be reviewed in an attempt to reconcile these viewpoints.

ANESTHESIA WITH ONE-LUNG VENTILATION

When both lungs are ventilated in the supine position, the cardiac output is divided so that 55% perfuses the right lung and 45% the left. If this flow distribution remained the same after the institution of one-lung ventilation, the procedure would be associated with a 50% pulmonary shunt and the arterial oxygen tension would be in the region of 50 mmHg.

Every experienced clinician is aware that in the majority of patients, arterial hypoxemia will not be encountered during one-lung ventilation whatever specific anesthetic technique is employed. One reason is that the blood flow distribution does not remain constant to the atelectatic lung, but instead is reduced so that more blood is diverted to the ventilated lung resulting in an improved pulmonary oxygen exchange (Figure 1).

T. H. Stanley and R. J. Sperry (eds.), Anesthesia and the Lung, 117–125.
© *1989 by Kluwer Academic Publishers.*

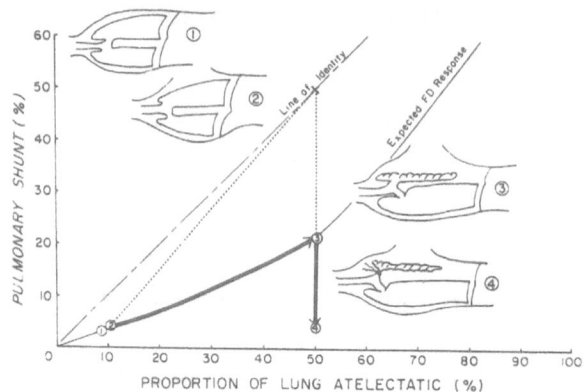

Figure 1. Pulmonary physiologic shunt measured in humans undergoing anesthesia for thoracic surgery. At 1, shunt is less than 5 percent with the patient in lateral position; this increases only slightly at 2, when the chest is opened. At 3, the upper lung is collapsed and ventilatory exchange is maintained through the lower lung only. Pulmonary shunt increases, not along the 45-degree line that would be expected in the absence of HPV, but instead along the line shown as expected flow diversion (FD) response in the presence of HPV. Precise correspondence of this example is fortuitous because there are mechanisms other than HPV influencing distribution of blood flow. At 4, the upper-lung hilum is cross-clamped, and the shunt returns to the value expected for the lower lung. (Reproduced by permission from Kerr LH et al. Observation during endobronchial anesthesia-II. Oxygenation. Br J Anaesth 46:84-92, 1974.)

TABLE 1: Arterial Oxygen Tension During Two- and One-Lung Ventilation with 100% Oxygen and Inhalational Anesthesia for Thoracic Surgery in Human Subjects

Study	No. of Subjects	Intraoperative P_{aO_2} Values* (mmHg)	
		Two-Lung Ventilation	One-Lung Ventilation
Torda et al. (36)	10	377 (472-282)	111 (165-57)
Kerr et al. (17)	9	452 (562-342)	248 (449-47)
Capan et al. (7)	11	376 (469-283)	155 (238-72)
Katz et al. (16)	17	421 (471-372)	210 (334-86)
	10	437 (524-350)	234 (336-132)
Rogers et al. (30)	10	445 (520-370)	278 (400-156)
Benumof (5)	6	484 (533-435)	116 (177-55)
	6	442 (500-384)	232 (329-135)

*Mean values, ± 1/SD; ranges are given in parentheses.

The data from various studies collected in Table 1 reveal that during one-lung ventilation, P_{ao2} values of less than 100 mmHg will be encountered in approximately 20% of patients and in 10% of patients values less than 60 mmHg are likely. Thus, in about one patient in four, arterial hypoxemia will be of concern and for one in ten may be a significant threat to life if uncorrected.

Evidently, if redistribution of blood flow is the primary mechanism preserving oxygenation during one-lung ventilation, the efficiency of the response is quite variable from one subject to another and/or from time to time. The questions is, therefore, what are the factors that determine the variability and can they be manipulated? A corollary of this question is to what extent is the choice of anesthetic agent a factor influencing this variability?

BLOOD FLOW DISTRIBUTION TO ATELECTATIC LUNG

While clinicians have been aware for many years that blood flow is reduced to the atelectatic lung, that HPV might be the mechanism responsible for reducing the blood flow in atelectasis was recognized surprisingly slowly. However HPV is responsible for reducing blood flow by about 50% to an atelectatic lung and the stimulus for HPV derives from the mixed venous oxygen tensions (1,25) but the effectiveness of the HPV response is influenced by temperature, sex, pH, PCO_2, age, cardiac output, left atrial pressure, mechanical ventilation and positive end-expiratory pressure as well as drugs and disease (22).

During one-lung ventilation for thoracic surgery, three additional factors also contribute to the distribution of blood flow; namely, the lateral posture (Figure 2) the influence of mechanical ventilation of the dependent lung and the effects of surgical trauma. The lateral posture results in a gravitationally determined reduction of blood flow to the non-dependent lung. Several studies have documented that this effect amounts to a 10-20% reduction of blood flow to the upper lung. Opposing this, however, is the effect of mechanical ventilation of the dependent lung.

Studies of _in vitro_ ventilated and perfused lung preparations reported that inhalational anesthetics inhibited HPV and subsequent work

120

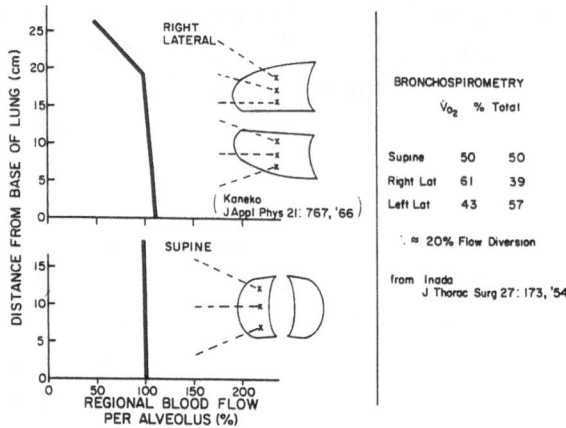

Figure 2.   Posture and pulmonary blood flow distribution.

demonstrated the dose/response relationships for inhibition by halothane, isoflurane and enflurane and showed that the ED_{50} concentration measured in MAC (minimum alveolar concentration) units was similar for all three agents with a value of about 0.5 MAC and 50% depression (32).   In striking contrast, none of the injectable agents were shown to have any influence on HPV, either in vivo or in vitro.

The results of the in vivo studies with inhalational agents have, however, been inconsistent leading more than one anesthesiologist to conclude that the influence of anesthesia on HPV is unimportant in vivo (4,33).   However, this denial of the problem ignores the important question as to why the in vivo result should be so different from and so variable compared to the in vitro studies.

An analysis of the variables was considered in my second lecture where the apparent inconsistencies in the reported studies was resolved; the direct action of inhalational agents is a consistent inhibition of HPV in humans and experimental animals (Figure 3).

Studies designed to test the influence of inhalational anesthetic agents on HPV in the absence of gross changes in cardiac output reveal that approximately 2 MAC of isoflurane or halothane will depress the HPV response by 50% but the sensitivity of the HPV response to inhibition by inhalational agents is strikingly different between the reports for in

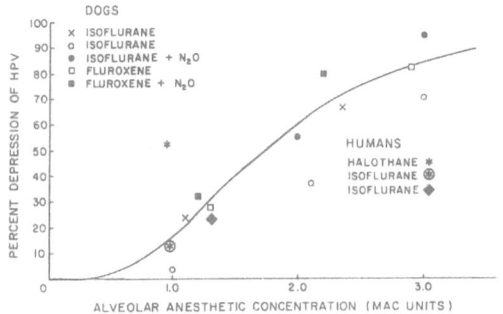

Figure 3. Inhibition of HPV by inhalational anesthetics.

vivo and in vitro preparations. The basis for this difference is unknown although it suggests that, fundamentally, HPV is very sensitive to depression by these agents, but that other factors in vivo reduce this sensitivity. And it is these other factors that contribute the individual variability that so characterizes the in vivo responses. The clinical experiences summarized in Table 1 suggest that diversion of blood flow from the atelectatic lung vary all the way from maximal effective HPV to no evidence for any HPV response. Part of this is the variability of the

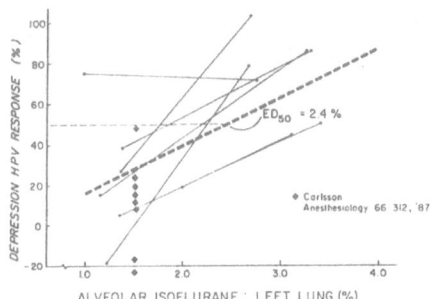

Figure 4. Individual variability of inhibition of HPV in dogs (solid circles) and humans (solid diamonds).

HPV response itself, but only about half of it appears likely to be accounted for in this way. Another important factor is the variability of the inhibition of HPV by the inhalational agents that is demonstrated in vivo (Figure 4).

With regard to the basis for this variability, it is interesting to note that the data provided by two recent human studies (4,33) suggest

that, while the response to isoflurane is characterized by a modest mean
depression but a wide variability, that for halothane (1 MAC) appears to
show much less variability, but a more marked depression (≈ 50%) of HPV
and this is the same pattern that has been observed in vitro (Figure 5).

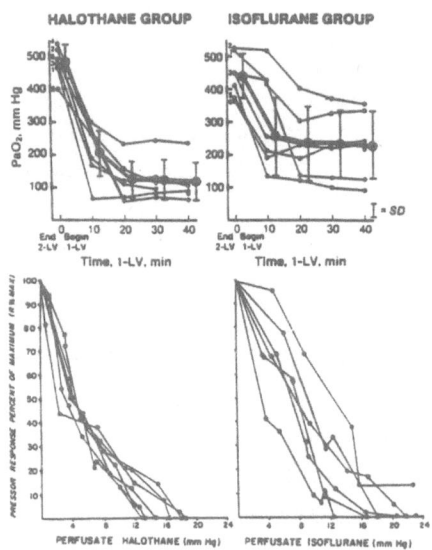

Figure 5. Patterns of response to halothane and isoflurane are similar in
vivo in humans (above) and in vitro in rats (below).

This result again suggests that other secondary effects such as trauma
have a profound influence on the outcome. Those individuals demonstrating
arterial hypoxemia during one-lung anesthesia are usually those in whom
the HPV response is inadequate or non-existent and, in some of these
patients, the cause is likely to be inhibition of HPV by inhalational
anesthetics. Switching to an injectable agent may be helpful. The use of
CPAP with oxygen to the non-dependent lung also provides a satisfactory
way of managing such patients clinically, but it is evident that the
surgical field is less satisfactory and the fundamental problem is still
present. A more satisfactory procedure would be to understand the
underlying processes sufficiently so that specific measures might be
utilized. An analysis of the several influences using the computer model
is shown in Table 2 and the importance of inhibition of HPV and the use of
ventilatory manipulation is well illustrated.

Table 2. Simulation of Effects of Posture, Thoracotomy and One-Lung Anesthesia on Pulmonary Hemodynamics and Gas Exchange*

Step	1	2	3	4	5	6	7
Posture	Supine	Lateral	Lateral	Lateral	Lateral	Lateral	Lateral
Ventilation**	Two	Two	Two	One	One	One	One
Thoracotomy	No	No	Yes	Yes	Yes	Yes	Yes
Anesthetic (MAC)	0	0	0	0	0	0	0
Constriction Fraction L	1	1	1	0.7	0.7	0.7	0.7
Fraction R	1	1	1	1	1	1	1
P_{ALV} (cmH$_2$O) L	2.5	2.5	2.5	0	0	5	0
R	2.5	2.5	2.5	2.5	2.5	2.5	10
P_{PL} (cmH$_2$O) L	-2	-5	0	0	0	5	0
R	-2	0	+2	+2	+2	+2	10
PAP (cmH$_2$O)	18.5	14.4	18.8	20.7	20.0	20.9	22.3
Left Lung Flow (% total)	45.0	33.8	35.1	21.1	26.7	19.7	33.8
P_{aO2} (mmHg)	400	400	400	150	115	170***	85

*In a hypothetical human subject with a left atrial pressure of 7 cmH$_2$O, a relative cardiac output of 0.8, and a hematocrit of 0.4. MAC = minimal alveolar concentration; L = left lung; R = right lung.
**Two-lungs or one-lung mode.
***P_{aO2} calculated assuming no gas exchange in left lung.

CONCLUSION

Atelectasis of an entire lung is generally not associated with hypoxemia because the blood flow decreases. The principal cause of this decrease is active hypoxic pulmonary vasoconstriction in the atelectatic lung stimulated by the replacement of the normal alveolar oxygen tension, of >100 mmHg, by the mixed venous oxygen tension of ≈ 40 mmHg.

This HPV response is variable quantitatively because pH, PCO_2, sex, age, disease and a variety of drugs and diseases serve to alter vascular tone and to reduce the effectiveness of HPV. The inhalational anesthetic agents depress this response in a dose-related manner, but the effect is quite variable in individual subjects. During the special circumstance of one-lung anesthesia for thoracic surgery, the direct surgical manipulation of the lung causes additional inhibition of HPV that varies with time and the type of trauma.

The emphasis of this presentation has, therefore, been the importance of understanding the causes of variability. It is the variability of individual responses that creates the challenge during clinical anesthesia. The pulmonary circulation is profoundly influenced during anesthesia and surgery, and the choice of the inhaled anesthetic agents are important contributors, both directly and indirectly.

REFERENCES

1. Bergofsky E.H.   Am J Med 57:378-394, 1974.
2. Bjertnaes L.J.   Acta Anaesth Scand 21:113-147, 1977.
3. Bjertnaes L.J.   Acta Anaesth Scand 22:570-588, 1978.
4. Benumof J.L.   Anesthesiology 43:525-532, 1975.
5. Benumof J.L.   Anesthesiology 67:910-915, 1987.
6. Bergman N.A.   In: General Anesthesia, Vol. I, 4th edition (Eds. T.C. Gray, J.E. Utting, J.F. Nunn), Butterworths, Boston, 1980, pp 477.
7. Capan L.M.   Anesth Analg 59:847-851, 1980.
8. Carlsson A.J.   Anesthesiology 66:312-316, 1987.
9. Chen L.   Anesthesiology 63:608-610, 1985.
10. Domino K.B.   Anesthesiology 64:423-429, 1986.
11. Domino K.B.   Anesthesiology 59:428-434, 1983.
12. Fishman A.P.   Circ Res 38:221-231, 1976.
13. Gothard J.W.W.   In: A Practice of Anesthesia, 5th edition (Ed. H.C. Churchill-Davidson), Year Book Medical Publishers, Chicago, 1984, p. 389.
14. Inada K.   J Thorac Surg 27:173-186, 1954.
15. Kaneko K.   J Appl Physiol 21:767-777, 1966.
16. Katz J.A.   Anesthesiology 56:164-171, 1982.
17. Kerr L.H.   Br J Anaesth 46:84-92, 1974.
18. Marin J.L.B.   Br J Anaesth 51:99-105, 1979.
19. Marshall B.E.   J Apply Physiol 51:1543-1551, 1981.
20. Marshall B.E.   In: Clinical Physiology Series (Eds. B.G. Covino, H.A. Fozzard, K. Rehder, G. Strichartz), Williams and Wilkins Company, Baltimore, 1985.
21. Marshall B.E.   In: Anesthesisa for Thoracic Procedures (Eds. B. E. Marshall, D.E. Longnecker, H.B. Fairley), Blackwell Scientific Publications, Boston, 1987, pp. 73-118.
22. Marshall B.E.   J Appl Physiol 64:68-77, 1988.

23. Marshall BE: In: Effects of Anesthesia, Clinical Physiology Series (Eds. B.G. Covino, H.A. Fozzard, K. Rehder, G. Strichartz), American Physiological Society, Bethesda, 1985, pp. 121-136.
24. Marshall B.E. In: Pulmonary Circulation in Health and Disease (Eds. J. Will, K. Weir, S. Cassin, C.A. Dawson, Academic Press, New York, 1987.
25. Marshall C. J Appl Physiol 55:711-716, 1983.
26. Marshall C. Anesthesiology 61:304-308, 1984.
27. Mathers J. Anesthesiology 46:111-114, 1977.
28. Miller F.L. Anesthesiology 63:22, 1985.
29. Pavlin E.G. In: Anesthesia, Vol. I, 2nd edition (Ed. R.D. Miller), Churchill-Livingstone, New York, 1986, p. 677.
30. Rogers S.N. Anesth Analg 64:946-954, 1985.
31. Saidman L.J. Anesthesiology 57:A472, 1982.
32. Sykes M.K. J Appl Physiol 39:103-108, 1975.
33. Sykes M.K. Br J Anaesth 50:1185-1196, 1978.
34. Sykes M.K. Br J Anaesth 49:293-299, 1977.
35. Sykes M.K. Br J Anaesth 49:301-307, 1977.
36. Torda T.A. Anaesthesia 29:272-279, 1974.
37. Voelkel N.F. Am Rev Resp Dis 133:1186-1195, 1986.

This work supported in part by grant from the National Institutes of Health GM29628.

OXIMETRY II: LIMITATIONS AND EFFECTS ON OTHER MONITORS

John W. Severinghaus, MD
University of California Medical School, San Francisco

LIMITATIONS OF PULSE OXIMETRY

Theoretic limitations: The optical signals are the pulsatile variations in light transmitted through tissue at 660 and 940 nM. The log of the ratio of these A.C. signals is a nonlinear empiric function of S_aO_2. The pulsatile signal is usually 0.5% - 10% of total light transmission from the light emitting diodes, not counting ambient light. Variations may be caused also by movement, ventilation, venous pressure waves and ambient flicker. The 660 nM wave length is on the steep part of the extinction curve of Hb making S_pO_2 very sensitive to LED wavelength drift (temperature, age, probe to probe variation). Since many pulse oximeters search for optimal signals by altering the intensity of the LEDs, and this power change alters LED wavelength, it is necessary to compensate for predicted wavelength changes in the calculations, introducing uncertainty. In view of these problems, the accuracy obtained in most instruments is remarkably good.

Pulse dependence: The major limitation is inadequate pulsatile signal, caused by hypotension, low pulse pressure or vasoconstriction. When pulse amplitude is too low, most pulse oximeters blank or read zero, but threshold are widely variable between manufacturers. Some instruments may continue to read but warn of inadequate signal. If oximeter heart rate is wrong, the S_aO_2 value is questionable.

Vasoconstrictors: A 30 kg emaciated 72 yr old female with intestinal obstruction undergoing adhesion lysis under narcotic - isoflurane anesthesia became hypotensive to systolic pressures of about 65. In addition to fluid loading, two 5 mg doses of ephedrine were given. Saturation fell over 3-5 min (Nellcor, non-disposable finger probe) from 98% to 40% while the heart rate detected by the oximeter continued to be correct. A radial arterial blood sample drawn when S_pO_2 = 40% showed Po_2 = 550 mmHg, and normal Pco_2 and pH. Over the following 15 min, with more fluid and blood administration, S_pO_2 returned to the high 90's. Patient core temperature was 34°C. The implication is that vasoconstriction *may* stop finger flow entirely, allowing tissue to slowly consume the O_2 in the stagnant arteries, without eliminating the pulsatile signal in the arteries. An alternative explanation is that vasoconstriction somehow induced pulsation of venous blood.

Ventilator induced pulse interference: With positive pressure ventilation, cycling venous and arterial pressure may block detection of saturation due to continuous searching for an optimal signal in some instruments.

Electro-cautery: Most oximeters are now relatively immune, but separation of the probe from the site of surgery and the ground pad helps.

Abnormal pulses: Some devices detect a large dichrotic notch, or fail with irregular rates. The S_pO_2 may be correct even if rate is not.

Forehead operation: Probes used on the forehead have tended to read too high in hypoxia and too low at normal levels, although CSI has found ways to overcome this problem. Infrared light penetrates more deeply than red light so the paths of the two wavelengths traverse different tissue and thus detect different degrees of pulsatility. The IR source must be located closer than the red LED to the detector to obtain accurate tracking of low saturation.

127

T. H. Stanley and R. J. Sperry (eds.), Anesthesia and the Lung, 127–131.
© 1989 by Kluwer Academic Publishers.

Response times: Circulation may delay finger responses more than 1 minute after pulmonary change. Averaging time varies, usually allowing a choice. Typical averaging time is 5-8 sec.

Accuracy: Manufacturers claim bias and precision of less than ±3% at normal levels, and this seems to be correct. At 55% S_aO_2 precision varies from ±3% to ± 8% and bias from +1.6% to -10.6% depending on the instrument (see table). There are variations between sites and between subjects that are not yet understood. Hypertensive and vasoconstricted subjects have shown large errors.

HbCO and HbMet: Pulse oximeters actually detect reduced Hb, which is normally about 3% (at 97% S_aO_2). When S_pO_2 reads low, P_aO_2 may be presumed to be low even if HbCO is present. HbCO is detected as HbO_2 and therefore does not alter the measured desaturated hemoglobin of a pulse oximeter. HbMet lowers the S_aO_2 reading, by about half the HbMet percentage at low levels. When using a multi-wavelength co-oximeter as a standard for testing the accuracy of pulse oximeters, arterial saturation, S_aO_2, is calculated as:

$$S_aO_2 = \frac{HbO_2}{100 - HbCO - HbMet}$$

Dyes, pigments, nail polish: Injected methylene blue and indocyanine green produce transient false desaturation. Skin pigment is usually not a problem since the nail bed and finger tips are usually less pigmented in blacks. Pigment does not cause error since it is not a pulsatile opacity. Nail polish reduces total light and may render the signal too small, but probes can be mounted side to side on a finger.

Ambient light: Some lights (esp. xenon OR lights) have caused false readings even without a subject connected. Opaque covering of the probe is helpful.

Ear vs finger: In general, signals from the ear are weaker, except when peripheral vasoconstriction or hypotension limits finger perfusion, but ear responses are much faster and at low saturations somewhat more accurate than finger data.

Alternative sites: In infants, flexible probes work through the palm, foot or even arm. The bridge of the nose and nasal septum have been used. The cheek may be used by placing an ear probe with either light source or detector inside the mouth. The wing of the nostril provides a useful site, and the tongue has been used. Use of "transflectance" from skin surfaces, particularly in the fetus, has been much tested but so far with little success. In general, we found the bias and precision to be better on the ear than on the finger at low saturation.

MRI interference: Magnetic resonance imaging does not seem to interfere with pulse oximetry, but the probe cable may introduce artifact into the field and generate granularity in the MRI image. Filtering of radio frequency signals picked up by the antenna-effect of the probe cable has been shown to reduce this problem but requires special probe extender/couplers.

Motion artifact: Probe motion may cause readings to fail or be incorrect. Ear and forehead probes may be more useful than finger probes in restless patients. One method of minimizing this is to couple an ECG signal to the oximeter to synchronize detection to heart rate (Nellcor N-200, CSI US).

Premature infant oxygen control: Pulse oximetry was thought incapable of detecting hyperoxia until it became clear that optimal S_pO_2 (and S_aO_2) in prematures is less than 90%, where oximetry has greater sensitivity than either arterial or transcutaneous Po_2 measurement. It is not known whether eye damage correlates better with Po_2 or S_aO_2.

Potential Dangers: There may be a possibility of pressure necrosis from some probes left on a single site too long (if a spring compresses the tissue, or tape is applied too tightly). Instances of 2nd and even 3rd degree skin burns have been reported with defective probes or designs (Datascope, Nellcor).

False alarms, false non-alarms Some oximeters may continue to indicate a saturation of 80-90% without adequate signal, when saturation is much lower. An instrument which alarms or drops to zero frequently due to motion or weak signals may fail to persuade the physician when real desaturation has occurred (wolf syndrome). Hypoventilation may go undetected by pulse oximetry if a patient is breathing supplementary oxygen.

IMPACT OF PULSE OXIMETRY ON OTHER MONITORING METHODS

I. Transcutaneous blood gases

Pulse oximetry and transcutaneous Po_2 measurement were initiated in the same year, 1972. However, the demands of the premature infant resulted in rapid application of transcutaneous Po_2 in nurseries within 5 years, whereas pulse oximetry development and application required 10 or more years. Because of its speed, simplicity, accuracy and freedom from calibration, from possible burns and from drift, pulse oximetry has virtually eliminated transcutaneous Po_2 from use in monitoring in adults, and is rapidly doing so in premature nurseries. At first, neonatologists believed that pulse oximetry could not disclose hyperoxia adequately. Now, however, they recognize that premature infant saturation should never exceed 95%, and should usually be held below 90%, a range in which the pulse oximeter is more dependable than transcutaneous Po_2 electrodes.

Transcutaneous Pco_2 measurement is a victim of the pulse oximeter as well, although it should be used more. $tcPco_2$ is accurate to ± 3 mmHg, can be operated at 40-42°C continuously without danger of burns, and is as accurate in adults as in babies. It is better than end tidal Pco_2 for estimating arterial Pco_2 because of the variable pulmonary a-A Pco_2 difference, and because it works without airway connection, for example in the recovery room or in patients who are sedated but not intubated.

The major missing factor in non-invasive monitoring is pH, and no present technology has proved useful to obtain it. There remains some hope that the pH of the tears under the eyelid may closely track arterial pH, but no instrument is available to test that possibility now. Eyelid Po_2 and Pco_2 instrumentation was developed and tested in the past 8 years, but appears to have failed due to a few reports of eye infections and reluctance of physicians to use such instrumentation.

II. Invasive blood gases

Pulse oximetry has also reduced the interest in and sales of invasive oxygen monitoring methods as well. The Oximetrix catheter oximeter was derived from the original reflectance oximetry work of Brinkman and Zijlstra in Groningen, Netherlands in the early 1950's, modified by Polanyi at the American Optical Company and by Shaw who introduced the HP multiwavelength oximeter. The Oximetrix is used occasionally to monitor mixed venous S_vO_2 as an index of the adequacy of both oxygenation and circulation, a useful concept. Unfortunately, the method requires a special balloon directed catheter costing about $150 per patient, and has problems of reflected light from heart and vessel walls if the tip touches them. This problem has greatly limited its use for arterial oxygen measurement since vessel walls are almost certain to be "seen" along with blood. Inherently, the reflectance method is highly accurate, and one may hope that means of optically shielding it from vessel walls can be found, perhaps by use of a black tube extending beyond the fiber tip but open to blood flow.

Another technology, optical measurement of Po_2, has been introduced by Dietrich Lübbers, and is primarily finding a role in continuous monitoring of Po_2 in pump oxygenators during cardiac bypass, since the disposable element is inherently inexpensive. The analytic instrument is not, costing about \$12,000, but yielding values for pH, Pco_2 and Po_2 in the pump blood stream. The Po_2 response is non-linear, but nearly hyperbolic, due to quenching in which the largest signal change occurs in a change from zero Po_2 to a few mmHg Po_2, making it insensitive to Po_2 at and above the normal range of arterial blood.

There are similar optical Po_2, Pco_2 and pH catheters under development and testing for arterial use. These will not suffer the reflection problems of the oximeters, but still have problems of drift, stability, non-linearity, clotting, calibration and sensitivity, as well as considerable expense.

MANDATION AND LEGISLATION

Should we use pulse oximeters routinely, and if so in which patients? Caplan et al reported [1] an ASA closed claim study which turned up 14 cardiac arrests in healthy patients under spinal anesthesia. In 12 IV sedation or narcotics had been given, and hypoventilation and hypoxia were probably responsible. Those presumably could have been prevented by pulse oximetry. Pulse oximeters would also immediately detect arrests occurring suddenly without sedation during spinal anesthesia and runs of ventricular tachycardia due to injecting epinephrine with halothane anesthesia.

The Closed Claims Study of the Professional Liability Committee of the ASA presented preliminary evidence [2] that respiratory problems constituted 31% of all insurance settlements, and that 55% of the inadequate ventilation had been judged to be due to poor monitoring, while 21% was thought due to poor vigilance, poor training or poor supervision. The panel concluded that in 133 of the 193 cases, or 69% of all, an available monitor *would* have prevented the complication. The average insurance payment in those preventable cases was \$400,000, almost twice the payment in the 70% judged not to be preventable by monitoring. If buying 100 pulse oximeters prevents one of those malpractice judgements, the cost equals the benefit.

Pulse oximetry has been shown to detect significant hypoxemia during recovery from anesthesia [3]. 14% of inpatients showed at least transient hypoxemia during recovery, whereas only 1% of outpatients became hypoxic in the recovery room. The reasons were many, including the more severely ill and more extensive surgery for inpatients, but the amount of premedication and fixed drugs was not significantly different.

Medline (June '88) lists 166 papers on pulse oximetry, mostly in the last 2 years. Many can be cited as showing benefits of pulse oximetry. These reports support the assertion that pulse oximetry should be used in all anesthetized and heavily sedated patients, not only in operating rooms, but in recovery, intensive care, and when any procedure is being done under sedation, whether endoscopic, plastic or dental.

Does that mean that pulse oximetry should be mandated? It is fairly easy to mandate something that is rapidly happening anyway, and I suppose legislatures will be only too happy to support it along with motherhood. Law follows practice, and 4 years have turned pulse oximetry from a rare practice to standard of practice in the operating room, but unfortunately not enough elsewhere. Mandated or not, it is evident that pulse oximetry reduces risks to both our patients and our pocketbooks.

FUTURE: Improvements and Other Uses of Pulse Oximetry

I suspect the pulse oximeter will soon be considered our basic monitor for all procedures where consciousness is impaired. There are several potential modifications of pulse oximeters under consideration, which might replace routine ECG and automated blood pressure monitors.

1. Pulse oximetry combined with capnometry: Because of the recent emphasis on the importance of end tidal CO_2 monitoring for detection of esophageal intubation, many pulse oximeter manufacturers are offering or planning combined instrumentation. In my view, the infrared end

tidal devices should measure anesthetic vapor concentration as well as Pco_2, with or without a combined pulse oximeter. The oximeter's uses are often in non-intubated patients in which end tidal gas concentration is unavailable or at best difficult to obtain, often in non-anesthetized but sedated or injured patients.

2. Substitution for the ECG: The routine use of the ECG for most anesthesia can be discontinued when a pulse oximeter is used. However, several manufacturers are finding that the pulse oximeter signal itself can be made more dependable if the computer is given an ECG signal for timing purposes. This suggests that the future pulse oximeter should contain an ECG input, preferably a two rather than three lead system, and should display the usual ECG trace or its equivalent.

3. Automated systolic pressure by cuff occlusion of the oximeter pulse: If a small cuff is placed on the finger or arm above the oximeter probe, when its pressure is linearly increased, pulse amplitude falls to zero at about systolic pressure. Since for many applications, this would suffice, and since this POX (Pressure, oximetric) can be read within about 6 sec as often as 5 times a minute, the addition of a pump, pressure gauge and display to pulse oximeters would extend their range of use.

4. Much effort is being invested in "reflectance" or "transflectance" surface pulse oximetry, both for fetal monitoring during labor, and for easier and less mobile sites in awake, restless patients. Forehead can be used accurately (CSI), and other sites on the head are promising, such as cheek, lips, nostrils, ear and tongue.

5. Telemetered pulse oximetry is needed, but not yet available, to permit patients to be cared for in their rooms, without being in intensive care situations, when they are recovering, or sedated, or in some danger of respiratory obstruction.

CONCLUSION

Pulse oximetry in my view is the most important monitoring tool made available to anesthesia. It will probably become the basic monitor for all patients in any jeopardy of ventilatory depression or obstruction or hypoxia. The future monitor as I see it will be a hybrid pulse oximeter detecting and displaying ECG and periodically inflating a cuff proximal to the oximeter probe to estimate systolic blood pressure. Oximetry could increase safety during post operative patient transport as well as during recovery.

REFERENCES:

1) Caplan, R A, R J Ward, K Posner, F W Cheney: Unexpected cardiac arrest during spinal anesthesia: A closed claims analysis of predisposing factors. Anesthesiology 68:5-11, 1988.

2) Caplan R A, K Posner, R W Ward and F W Cheney: Respiratory Mishaps: Principal areas of risk and implications for anesthetic care. Anesthesiology 67:3A469 (abs), 1987.

3) Morris R W, A Buschman, D L Warren, J H Philip and D B Raemer: The prevalence of hypoxemia detected by pulse oximetry during recovery from anesthesia. J Clin Monitoring 4:16-20, 1988.

ANESTHESIA FOR THORACIC SURGERY: PART I—DOUBLE-LUMEN TUBE INTUBATION

JONATHAN L. BENUMOF, M.D.

Anesthesia Research Lab, T-001, University of California San Diego,
La Jolla, California 92093

INTRODUCTION

Double-lumen tube intubation is the method of choice of separating the
two lungs to facilitate the performance of thoracic surgery in the vast
majority of cases.   Proper insertion and positioning of the double-lumen
tube is often the most important determinant as to whether these cases [in
particular one-lung ventilation (1LV) cases] proceed smoothly.   If the
double-lumen tube is in the right position, the nondependent lung will
collapse completely and easily, the surgeon will be able to work
efficiently without damaging the nondependent lung, and the dependent lung
will be unobstructed and easy to ventilate.   This lecture discusses the
proper insertion and positioning of double-lumen tubes.

CORRECT POSITIONING OF DOUBLE-LUMEN TUBE: CONVENTIONAL AND FIBEROPTIC
BRONCHOSCOPY TECHNIQUES (1)

When surgery is performed on the right lung a left-sided double-lumen
tube (DLT) is used (Figure 1).   When surgery of the left lung is performed
(Figure 1), either a left- or right-sided DLT may be used.   However, since
the margin of safety in positioning a right-sided tube is much less than
for a left-sided tube, use of a right-sided DLT for left lung surgery
introduces the risk of inadequate ventilation of the right upper lobe (RUL)
if the RUL ventilation slot is not closely opposed to the RUL orifice
(Figure 2, middle and bottom panels).(2)   To avoid this complication, I use
a left-sided DLT for all cases requiring 1LV.   If clamping of the left
mainstem bronchus is necessary, the DLT can be withdrawn at that time
(after deflating the cuffs) into the trachea and then used as a single-
lumen tube (deflate only the left lumen cuff and use both of the lumens to
ventilate the right lung) (Figure 1).   A right-side DLT is indicated only
when a left-sided DLT is contraindicated, such as when there is a large
exophytic lesion in the left mainstem bronchus or there is a tight left
mainstem bronchus stenosis.   Clear, nontoxic plastic, low pressure cuff,
disposable Robertshaw type DLT should be used.

133

T. H. Stanley and R. J. Sperry (eds.), Anesthesia and the Lung, 133–139.
© 1989 by Kluwer Academic Publishers.

134

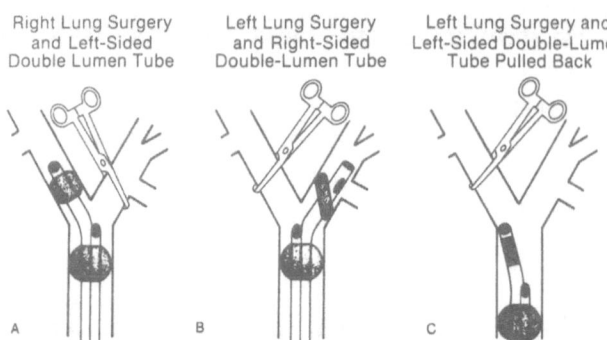

Right Lung Surgery and Left-Sided Double Lumen Tube

Left Lung Surgery and Right-Sided Double-Lumen Tube

Left Lung Surgery and Left-Sided Double-Lumen Tube Pulled Back

A   B   C

Figure 9–8. Use of left-sided and right-sided double-lumen tubes for left and right lung surgery (as indicated by the clamp). When surgery is going to be performed on the right lung, a left-sided double-lumen tube should be used (A). When surgery is going to be performed on the left lung, a right-sided double-lumen tube can be used (B). However, because of uncertainty as to the alignment of the right upper lobe ventilation slot to the right upper lobe orifice, a left-sided double-lumen tube can also be used for left lung surgery (C). If the left lung surgery requires a clamp to be placed high on the left mainstem bronchus, the left endobronchial cuff should be deflated, the left-sided double-lumen tube pulled back into the trachea, and the right lung ventilated through both of the lumens (use the double-lumen tube as a single-lumen tube).

FIGURE 1.   Reproduced with permission from Reference #1.

The Margin of Safety (MS) in Positioning Double-Lumen Endotracheal Tubes

Left-Sided Tube

Outermost Acceptable Position

Innermost Acceptable Position

Proximal Left Cuff to Tip

MS

LUL

LMS

Proximal Surface of Left Endobronchial Cuff Just Below Tracheal Carina

Tip of Left Lumen at Left Upper Lobe

Proximal Left Cuff to Tip — MS

LMS

MS = LMS – Proximal Left Cuff to Left Tip

Mallinkrodt Right-Sided Tube

Outermost Acceptable Position

Innermost Acceptable Position

RUL

MS RMS

Proximal Surface of Right Endobronchial Cuff Just Below Tracheal Carina

Width of Cuff

Distal Surface of Cuff at RUL

RUL

MS RMS Width of Right Cuff

MS = RMS – Width of Right Cuff

FIG. 1. This schematic shows the definitions of most proximal and most distal acceptable positions of left- and right-sided double-lumen tubes and the margin of safety in positioning these double-lumen tubes. Top panel = all left-sided double-lumen tubes; middle panel = Mallinkrodt right-sided double-lumen tube; bottom panel = Rusch right-sided double-lumen tube; LMS = length left mainstem bronchus; RMS = length right mainstem bronchus; MS = margin of safety in positioning double-lumen tube; LUL = left upper lobe; RUL = right upper lobe.

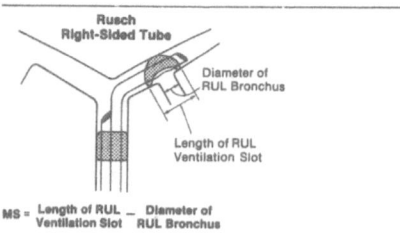

Rusch Right-Sided Tube

Diameter of RUL Bronchus

Length of RUL Ventilation Slot

MS = Length of RUL Ventilation Slot – Diameter of RUL Bronchus

FIGURE 2.   Reproduced with permission from Reference #2.

The Robertshaw type DLT is passed with the distal curvature initially concave anteriorly (Figure 3, panel 1). After the tube tip passes the larynx the tube is rotated ninety degrees so that the proximal curve is concave anteriorly (Figure 3, panel 2) to allow endobronchial intubation on the appropriate side. The tube is then pushed in until most of it is in (common two-lumen molding is at the level of the teeth) and/or a moderate resistance to further passage is encountered. Once the tube tip is thought to be endobronchial, both the tracheal and endobronchial cuffs should be inflated and bilateral ventilation checked. Then one connecting tube should be clamped (Figure 3, panel 3) and the disappearance of breath sounds on that side and the continuance of breath sounds on the other side should be listened for to ensure proper positioning of the tube.

If the position of the DLT is correct, then the anesthetist should be able to make four observations during unilateral clamping. First, the breath sounds should only be heard on the contralateral side and the breath sounds should disappear on the ipsilateral (clamped) side. Second, the contralateral lung should feel reasonably compliant. Third, only the contralateral chest should rise and fall with ventilation giving the chest a rocking boat motion. Fourth, the respiratory gas moisture should disappear on inhalation and reappear on exhalation on the ventilated side, and the respiratory gas moisture should be stationary on the clamped side.

There are three very gross malpositions for a DLT (Figure 4). The DLT can be in too far in the left or the right mainstem bronchus, or it may be inserted too little so that both lumens are in the trachea. In each malposition the left cuff, when inflated, blocks the right lumen and this can be taken advantage of to diagnosis the DLT malposition. When the left cuff is inflated and the left lumen is clamped (ventilation is only through the right lumen), the left cuff will block the right lumen in all three malpositions and the breath sounds will be either absent or very diminished. When the left cuff is then deflated, breath sounds will only be heard on the left side when the DLT is in too far on the the left; breath sounds will be heard on both sides when the DLT is out too far; and breath sounds will only be heard in the right lung when the DLT is in too far on the right.

Unfortunately, the above scheme of left lumen clamping, left cuff inflation-deflation, and auscultation maneuvers to determine DLT malposition is not usable and/or reliable all of the time. The reasons for the failure of the method consist of: 1) once the patient is prepared and draped, the chest is no longer available for auscultation; 2) use of breath sounds as an endpoint is often not sensitive enough because of either

Passage of Left-Sided Double-Lumen Tube

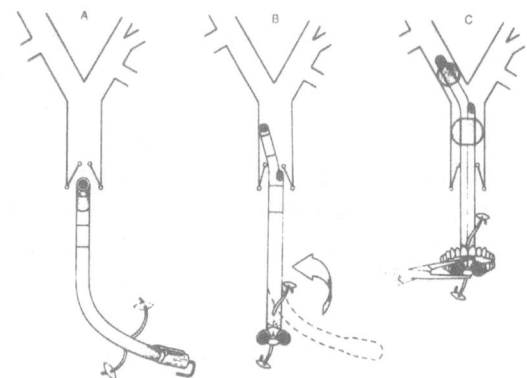

Figure 9–9. This schematic diagram depicts the passage of the left-sided double-lumen tube in a supine patient. A. The tube is held with the distal curvature concave anteriorly and the proximal curve concave to the right and in a plane parallel to the floor. The tube is then inserted through the vocal cords until the left cuff passes the vocal cords. The stylet is then removed. B. The tube is rotated 90° counter-clockwise so that the distal curvature is concave anteriorly and the proximal curvature is concave to the left and in a plane parallel to the floor. C. The tube is inserted until either a moderate resistance to further passage is encountered or the end of the common molding of the two lumens is at the teeth. Both cuffs are then inflated, and both lungs are ventilated. Finally, one side is clamped while the other side is ventilated and vice versa (see text for further explanation).

FIGURE 3. Reproduced with permission from Reference #1.

Double-Lumen Tube Malpositions

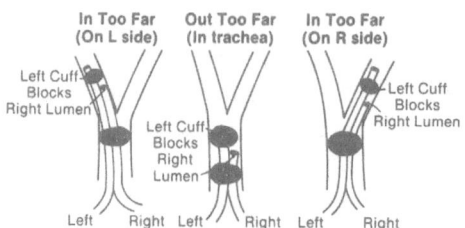

Procedure	Breath Sounds Heard		
Clamp Right Lumen Both Cuffs Inflated	Left	Left and Right	Right
Clamp Left Lumen Both Cuffs Inflated	None or Very ↓↓	None or Very ↓↓	None or Very ↓↓
Clamp Left Lumen Deflate Left Cuff	Left	Left and Right	Right

Figure 9–12. There are three major (involving a whole lung) malpositions of a left-sided double-lumen endotracheal tube. The tube can be in too far on the left (both lumens are in the left mainstem bronchus), out too far (both lumens are in the trachea), or down the right mainstem bronchus (at least the left lumen is in the right mainstem bronchus). In each of these three malpositions the left cuff, when fully inflated, can completely block the right lumen. Inflation and deflation of the left cuff while the left lumen is clamped creates a breath sound differential diagnosis of tube malposition. (See text for full explanation). (L = left; R = right; ↓ = decreased.)

FIGURE 4. Reproduced with permission from Reference #1.

preexisting or anesthesia-induced lung disease; 3) the tube may move during the middle of a case (surgeon traction, patient coughing, patient turning); 4) the tube may be just barely malpositioned; and 5) some combination of the above.

Whenever there is any doubt as to where the DLT is, it may be resolved by the use of fiberoptic bronchoscopy (FOB). A pediatric FOB (outside diameter less than 4.0 mm) can be passed down the lumens of all sized (35, 37, 39, 41 Fr) DLTs. A 4.9 mm outside diameter FOB will not pass down the 35 French and is a tight squeeze through a 37 French tube. The simplest method of determining DLT position is to pass the FOB down the right lumen, much as one might pass a suction catheter.

Looking down the right lumen, the endoscopist should see a clear straight-ahead view of the tracheal carina, the left lumen going off to the left side, and the upper surface of the blue left endobronchial cuff just below the tracheal carina (Figure 5, two right panels). Looking down the right lumen, the endoscopist should not see the left cuff herniating over the carina or the carina pushed over to the right and compromising the right mainstem bronchial orifice (Figure 5, two right panels). Looking down the left lumen (which is not usually done), the endoscopist should see a clear straightahead view of the bronchial carina and only a slight left-luminal narrowing (Figure 5, two left panels). The FOB is used anytime during the case there is a doubt about position of the DLT.

The importance of seeing the upper surface of the blue left endobronchial cuff just below the tracheal carina needs to be emphasized.(2) The outermost acceptable position of a left-sided DLT occurs when the left endobronchial cuff is just below the tracheal carina (Figure 2, top panel). If a left-sided DLT is pulled out any further, the left endobronchial cuff will obstruct the trachea and the right mainstem bronchus. The innermost acceptable position occurs when the distal tip of the left lumen is at the left upper lobe (LUL) bronchus, because further insertion will obstruct the LUL. The distance between the right and left lumen tips for the Nat. Cath. Corp. tube (=70 mm) is longer than the length of the left mainstem bronchus (=50 mm in adult males and females). Thus, it is possible for the right lumen to be above the tracheal carina while the left lumen tip obstructs the LUL. The distance between the upper surface of the left endobronchial balloon and the left tip is 25 mm (which is shorter than the shortest left mainstem bronchus). Thus, when the upper surface of the left endobronchial balloon is just below the tracheal carina, it is not possible for the left tip to obstruct the LUL.

Use of Fiberoptic Bronchoscope to Determine Precise Left-Sided Double-Lumen Tube Position

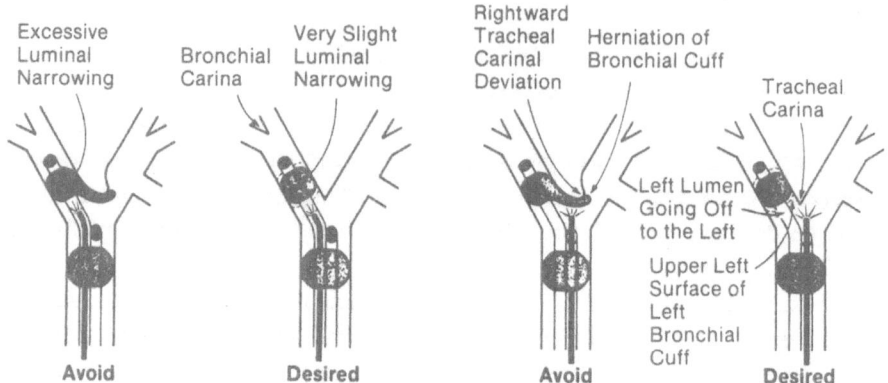

Excessive Luminal Narrowing

Bronchial Carina

Very Slight Luminal Narrowing

Rightward Tracheal Carinal Deviation

Herniation of Bronchial Cuff

Tracheal Carina

Left Lumen Going Off to the Left

Upper Left Surface of Left Bronchial Cuff

Avoid **Desired** **Avoid** **Desired**

View Down Left (Bronchial) Lumen **View Down Right (Tracheal) Lumen**

Figure 9–15. This schematic diagram depicts the complete fiberoptic bronchoscopy picture of left-sided double-lumen tubes (both the desired view and the view to be avoided from both of the lumens). When the bronchoscope is passed down the right lumen of the left-sided tube, the endoscopist should see a clear straight-ahead view of the tracheal carina and the upper surface of the blue left endobronchial cuff just below the tracheal carina. Excessive pressure in the endobronchial cuff, as manifested by tracheal carinal deviation to the right and herniation of the endobronchial cuff over the carina, should be avoided. When the bronchoscope is passed down the left lumen of the left-sided tube, the endoscopist should see a very slight left luminal narrowing and a clear straight-ahead view of the bronchial carina off in the distance. Excessive left luminal narrowing should be avoided.

FIGURE 5. Reproduced with permission from Reference #1.

Use of Fiberoptic Bronchoscope to Insert Left-Sided Double-Lumen Tube

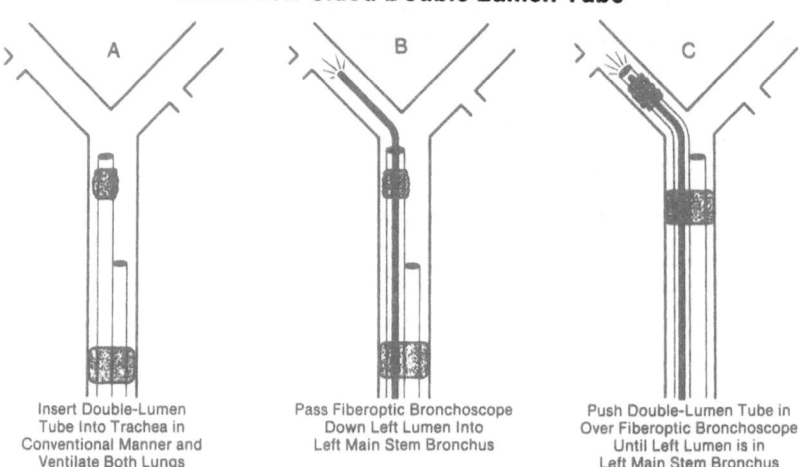

Insert Double-Lumen Tube Into Trachea in Conventional Manner and Ventilate Both Lungs

Pass Fiberoptic Bronchoscope Down Left Lumen Into Left Main Stem Bronchus

Push Double-Lumen Tube in Over Fiberoptic Bronchoscope Until Left Lumen is in Left Main Stem Bronchus

Figure 9–13. This schematic diagram portrays use of the fiberoptic bronchoscope to insert a left-sided double-lumen tube. The double-lumen tube can be put into the trachea in a conventional manner, and both lungs can be ventilated by both lumens (A). The fiberoptic bronchoscope may be inserted into the left lumen of the double-lumen tube through a self-sealing diaphragm in the elbow connector to the left lumen; this allows continued positive pressure ventilation of both lungs through the right lumen without creating a leak. After the fiberoptic bronchoscope has been passed into the left mainstem bronchus (B), it is used as a stylet for the aftercoming left lumen (C). The fiberoptic bronchoscope is then withdrawn. Final precise positioning of the double-lumen tube is performed with the fiberoptic bronchoscope in the right lumen (see Fig. 9–14).

FIGURE 6. Reproduced with permission from Reference #1.

USE OF FIBEROPTIC BRONCHOSCOPE TO INSERT THE BRONCHIAL LUMEN OF A DOUBLE-LUMEN TUBE INTO A MAINSTEM BRONCHUS

The insertion of the bronchial lumen of a double-lumen tube into the appropriate mainstem bronchus may be aided by the use of a fiberoptic bronchoscope (Figure 6). The double-lumen tube is first placed in the trachea in a conventional manner (laryngoscopy, manual tube insertion) until the tracheal cuff just passes the vocal cords, the tracheal cuff is inflated, and both lungs are ventilated with both lumens (use the double-lumen tube as if it were a single-lumen tube). A pediatric fiberoptic bronchoscope can then be inserted into the bronchial lumen through a self-sealing diaphragm in the elbow connector to the bronchial lumen (which permits continued positive-pressure ventilation through that lumen around the fiberoptic bronchoscope) and passed into the appropriate mainstem bronchus. The tracheal cuff is then deflated and the bronchial lumen is passed over the fiberoptic bronchoscope stylet into the appropriate mainstem bronchus. The fiberoptic bronchoscope is then withdrawn from the bronchial lumen and passed down the tracheal lumen to determine the precise double-lumen tube position (see the previous section).

Alternatively, once the double-lumen tube is in the trachea, the fiberoptic bronchoscope can be inserted into the tracheal lumen through a self-sealing diaphragm in the elbow connector to the tracheal lumen (which permits continued positive-pressure ventilation through that lumen around the fiberoptic bronchoscope) and passed just proximal to the tracheal carina. While the carina and the two mainstem bronchial orifices are in view, the double-lumen tube can be advanced and the degree of lateral rotation adjusted so that the left lumen enters the left mainstem bronchus. Final precise positioning (see the previous section) can be done with the fiberoptic bronchoscope remaining in the tracheal lumen.

REFERENCES
1. Benumof, J.L. Anesthesia for Thoracic Surgery. W.B. Saunders Co., Philadelphia, 1987.
2. Benumof, J.L. Anesthesiology 67:729-738, 1987.

ANESTHESIA FOR THORACIC SURGERY: PART II—MANAGEMENT OF ONE-LUNG
VENTILATION

JONATHAN L. BENUMOF, M.D.

Anesthesia Research Lab, T-001, University of California San Diego,
La Jolla, California 92093

INTRODUCTION
    The choice of anesthetic drug and technique is one of the factors that
may influence the distribution of blood flow during one-lung ventilation
(1LV), and is a factor that is under the control of the anesthesiologist.
The first half of this lecture will consider the "Effect of Inhalation
Anesthetics on Arterial Oxygenation and Intrapulmonary Shunt During One-
Lung Ventilation." Since the two lungs are separated by a double-lumen
tube during 1LV, it is possible to treat the two lungs differently. The
second half of this lecture "Management of Each Lung Separately During One-
Lung Ventilation" outlines the initial management of 1LV and what to do if
hypoxemia ensues (such as nondependent lung CPAP, dependent lung PEEP,
differential lung ventilation).

EFFECT OF INHALATION ANESTHETICS ON ARTERIAL OXYGENATION AND INTRAPULMONARY
SHUNT DURING ONE-LUNG VENTILATION
Distribution of blood flow during two-lung ventilation and
lateral decubitus position
    The fractional blood flow to the left and right (and larger) lungs in
the upright and supine positions is 45 and 55%, respectively. However, 1LV
is usually performed in the lateral decubitus position and gravitational
forces will alter the distribution of blood flow between the two lungs
(from the supine distribution) so that the nondependent lung receives
relatively less and the dependent lung receives relatively more blood flow.
Thus, when the left lung is the nondependent lung the fractional blood flow
between the left and right lungs is 35 and 65%, respectively, and when the
right lung is the nondependent lung the fractional blood flow between the
left and right lung is 45 and 55%, respectively. The left hand side of
Figure 1 shows typical two-lung ventilation (2LV) conditions in the lateral

141

T. H. Stanley and R. J. Sperry (eds.), Anesthesia and the Lung, 141–148.
© 1989 by Kluwer Academic Publishers.

decubitus position. The average nondependent and dependent lung blood flow distribution would be 40% (35+45/2) and 60% (65+55/2), respectively (Figure 1, left panel).

Distribution of blood flow during one-lung ventilation, lateral decubitus position

When 1LV is employed the nondependent lung is the nonventilated and collapsed lung and the dependent lung is the ventilated lung. Consequently, 1LV creates an obligatory shunt through the nonventilated lung which is not present during 2LV. Thus, it is not surprising that, for the same F_IO_2 and hemodynamic and metabolic status, 1LV results in a much decreased P_aO_2. However, and fortunately, there are both passive mechanical and active vasoconstrictor mechanisms that are usually operant that minimize the blood flow to the nonventilated lung and, thereby, prevent the P_aO_2 from decreasing as much as might be expected.

Blood flow to the nondependent nonventilated lung.(1) The passive mechanical mechanisms decreasing blood flow to the nondependent lung consist of gravity and surgical interference with blood flow. Gravity contributes to the vertical gradient in the distribution of pulmonary blood flow during 1LV in the lateral decubitus position just as it does during 2LV in the lateral decubitus position. The gravity component of blood flow reduction to the nondependent lung should be constant with respect to both time and magnitude. The surgical interference of nondependent lung blood flow involves compression and retraction of the nondependent lung and ligation of nondependent lung blood vessels. The surgical interference component of nondependent lung blood flow reduction should be variable with respect to both time and magnitude.

The most significant reduction in blood flow to the nondependent lung is caused by an active vasoconstrictor mechanism. The normal response of the pulmonary vasculature to atelectasis is an increase in pulmonary vascular resistance (PVR) (in just the atelectatic lung) and the increase in atelectatic lung PVR is thought to be due almost entirely to hypoxic pulmonary vasoconstriction (HPV). The selective increase in atelectatic lung PVR diverts blood flow away from the atelectatic lung towards the remaining normoxic or hyperoxic ventilated lung. The diversion of blood flow minimizes the amount of shunt flow that occurs through hypoxic lung. It is not surprising then, that numerous clinical 1LV studies have found that the shunt through the nonventilated lung is usually only 20-25% of the cardiac output as opposed to the 35-45% shunt that might be expected if there was no HPV in the nonventilated lung. Thus, HPV is an autoregulatory

Effect of 1 MAC Isoflurane Anesthesia on Shunt During One Lung Ventilation (1LV) of Normal Lungs

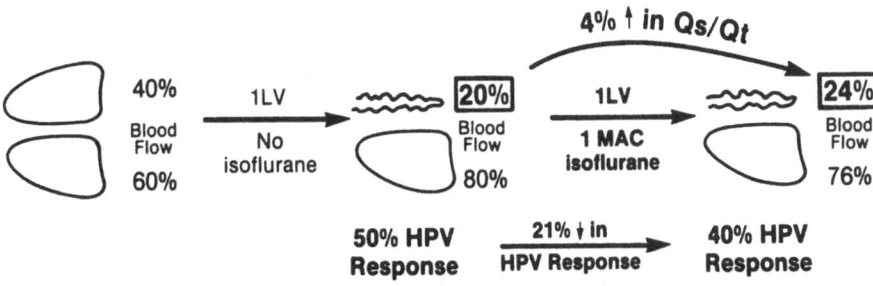

$\boxed{\% \downarrow \text{HPV}}$ = 22.8 (% Alveolar Isoflurane) - 5.3 = 22.8 (1.15) - 5.3 = $\boxed{21\%}$

Figure 8–4. This schematic diagram shows that the two-lung ventilation nondependent/dependent lung blood flow ratio is 40/60 per cent (left-hand side). When two-lung ventilation is converted to one-lung ventilation (as indicated by atelectasis of the nondependent lung), the HPV response decreases the blood flow to the nondependent lung by 50 per cent, so that the nondependent/dependent lung blood flow ratio is now 20/80 per cent (middle). According to the data of·Domino et al,[52] administration of 1 MAC isoflurane anesthesia should cause a 21 per cent decrease in the HPV response, which would decrease the 50 per cent blood flow reduction to a 40 per cent blood flow reduction HPV response. Consequently, the nondependent/dependent lung blood flow ratio would now become 24/76 per cent, representing a 4 per cent increase in the total shunt across the lungs (right-hand side). (Reproduced with permission from Benumof JL: Isoflurane anesthesia and arterial oxygenation during one-lung ventilation. Anesthesiology 64:419–422, 1986.)

Figure 1 reproduced with permission from reference within legend as well as reference #2 in this lecture.

mechansism that protects the P_aO_2 by decreasing the amount of shunt flow that can occur through hypoxic lung.

The middle panel of Figure 1 shows what happens to fractional lung blood flows, and $\dot{Q}_s/\dot{Q}_t$ when 2LV is changed to 1LV in the lateral decubitus position and there is no isoflurane anesthesia (gravity and HPV are the only forces affecting the 1LV blood flow distribution). Since HPV can decrease blood flow to a single lung by 50%,(2) the flow to the nondependent lung decreases to 20% of the cardiac output.(1)

Anesthetic drugs may inhibit HPV.(3) Many experimental studies in animals indicate that the halogenated inhalational anesthetics exhibit a dose dependent inhibition of regional HPV, whereas the intravenous anesthetics do not. In one recent animal study, the authors summarized their findings in an equation that related the dose of halogenated drug anesthesia to the amount of expected inhibition of HPV (equation at top of Figure 1).(4) With 1 MAC isoflurane anesthesia the HPV response should be decreased by 21%. A 21% decrease in the HPV response would decrease the nondependent lung HPV response from a 50% to a 40% nondependent lung blood flow reduction, which would increase nondependent lung blood flow from 20% to 24% of total blood flow, causing shunt to increase only 4% of the cardiac output (Figure 1, right hand panel).(5) An increase in shunt of 4% of the cardiac output is unlikely to be of much clinical significance and may not be detected with clinical methodology.

Indeed, recent studies in patients undergoing thoracotomy in the lateral decubitus position indicate that halothane, isoflurane, and enflurane in approximately 1 MAC dose, do not decrease P_aO_2 any more than intravenous anesthesia during stable 1LV conditions.(6-9) Although these studies did not examine whether HPV in the nondependent lung was inhibited or not, the results were consistent with the contention that these drugs did not have a major inhibitory effect on nondependent lung HPV. Since these drugs have a number of desirable properties (permit the use of a higher F_IO_2, are rapidly eliminated, have a salutory effect on bronchomotor tone, and have few negative cardiovascular effects at a 1 MAC dose), and do not decrease P_aO_2 any more than intravenous anesthesia during human 1LV conditions, they are desirable anesthetics to use during 1LV.

MANAGEMENT OF EACH LUNG SEPARATELY DURING ONE-LUNG VENTILATION(10-12)

The one-lung ventilation situation. The dependent lung usually has an increased amount of blood flow due to both passive gravitational effects and active nondependent lung HPV. However, the dependent lung may also develop a larger hypoxic compartment intraoperatively for several reasons. First, the dependent lung usually has a reduced lung volume due to the combined factors of induction of general anesthesia and circumferential (and perhaps severe) compression by the mediastinum (M) from above, by the abdominal contents pressing against the diaphragm (D) from the caudad side, and by suboptimal positioning effects (P) (rolls, packs, shoulder supports) pushing in from the dependent side and axilla (Figure 2, upper left panel). Second, absorption atelectasis can also occur in regions of the lung that have low $\dot{V}/\dot{Q}$ ratios when they are exposed to high F_IO_2. Third, difficulty in removal of secretions may cause the development of low $\dot{V}/\dot{Q}$ and atelectatic areas in the dependent lung. Finally, maintaining the lateral decubitus position for a prolonged period of time may cause fluid to transudate into the dependent lung (which may be vertically below the atrium), and cause a further decrease in dependent lung volume. The development of low $\dot{V}/\dot{Q}$ and/or atelectatic areas in the dependent lung will increase dependent lung PVR, thereby decreasing dependent lung blood flow and increasing nondependent lung blood flow.

Conventional management of 1LV. The proper management of 1LV is based on the above 1LV pathophysiology. First, although the theoretical possibilities of absorption atelectasis and oxygen toxicity exist, the benefits of ventilating the dependent lung with 100% oxygen far exceed the risks. A high F_IO_2 in the single ventilated lung may increase the P_aO_2 from arrhythmogenic and life-threatening levels to safer levels. In addition, a high F_IO_2 in the dependent lung will vasodilate the dependent lung, thereby increasing the dependent lung capability of accepting blood flow redistribution due to nondependent lung HPV. Direct oxygen toxicity will not occur during the span of the operative period and absorption atelectasis in the dependent lung is unlikely to occur in view of the remaining 1LV management characteristics listed below. Second, the dependent lung should be ventilated with a tidal volume of 10 ml/kg. Use of a tidal volume less than 10 ml/kg might promote dependent lung atelectasis. Use of a tidal volume greater than 10 ml/kg might increase dependent lung airway pressure and PVR, and thereby increase nondependent lung blood flow (decrease nondependent lung HPV). Third, the respiratory rate should be set so that the P_aCO_2 remains at 40 mm Hg (usually requires a 20% increase above the rate used for 2LV). Hypocapnia should be avoided because the increase in airway pressure in the dependent lung necessary to produce hyperventilation may increase dependent lung PVR. Furthermore, hypocapnia may inhibit HPV in the nondependent lung. Finally, no PEEP should be used initially because of concern of unnecessarily increasing dependent lung PVR (see selective dependent lung PEEP section below).

Very occasional ventilation of the nondependent lung (one breath every 5-10 minutes) causes some oxygen or oxygen-enriched gas to remain in the nonventilated lung and blood flowing through this lung can continue to take up some oxygen for a period of some minutes. Of course the effect of an occasional positive pressure breath to the nondependent lung on P_aO_2 will be uncertain with regard to magnitude and temporal profile, and requires the nondependent lung to be at least partially inflated for a period of some minutes.

Selective dependent lung PEEP. Since the ventilated lung often has a decreased lung volume during 1LV, it is not surprising that several attempts have been made to improve P_aO_2 by treating the ventilated lung with PEEP. However, it is important to realize that while selective dependent lung PEEP may improve $\dot{V}/\dot{Q}$ relationships in the dependent lung, it may also increase dependent lung PVR and shunt blood flow up to the nonventilated nondependent lung causing no change or even a decrease in P_aO_2 (Figure 2, right upper panel).

Selective nondependent lung CPAP. PEEP can be selectively applied to just the nonventilated nondependent lung. Since under these conditions the nonventilated lung is only slightly but constantly distended by oxygen, a

146

ONE LUNG VENTILATION: THE SITUATION

ONE LUNG VENTILATION: DOWN LUNG PEEP

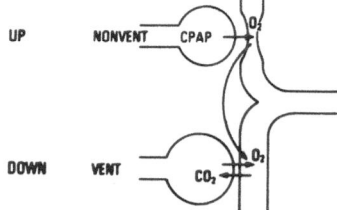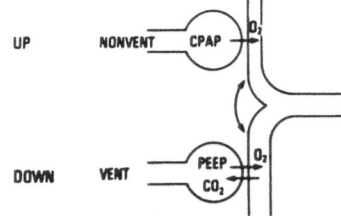

ONE LUNG VENTILATION: UP LUNG CPAP

ONE LUNG VENTILATION: DIFFERENTIAL LUNG $\frac{CPAP}{PEEP}$

Figure 2. The upper left panel schematically depicts the one-lung ventilation situtation. The UP lung is the nondependent lung and the DOWN lung is the dependent lung. The nondependent lung is nonventilated and the dependent lung is ventilated. M = mediastinum; P = positioning effects. The right upper panel schematically depicts the effects of selective PEEP to the dependent lung during one-lung ventilation. The lower left panel schematically depicts the effect of nondependent lung CPAP during one-lung ventilation. The lower right panel schematically depicts the effects of differential lung CPAP/PEEP during one-lung ventilation.

better term for this ventilatory pattern arrangement would be nonventilated lung continuous positive airway pressure (CPAP). Recently, two reports, one in humans[11] and one in dogs,[12] have shown that the application of CPAP to the nonventilated lung significantly increased P_aO_2. The latter study was performed with the dogs in the lateral decubitus position and showed that low levels of CPAP (5-10 cm H_2O) to the nonventilated lung increased P_aO_2 and decreased shunt, while blood flow to the nonventilated lung remained unchanged. Therefore, low levels of CPAP simply maintained the patency of nondependent lung airways allowing some oxygen distention of the gas exchanging alveolar space in the nondependent lung (Figure 2, lower left panel). On the other hand, 15 cm H_2O of CPAP caused similar P_aO_2 and shunt changes while blood flow to the nonventilated lung decreased significantly. Therefore, high levels of nonventilated lung CPAP act by permitting oxygen uptake in the nonventilated lung as well as by causing blood flow diversion to the ventilated lung where both oxygen and carbon dioxide exchange can take place (Figure 2, lower left panel). Since low levels are as effective as high levels of nonventilated lung CPAP and have less surgical interference and hemodynamic implications, it is logical to use low levels of nonventilated CPAP first. Low levels of nonventilated CPAP usually correct severe hypoxemia (P_aO_2 <50 mm Hg) provided the DLT is positioned correctly. In both the human and dog studies, O_2 insufflation at zero airway pressure did not improve P_aO_2 and shunt significantly, and this was probably due to the inability of zero transbronchial airway pressure to maintain airway patency. Several easy to assemble selective nondependent lung CPAP systems have been described recently.

Differential lung PEEP, CPAP. From the above considerations, it seems that the ideal method to improve P_aO_2 during 1LV is the application of differential lung PEEP or PEEP/CPAP. In this situation, PEEP is applied to the ventilated lung in the conventional manner to improve ventilated lung volume and $\dot{V}/\dot{Q}$ relationships. Simultaneously, the nonventilated lung receives CPAP to improve oxygenation of the blood perfusing the nonventilated lung. Therefore, with differential lung PEEP or PEEP/CPAP, the distribution of blood flow is not a critical issue because all pulmonary perfusion can participate in oxygen uptake from both oxygen expanded lungs (Figure 2, lower right panel).

Summary of Special One-Lung Management Maneuvers. The foregoing discussion indicates that the sequence of treating hypoxemia during 1LV in the lateral decubitus position should be as follows. First, 5 cm H_2O of CPAP should be applied to the nonventilated nondependent lung. Nondependent lung CPAP should be applied during the deflation phase of a large tidal volume breath to overcome critical opening pressures in the atelectatic lung. In the vast majority of cases of hypoxemia during one-lung ventilation, this one simple single maneuver eliminates the hypoxemia. If oxygenation still does not improve, then 5 cm H_2O of PEEP to the ventilated dependent lung should then be applied. Finally, if oxygenation is still not satisfactory, nondependent lung CPAP should be increased to 10-15 cm H_2O; dependent lung PEEP may follow to the same level in the rare case this is necessary. The differential lung CPAP/PEEP search is conducted in this way to find the optimal end-expiratory pressure for each lung and minimum $\dot{Q}_s/\dot{Q}_t$ for the patient as a whole. However, in view of the usual efficacy of nonventilated nondependent lung CPAP, use of differential lung PEEP/CPAP should rarely be necessary. If severe hypoxemia is still present following the use of differential lung CPAP/PEEP, it should be remembered that the nondependent lung may be intermittently ventilated with positive pressure with oxygen (i.e., use two-lung ventilation). Finally,

most of the $\dot{V}/\dot{Q}$ imbalance is eliminated during a pneumonectomy by
tightening a ligature around the nonventilated lung pulmonary artery as
early as possible, which directly eliminates all shunt flow through the
nonventilated lung.

REFERENCES

1. Marshall, B.E., Marshall, C. J. Appl. Physiol. 59:189-196, 1980.
2. Benumof, J.L. Chapters 4 and 8 in: Anesthesia for Thoracic Surgery
   (single-authored by J.L. Benumof) W. B. Saunders, Philadelphia, 1987.
3. Benumof, J.L. Anesth Analg 64:821-833, 1985.
4. Domino, K., Borowec, L., Alexander, C.M., Williams, J.J., Chen, L.,
   Marshall, C., Marshall, B.E. Anesthesiology 64:423-429, 1986.
5. Benumof, J.L. Anesthesiology 64:419-422, 1986.
6. Rogers, S.N., Benumof, J.L. Anesth Analg 64:946-954, 1985.
7. Benumof, J.L., Augustine, S.D., Gibbons, J. Anesthesiology
   67:910-915, 1987.
8. Carlsson, A.J., Bindslev, L., Hedenstierna, G. Anesthesiology
   66:312-316, 1987.
9. Carlsson, A.J., Hedenstierna, G., Bindslev, L. Acta Anaesthesiol
   Scand 31:57-62, 1987.
10. Benumof, J.L. Anesthesiology 56:161-163, 1982.
11. Capan, L.M., Turndorf, H., Patel, C., Ramanthan, S., Acinapura, A.,
    Chalon, J. Anesth Analg 59:847-851, 1980.
12. Alfery, D.D., Benumof, J.L. Anesthesiology 55:381-385, 1981

ANESTHETIC MANAGEMENT OF THE PATIENT WITH REACTIVE
AIRWAYS

STEVEN J. ALLEN

Department of Anesthesiology, Center for Microvascular and
Lymphatic Studies, The University of Texas Medical School at
Houston, 6431 Fannin, Houston, Texas

The American Thoracic Society has defined asthma as "a
syndrome characterized by increased responsiveness of the tracheo-
bronchial tree to a variety of stimuli." Asthma currently affects 5%
of the population. Perioperative bronchospasm may develop into a
significant problem for the anesthesiologist. More intraoperative
deaths have been noted to occur in asthmatic patients compared to
nonasthmatics. Respiratory complications occur more frequently in
asthmatic patients. Contemporary optimal management of patients
with asthma requires knowledge of 1) the pathophysiology, 2) the
triggering or bronchodilating effect of anesthetic agents and
maneuvers, as well as 3) the various bronchodilator drugs.

PATHOPHYSIOLOGY OF BRONCHOSPASM

Triggers. Studies in recent years have markedly expanded
our understanding of what factors may trigger bronchospasm.
These factors not only include antigens (extrinsic asthma) but a
number of "nonspecific" agents that do not trigger through immunologic mechanisms. This latter class of bronchospasm triggers
(intrinsic asthma) includes aerosols of distilled or hypertonic water,
sulfur dioxide, ammonia, aspirin (and other nonsteroidal anti
inflammatory agents), sulfites, beta blockers, exercise, emotional
disturbance, as well as others. The ability of triggers to stimulate
bronchospasm depends on the state of reactivity of the airways.
The hallmark of asthmatics is their increased bronchial reactivity
which may increase over time due to illness or other factors.

T. H. Stanley and R. J. Sperry (eds.), Anesthesia and the Lung, 149–163.
© 1989 by Kluwer Academic Publishers.

Cells and mediators. The mechanism(s) by which triggers induce asthma are not clear. The mast cell has long been implicated in asthma. Release of mast cell mediators results in onset of bronchospasm. However, other cells such as eosinophils and macrophages may be as important.

The mast cell appears to be key to allergic induced (immediate hypersensitivity) reaction. In the lung, mast cells are found in the bronchial lumen, under the airways' basement membrane, near blood vessels, throughout the smooth muscle bundles, and in the alveolar septa. As a prelude to an allergic reaction, IgE antibodies must bind to the surface of the mast cell. When an antigen is recognized by the mast cell bound IgE antibody, the mast cell is stimulated to release preformed compounds and produce mediators. The effect of mast cell derived mediators are immediate and myriad. They include increased vascular permeability, smooth muscle contraction, mucus secretion, and leukocyte chemoattraction. Over time, further changes occur including mucosal edema and cellular infiltration, desquamation of epithelial cells, thickening of basement membrane, and hyperplasia of goblet cells. These later events may be due to mast cell contents or to other cells attracted to the site. Mast cells may also degranulate in response to other stimuli besides immunologic agents. Hypoxia, opiates, certain drugs, neuropeptides and changes in local osmolarity can cause mast cell degranulation in vitro. The presence of bronchospasm also appears to increase the bronchial reactivity further, thus making another attack more likely.

Asthmatic patients who are bronchoscoped following antigenic challenge show extensive mucosal edema. Airway mucosal edema is due to increased vascular permeability. Histamine, prostaglandin (PG) E2, Leukotriene (LT) C4, LTD4, platelet activating factor, and bradykinin can induce mucosal edema. However, the contribution of mucosal edema to bronchospasm is not clear. The airway mucosa often contains infiltrates of eosinophils, neutrophils, macrophages, lymphocytes, and plasma cells. In the lumen itself, the secretions may contain eosinophils, neutrophils, and desquamated epithelial cells. Again, the clinical significance of these cellular infiltrates is not clear.

Mucus secretion plays a major role in the clinical picture of asthma. Allergic mediators increase mucus and stimulate active fluid secretion by the surface epithelium. However, airway mucus transport rates are lower in asthmatics; investigators have found a substance in the sputum of asthmatics that inhibits ciliary beating.

In severe asthma attacks, the airway epithelial surface may become denuded and covered by goblet cells. The mechanism for the sloughing of epithelial cells is not known.

CLINICAL PRESENTATION

Airway narrowing causes most of the clinical manifestations in asthmatic attacks. Airway narrowing in asthmatics probably involves all of the tracheobronchial tree. In the early response to antigen, airway narrowing is due to bronchial smooth muscle constriction and is generally promptly reversible with beta adrenergic drugs. However, in the late antigen response, mucus and mucosal edema contribute to airway narrowing and bronchodilators have less of an effect. In fact, the mucus retention leads to the characteristic obstruction of smaller airways seen in severe asthma.

Pulmonary mechanics. The airway narrowing results in relative obstruction of airflow throughout the tracheobronchial tree. Of importance to the anesthesiologist is that patients may have marked bronchospasm and still be asymptomatic. However, any further worsening of the airway narrowing may result in critical deterioration. The obstruction to airflow imposed by airway narrowing may result in air trapping. Thus, during an acute attack, both residual volume (RV) and functional residual capacity (FRC) are increased. In most instances these abnormalities return to normal after the attack subsides, but may persist long after the airway narrowing has resolved in some patients. Total lung capacity (TLC) probably does not change significantly during attacks. Similarly, elastic recoil is relatively unaffected in asthma.

Alterations in pulmonary circulation. The degree of bronchospasm varies throughout a patient's airway. This results in uneven distribution of ventilation. Hypoxic pulmonary vasoconstriction (HPV) develops in lung units where ventilation is inadequate and results in redistribution of pulmonary blood flow to lung units where ventilation is better. However, this response appears to fatigue over time with corresponding worsening of hypoxemia. Due to HPV, pulmonary hypertension may develop during severe asthma and may be evident on EKG by a reversible "p pulmonale" pattern.

Alterations in gas exchange. The uneven ventilation distribution may lead to mild hypoxemia which is a common finding in severe asthmatic attacks. Bronchodilators such as isoproterenol may worsen hypoxemia by interfering with HPV. In fact, investigators have documented worsening PaO2 as bronchospasm improves. The tachypnea associated with asthma often results in hypocapnia and respiratory alkalosis. The development of normocapnia or hypercapnia is an ominous sign of respiratory collapse and requires intervention.

The cardiovascular effects of asthma are not trivial. The more negative pleural pressure required for ventilation results in enhancement of the central blood volume. Pulmonary vascular resistance may be increased by 1) HPV (see above), 2) hyperinflation of the lung, and 3) acidosis. Thus, right ventricular function may be compromised by afterload sufficiently to result in a decrease in cardiac output. Similarly, the more negative pleural pressure results in a relatively greater afterload for the left ventricle. These may be possible mechanisms for the exaggerated decrease in blood pressure during inspiration (pulsus paradoxus) that is often seen in severe asthma.

PHARMACOLOGY OF BRONCHODILATORS

Beta agonists are currently the drugs of choice in the treatment of asthma. Bronchial smooth muscle possesses beta-2 receptors which, when stimulated, produce bronchodilatation. Newer agents are more selective of beta-2 sites and have a longer duration of action than the older drugs used for asthma. The agents may be given by inhalation, IV, orally, or IM. Inhalation appears to be the best route of administration for producing rapid

onset and few systemic side effects. Inhalation may be
accomplished by a metered-dose inhaler or by aerosolization with
compressed gas. Epinephrine and isoetharine are available for
inhalation and subcutaneous (epinephrine only) administration.
They are much shorter acting than the newer beta-2 selective
agents and are associated with more adverse side effects.
Isoproterenol (Isuprel) is also a nonspecific beta agonist and is
available for inhalation. It may be used intravenously in children.
However, the associated tachycardia and ventricular ectopy limit the
use of IV isoproterenol in adults. Albuterol (Proventil, Ventolin) is
beta-2 selective and may be administered orally or inhalationally.
Terbutaline (Brethine) is a selective beta-2 agent and is available
for inhalation, oral, and subcutaneous administration. Bitolterol
(Tornalate) is the latest selective beta-2 agent and is available for
inhalation. Metaproterenol (Alupent) is not as selective a beta-2
drug as terbutaline, and results in more cardiac stimulation.

Corticosteroids have increased in popularity for early treatment
of asthmatic attacks that do not respond to adrenergic agents.
Steroids probably induce their antiasthmatic effect by reducing the
inflammatory reaction that is inherent in the pathophysiology of
airway narrowing. The drugs may be given in high doses for short
terms (< 2 weeks) and toxicity is rare. Inhaled steroids include
beclomethasone (Vanceril), Flunisolide (Aerobid), and triamcinolone
(Azmacort). These may be combined with alternate day oral
Prednisone.

Ipratropium (Atrovent) is an anticholinergic drug that
enhances the bronchodilating action of adrenergic agents. It is
administered by inhalation. Similarly, atropine has been reported
to improve asthmatic patients when given by inhalation. Although
anticholinergics may increase the tenacity of secretions, this is more
than offset by their bronchodilating action.

Theophylline, once used extensively to treat bronchospasm,
has dropped in popularity in recent years due to associated toxicity
and the realization that it is not particularly effective when
compared to the newer adrenergic agents. One study involved 40
asthmatic patients treated with an inhalation beta agonist every

three hours. The addition of therapeutic levels of theophylline did not improve the bronchospasm but did increase the frequency of side effects. Blood levels below 10 mcg/ml are not generally associated with toxicity. Theophylline blood levels between 10 and 20 mcg/ml is often associated with jitteriness as well as behavioral changes. Above 20 mcg/ml, nausea, vomiting, diarrhea, insomnia, cardiac rhythm irregularities, seizures, and death may occur.

Cromolyn (Intal) acts to stabilize mast cells and inhibit release of asthma mediators. It is of no use in an acute episode once the mast cells have degranulated. Cromolyn is administered by an inhaler and must be taken regularly for effective prophylaxis.

New Drugs. Azlestine is an investigational calcium entry blocker that acts as a bronchodilator with antihistamine and anti-inflammatory properties. Ketotifen is another investigational drug that is similar to Azlestine. It appears to prevent down regulation of beta receptors. Procaterol is a new beta 2 agonist undergoing clinical trials.

PERIOPERATIVE MANAGEMENT OF PATIENT WITH HISTORY OF BRONCHOSPASM

Preoperative evaluation of the patient with asthma requires an understanding of severity of disease and effectiveness of current management, as well as whether further therapy should be instituted prior to surgery. The goal of preoperative evaluation is to formulate a plan that will prevent or ameliorate airway narrowing. Preoperative evaluation begins with a careful history to elicit the severity of disease. Patients may be grouped according to their precipitating factors, degree to which daily activities are limited, number of hospitalizations, medications, and previous anesthesia history.

Pulmonary function tests. There are three parameters that are generally used to quantitate the degree of airway narrowing.

Forced vital capacity (FVC) is the maximal volume that can be forcibly exhaled after inspiration to total lung capacity. When FVC is plotted over time, the volume expired over the first second (FEV1) and the forced expiratory flow 25-75% (FEF 25-75%) may be calculated. An asthma attack is associated with an obstructive pattern demonstrating delayed expiration with a consequent decrease FVC, FEV1, FEV1/FVC, and FEF 25-75%. The FEF 25-75% is felt to be a more sensitive indicator of airway narrowing in the smaller bronchioles.

Peak (maximum) expiratory flow rate (PEFR) can be calculated from a spirogram or by using a peak expiratory flow meter. PEFR is markedly decreased in asthma attacks. For example, normal PEFR is > 600 L/min which may be reduced to 100 L/min in a severe asthma attack.

Patients with a history of asthma may be divided into three groups. Individuals in the first group have had no attacks in recent years, take no bronchodilator medications, and physical examination reveals no wheezing. The second group have recurrent attacks and take prophylactic bronchodilator medications but are not actively wheezing. The third group consists of patients who are actively wheezing at the time of examination or who report deterioration in their pulmonary status.

The first group requires no other work-up. The third group needs preoperative PFTs to document their baseline and should not undergo elective surgery until their bronchodilator therapy has been optimized. Controversy exists concerning the preoperative management of the second group. Some authors recommend obtaining pre and post bronchodilator PFT's in these patients. These clinicians recommend delay of elective surgery and further bronchodilator therapy to optimize the patient's status. As any patient with a history of asthma may develop intraoperative bronchospasm, all such patients should be administered a technique that has the least risk of triggering an attack.

ANESTHETIC MANAGEMENT

Regional anesthesia remains the technique of choice for patients with a history of asthma, although one study found that 1.9% of asthmatic patients receiving regional anesthesia still developed bronchospasm during surgery. However, there are many instances where a regional anesthetic is not appropriate. The

administration of general anesthesia contains such a number of
potential triggers that bronchospasm cannot always be prevented.
The anesthesiologist must understand the relative bronchospasm
inducing property of various anesthetic techniques and drugs so
that morbidity is minimal.

Premedication.   Few studies have been performed to ascertain
the relative benefit of one premedicant regimen over another.
However, practical considerations dictate careful administration of
any respiratory depressants, such as narcotics, to patients with
significant bronchospastic disease.   Diazepam does not increase
airway resistance in patients with asthma.   Hydroxyzine and
droperidol are probably safe as well.   If the patient has been
receiving corticosteroid therapy, a plan for continuation should be
developed.

Induction.   Concern has been expressed in the literature over
the triggering potential of thiopental.   The evidence suggests that
too little thiopental (light anesthesia) is the more likely culprit
rather than thiopental itself.   However, reflex triggered bronchospasm may still occur even with appropriate dosing of thiopental
and administration of potent volatile anesthetics may be necessary.
After intubation, it may be difficult to determine whether a patient
has a "tight chest" (with subsequent difficulty in manual
ventilation) due to light anesthesia or bronchospasm.   Succinylcholine will relieve the difficulty in ventilation due to light
anesthesia but it will have no effect on true bronchospasm.
Ketamine has the advantage of possessing sympathomimetic action
and enhance bronchodilatation in asthmatics.   Lidocaine 1 mg/kg IV
has been found to be beneficial in the induction of asthmatic
patients.   Intravenous local anesthetics ameliorate reflex-induced
bronchospasm, probably by a central mechanism.   Aerosol administration of lidocaine is felt by some to increase the risk of
bronchospasm while others believe it is the most effective.   Some
authors recommend IV atropine prior to stimulating the airway to
block cholinergic mediated bronchoconstriction.

Inhalation agents.   Halothane, enflurane, and isoflurane are
equally effective bronchodilators.   The concomitant use of halothane

and aminophylline may produce cardiac arrhythmias; enflurane or isoflurane may be a safer alternative.

Nitrous oxide/narcotic. There is a paucity of studies evaluating narcotics in asthmatic patients. In contrast to the volatile agents, narcotics do not possess bronchodilating properties. Further, the administration of morphine results in elevated plasma histamine levels which may trigger or exacerbate bronchospasm. Although the newer narcotics are not associated with histamine release, the risk of postoperative respiratory depression reduces their popularity.

Muscle relaxants and antagonists. d-tubocurarine is associated with histamine release and, theoretically, would be less desirable than a sympathomimetic muscle relaxant such as pancuronium. However, the data is conflicting and both asthmatic and nonasthmatic patients have developed bronchospasm with pancuronium. Atracurium is also associated with histamine release, but the risk of bronchospasm with this drug is still unclear. Succinylcholine appears as safe as any other muscle relaxant in asthmatics. Neostigmine increases cholinergic activity and may induce bronchospasm which is usually prevented by atropine.

Recommendations. An optimal anesthetic plan designed to prevent the development of bronchospasm must be tailored to each patient. However, for the elective patient at risk who has no other medical problems, the following suggestions may be useful:

After monitors have been placed, administer
  - atropine 1 mg or iprotropium (36-72 mcg) by inhalation and/or
  - metaproterenol 0.65 mg or albuterol (90 mcg) by inhalation

While breathing 100% O_2,
  - thiopental 3-5 mg/kg or ketamine 1-2 mg/kg IV and/or
  - mask induction with enflurane or isoflurane and/or
  - lidocaine 1.5 mg/kg IV bolus and 2 mg/min infusion

Intubation when patient deeply anesthetized

Management of Intraoperative Bronchospasm.   Wheezing and
increased inflation pressures are the signs of the onset of bronchospasm.   Adequacy of oxygenation and ventilation are the first
priorities.   The work of breathing may increase several fold and
spontaneous ventilation may not be adequate.   Ventilation by
mechanical means may be difficult to maintain due to 1) the high
inflation pressures required to move air past the narrow airways
and 2) the long expiratory phase needed to prevent air trapping.
Many ventilators available on anesthetic machines will not be
suitable and manual ventilation may be necessary.   Positive end
expiratory pressure (PEEP) may worsen air trapping and is generally avoided in acute asthma.   Oxygenation may worsen with
bronchospasm.   ABG's or pulse oximetry may be helpful in
adjusting the FiO_2.

Suppression of bronchospasm may be accomplished by 1) giving
IV lidocaine or ketamine, 2) increasing the concentration of the
volatile anesthetic or 3) administering a nonanesthetic bronchodilator.   IV lidocaine has been reported to reverse intraoperative
bronchospasm with a single bolus of 100 mg.   Similarly, ketamine
has been effective even in the presence of halothane anesthesia.
Increasing the volatile anesthetic concentration may improve the
bronchospasm but the cardiovascular depression may be
unacceptable.

Adminstration of beta-2 selective adrenergic agents such as
albuterol are often effective in treating intraoperative bronchospasm.   An adapter for the metered dose inhaler can be placed in
the anesthesia circuit.   Terbutaline 0.25 mg SQ may also be
effective.   Despite its popularity in anesthetized patients with
bronchospasm, theophylline is short on benefit and long on adverse
side effects.   Interestingly, most of the studies in the anesthetic
literature concerning theophylline concern the side effects of the
drug.   Theophylline has been reported to antagonize the action of
morphine, benzodiazepines, and barbituates.

Corticosteroids have been used intraoperatively for treatment
of acute bronchospasm.   Although a minimum of 3-4 hours would be
expected after injection before any benefit might be seen, there are

reports of almost immediate response. As a single dose of steroids poses little risk to the patient, there is little reason not to administer in a critical situation. All intraoperative wheezing is not bronchospasm. Other causes include aspiration, pulmonary edema, endobronchial intubation, tension pneumothorax and systemic allergic reactions.

Emergence. The endotracheal tube in a lightly anesthetized patient with asthma poses the greatest stimulus for inducing or exacerbating bronchospasm. Thus, many clinicians extubate while the patient is deeply anesthetized. In a patient who has active wheezing, one has to decide whether the endotracheal tube is better left in or taken out. In severely affected patients, continued intubation and mechanical ventilation may be necessary to maintain adequate gas exchange until the airway narrowing improves. Even if extubation occurs uneventfully, the severe asthmatic can develop life threatening bronchospasm at anytime during the immediate postoperative period, and therefore, requires close observation until fully recovered.

EMERGENCY SURGERY

Anesthetizing the patient with asthma for an emergency procedure is complicated by a number of factors. It may not be possible to find out the severity of disease or even the medications taken for asthma. There is often insufficient time to attempt optimization of bronchodilator therapy prior to surgery. Maneuvers to protect the airway in emergency patients increase the risk for developing bronchospasm. Regional anesthesia remains the technique of choice in asthma patients undergoing emergency surgery. However, the risk of this technique in these patients is not the block but the attendant sedation with its potential respiratory depression.

Intubation. Many, if not all, patients presenting for emergency surgery are at risk for aspiration of gastric contents. The lungs must be protected if airway reflexes are to be impaired by anesthetics. There are two techniques for intubation that allow for protection of the airway, awake and rapid sequence. Both have

disadvantages, particularly for patients with asthma. Awake
intubation in a patient with a full stomach will stimulate laryngeal
and tracheal reflexes which may induce bronchospasm. Rapid
sequence induction and intubation may result in a lightly anesthetized patient at the time of intubation and induce bronchospasm. A
slow induction may allow a more completely anesthetized patient but
may also increase the risk of aspiration, which, in a severe
asthmatic, may be life-threatening.

Induction.   Thiopental is not associated with a increase in
bronchospasm. However, ketamine may be an alternative when
hypovolemia is suspected. Ketamine possesses sympathomimetic
properties and is associated with improvement of bronchospasm.
Onset of bronchodilating action is immediate if the drug is given IV
and lasts 6-8 minutes. It has been used to treat status asthmaticus. Ketamine is not without adverse side effects. The
sympathomimetic properties of ketamine may be additive to those of
other anti asthma drugs. Seizures have been reported in patients
receiving aminophylline who were given ketamine. Because of the
increased secretions seen with ketamine, atropine should be
administered prior to induction if tachycardia is not a problem.
Regardless of the induction agent chosen, intravenous lidocaine 1
mg/kg should be given prior to laryngoscopy for reasons described
above.

Emergence.   In order to prevent reflex induced
bronchospasm, elective asthmatic patients are often extubated while
deeply anesthetized. This is not a suitable option in patients who
require airway protection. Pretreatment prior to extubation with
intravenous lidocaine or ephedrine may help prevent problems.

ASTHMA AND PREGNANCY

The effect of pregnancy on preexisting asthma is variable. In
fact, one third of asthmatic women will worsen, one third improve
and the rest remain unchanged. A particular problem that arises in
women at term is that beta-2 agents are not only bronchodilators,
but tocolytics as well. Thus, albuterol and terbutaline could
potentially inhibit the progress of labor. Anticholinergic drugs

such as ipratropium may be of benefit. There is a report of
improvement of asthma following the institution of epidural
anesthesia. The authors felt that some degree of broncospasm was
due to the mother's anxiety of the pain of labor, which, once
relieved, no longer contributed to airway narrowing.

Emergency Caesarean sections generally require a general
anesthetic. In order to prevent fetal depression, the anesthetic is
usually kept light. However, a light anesthetic may induce bronchospasm in the mother. A suitable anesthetic plan has not been
generally accepted for this situation. Fetal toxicity has been
reported with the use of IV theophylline in the mother. Halothane
or isoflurane appear to be reasonable alternatives. Uterine relaxation induced by a volatile inhalation agent may be treated with
pitocin infusion.

ASTHMA AND COEXISTING HEART DISEASE

Patients with both asthma and coronary artery disease pose a
difficult management problem. Therapies that are effective for
treating one condition may exacerbate the other. Beta adrenergic
drugs and the theophylline derivatives may enhance dysrhythmias
or alter metabolism of cardiac drugs. On the other hand, beta
blockers are popular agents in the treatment of cardiac disease and
hypertension. This class of drugs may induce bronchospasm. If
bronchospasm does develop intraoperatively, IV lidocaine as a bolus
followed by an infusion can be effective. Preliminary work
suggests that calcium entry blockers may be the best alternative for
treatment of bronchospasm in these patients.

MANAGEMENT OF STATUS ASTHMATICUS

Status asthmaticus is defined as unresolving bronchospasm that
is severe enough to be considered life-threatening. Thus, patients
in status should be monitored in an intensive care setting. Because
of their expertise in airway and ventilator management, anesthesiologists may be called upon to assist with the care of a patient in
status. A brief review of therapeutic points is presented below.

Oxygen. Hypoxemia is a major contributing factor to patients who die of asthma. Supplemental oxygen should always be administered and the adequacy of patient oxygenation monitored by either pulse oximetry or ABG's. Humidification of delivered gas is highly desirable and heated saline is preferable.

Fluids. A decrease in the extracellular fluid volume is common in patients with severe asthma and may be reflected by increased hematocrit and BUN. This relative volume deficit may contribute to the tenacity of sputum and enhance airway obstruction. Hydration with intravenous fluids is usually indicated.

Baseline data. Peak flow measurement in order to quantify effects of therapy
> Chest X-ray to check for pneumonia, atelectasis,
>> pneumothorax
> ABG's
> H&H and electrolytes
> ECG to follow right ventricular strain
> Sputum Gram stain and culture

Intubation and mechanical ventilation is instituted usually for progressive alveolar hypoventilation and/or exhaustion. As these patients may suddenly develop apnea, intubation should be performed before respiratory arrest occurs. Once connected to a mechanical ventilator, minute ventilation is adjusted to correct respiratory acidosis. Profoundly elevated inspiratory pressure is often required in order to deliver an appropriate tidal volume. Further, the airway narrowing requires a prolonged expiratory phase to avoid aggravation of air trapping. Pulmonary toilet is helpful in treating and preventing the obstruction of airways with secretions.

Drugs. By definition, status asthmaticus is diagnosed when the patient has not responded to bronchodilators. Thus, beta adrenergics and theophylline have already been administered to maximal doses in these patients. The next step is corticosteroids. 1000 mg hydrocortisone is administered IV followed by 4 mg/kg Q4H. Benefit is usually not evident for several hours.

There appear to be cholinergic receptors that result in the production of mediators. <u>Atropine and ipratropium</u> given inhalationally may improve the occasional patient.

<u>Antibiotics</u> are given to treat documented infection.

<u>General anesthesia</u>. When conventional therapy fails, general anesthesia has been advocated in selected patients. Halothane, enflurane, and isoflurane have been used successfully to treat refractory status. As many of these patients are receiving maximal doses of potentially cardiac stimulating drugs, enflurane and isoflurane may be preferable. There is one reported case of 50 hours of general anesthesia for the successful treatment of status asthmaticus.

<u>Fiberoptic bronchoscopic bronchial lavage</u> with large amounts of saline is advocated by some clinicians for the removal of tenacious secretions in refractory status. There does not appear be to wide spread acceptance of this potentially dangerous technique.

SUGGESTED READING

1. Drazen, J.M., Boushey, H.A., Holgate, S.T., Kaliner, M., O'Byrne P., Valentine, M., Widdicombe, J.H., Phil, D. and Woolcock, A. J. Allergy Clin. Immunol. 80:428-437, 1987.
2. Fung, D.L. Clin. Rev. Allergy 3:127-141, 1985.
3. Hopewell, P.C. and Miller, R.T. Clinics in Chest Med. 5:623-634, 1984.
4. Kingston, H.G.G. and Hirshman C.A. Anesth. Analg. 63:844-855, 1984.
5. Larach, D.R. and Zelis, R. Surg. Pharmacol. 151:527-537, 1986.
6. Parnass, S.M., Feld, J.M,. Chamberlin, W.H. and Segil, L.J. Anesth. Analg. 66:193-195, 1987.
7. Younker, D., Clark, R., Tessem, J,. Joyce, T.H. and Kubicek, M. Can. J. Anesth. 34:609-612, 1987.

DIFFERENTIAL LUNG VENTILATION

JONATHAN L. BENUMOF, M.D.

Anesthesia Research Lab, T-001, University of California San Diego,
La Jolla, California 92093

INTRODUCTION

In the vast majority of patients with bilateral lung disease, the
application of PEEP to both of the lungs increases the functional residual
capacity of both lungs, thereby reversing atelectasis and increasing the
ventilation-perfusion ratio of both lungs (Figure 1). Similarly, in the
vast majority of patients with unilateral lung disease, the application of
PEEP to both of the lungs increases the functional residual capacity of the
diseased lung toward normal while not excessively increasing the functional
residual capacity of the normal lung (Figure 2). However, in some patients
with unilateral lung disease, PEEP to both of the lungs may fail to expand
the diseased lung and excessively distend the normal lung. The distension
of the normal lung may selectively increase pulmonary vascular resistance
in the nondiseased lung and shunt blood flow to the diseased lung, thereby
increasing the right-to-left shunt and causing a paradoxic decrease in the
arterial oxygen tension (Figure 3).(1,2) Similarly, in some patients with
bilateral lung disease, in which the disease is in the basilar regions
(with normal apical regions), PEEP to both lungs may fail to expand the
bases and may excessively distend apical regions (Figure 4). The excessive
distension of apical regions may selectively increase pulmonary vascular
resistance in the apical regions and shunt blood flow to the atelectatic
and low ventilation-perfusion ratio basilar regions, thereby increasing the
right-to-left shunt and causing a paradoxic decrease in the arterial oxygen
tension.(3,4)

DIFFERENTIAL LUNG VENTILATION

In situations in which PEEP increases the right-to-left shunt and
decreases the arterial oxygen tension (unilateral or asymmetric lung
disease and bilateral basilar disease), differential lung ventilation and
PEEP can result in much more selective application of PEEP to the diseased
area. In the first instance (unilateral lung disease), the application of

165

T. H. Stanley and R. J. Sperry (eds.), Anesthesia and the Lung, 165–171.
© 1989 by Kluwer Academic Publishers.

CONVENTIONAL TWO LUNG PEEP

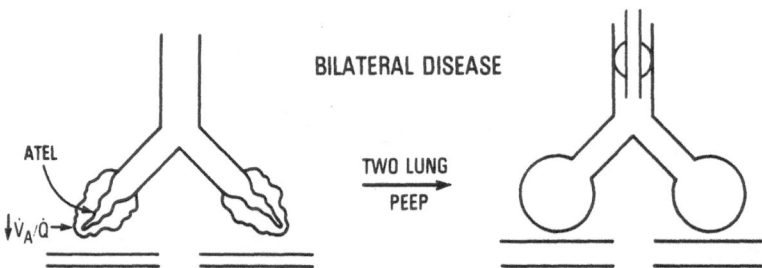

Figure 19–4. Application of PEEP to both lungs through a single-lumen tube in patients with bilateral lung disease usually results in a reversal of low ventilation to perfusion relationships and atelectasis in both lungs. (ATEL = atelectasis; ↓ V/Q = low ventilation-perfusion ratio.)

FIGURE 1. Reproduced with permission from Benumof JL: Anesthesia for Thoracic Surgery. Philadelphia, W.B. Saunders Co., 1987.

CONVENTIONAL TWO LUNG PEEP

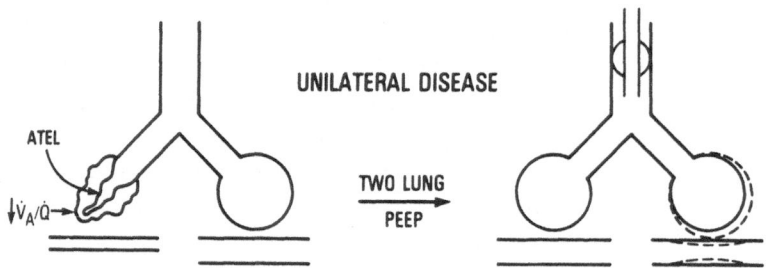

Figure 19–5. Application of PEEP to both lungs through a single-lumen tube to patients with unilateral lung disease usually results in a reversal of low ventilation to perfusion relationships and atelectasis in the one diseased lung. (ATEL = atelectasis; ↓ $\dot{V}_A/\dot{Q}$ = low ventilation-perfusion ratio.)

FIGURE 2. Reproduced with permission from Benumof JL: Anesthesia for Thoracic Surgery. Philadelphia, W.B. Saunders Co., 1987.

PEEP to the two lungs (via a double-lumen tube) in an inverse proportion to their compliances should result in equal and normal functional residual capacities in both lungs (Figure 5).(5) In this way a high level of PEEP is applied to only the diseased area in a much more economic and efficient manner. Since the PEEP is just being applied to part of the lung, the effects on cardiac output are much decreased. In the second instance (bilateral basilar disease), reversal of atelectasis and improvement in ventilation-perfusion ratio in both lungs can be accomplished by placing the patient in the lateral decubitus position, ventilating each lung separately (via a double-lumen tube), and applying PEEP to only the dependent lung (Figure 6).(6) The nondependent lung will improve its function by experiencing a low pulmonary vascular pressure, which results in a low blood flow and shunt in the nondependent lung and a propensity to

SELECTIVE APPLICATION OF PEEP TO NORMOXIC LUNG

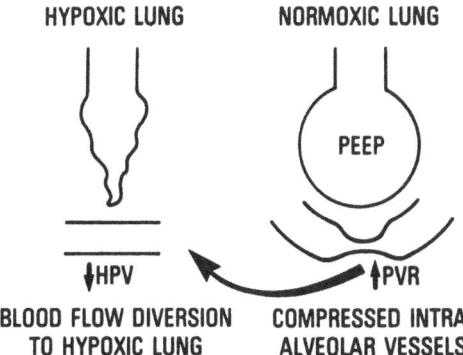

HYPOXIC LUNG   NORMOXIC LUNG

PEEP

↓HPV   ↑PVR

BLOOD FLOW DIVERSION   COMPRESSED INTRA-
TO HYPOXIC LUNG   ALVEOLAR VESSELS

Figure 19–6. Application of PEEP to both normoxic and hypoxic regions may fail to expand the hypoxic lung regions. This results in the selective application of PEEP to just the normoxic lung. The selective application of PEEP to only the normoxic lung can compress the small intra-alveolar vessels in the normoxic lung and increase normoxic lung pulmonary vascular resistance (PVR). The increase in normoxic lung PVR can cause diversion of blood flow to the hypoxic lung and effectively decrease hypoxic pulmonary vasoconstriction (HPV) in the hypoxic lung.

FIGURE 3. Reproduced with permission from Benumof JL: Anesthesia for Thoracic Surgery. Philadelphia, W.B. Saunders Co., 1987.

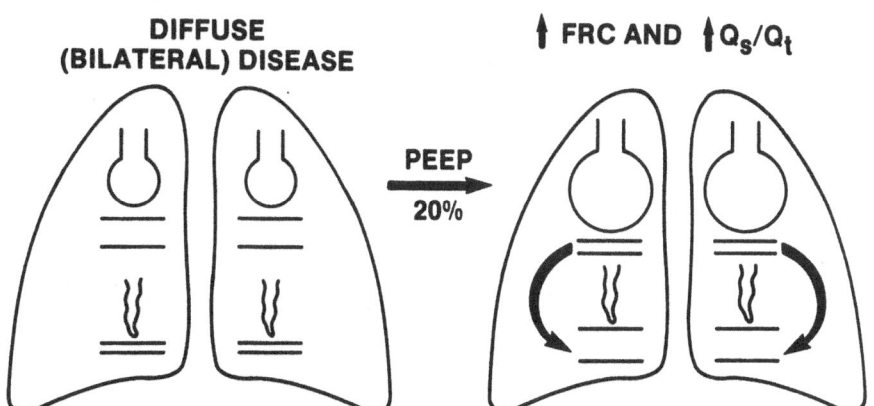

DIFFUSE (BILATERAL) DISEASE   ↑ FRC AND ↑Q_s/Q_t

PEEP
20%

Figure 19–7. The application of PEEP to both lungs, when both lungs contain diseased basilar regions, may result in distension of the apical regions, causing a selective increase in pulmonary vascular resistance in the apical regions, which results in a diversion of blood flow from the apical regions to the basilar regions. This may occur 20 per cent of the time that PEEP is applied to this kind of situation.[54,55] The distension of the apices results in an increase in functional residual capacity (FRC), and the diversion of blood flow to the basilar regions results in an increase in shunt ($\dot{Q}_s/\dot{Q}_t$).

FIGURE 4. Reproduced with permission from Benumof JL: Anesthesia for Thoracic Surgery. Philadelphia, W.B. Saunders Co., 1987.

resorb fluid rather than transudate fluid in the nondependent lung. The dependent lung will improve its function by virtue of the application of selective PEEP to that lung. Again, the selective application of PEEP to only one lung minimizes effects on venous return and preserves the cardiac output.

The main criterion for initiation of differential lung ventilation is when PEEP to all of the lung causes an increase in shunt and a decrease in the arterial oxygen tension.(5,6) Measurement of functional residual capacity cannot be used as a criterion, since functional residual capacity may be normal or increasing with the application of PEEP owing to distension of only the normal areas of lung (either the one lung or the apical regions), even though there is continued failure to expand the diseased areas of lung (either the other lung or the basilar regions) (Figures 3 and 4). Of course, the chest roentgenogram must show either severe unilateral asymmetric lung disease or severe bilateral basilar disease. An additional specific indication for initiation of differential lung ventilation, which is independent of the PEEP-induced shunting issue, is the presence of bronchopleural fistula that prevents positive-pressure ventilation because of loss of tidal volume through the fistula.

There are several methods for demonstrating a PEEP-induced increase in shunt with unilateral lung disease. First, shunt can be measured before and after the application of PEEP. Second, pulmonary angiograms, which provide a qualitative measure of regional lung blood flow, can be obtained via a pulmonary artery catheter injection.(2) Third, lung perfusion scans, which provide a quantitative measure of regional blood flow, can be performed with radioisotopes.(7)

The specific management of differential lung ventilation and PEEP for the patient with unilateral lung disease is as follows. Since it may be necessary to determine the position of the double-lumen tube with precision at any time (e.g., following any significant patient movement), a fiberoptic bronchoscope should be at the bedside. The most diseased lung should be placed in a nondependent position. The compliance of each lung should then be measured separately. The amount of PEEP applied to each lung should initially be inversely proportional to the compliance of each lung. For example, if one lung has one-third the compliance of the other lung, then it would be reasonable to initially apply 15 cm H_2O to the diseased lung and 5 cm H_2O to the nondiseased lung (Figure 5). The tidal volume to each lung should be equal; equal tidal volumes will, of course, result in different peak inspiratory pressures. The application of PEEP inversely proportional to lung compliance and use of equal tidal volumes

Differential Lung PEEP

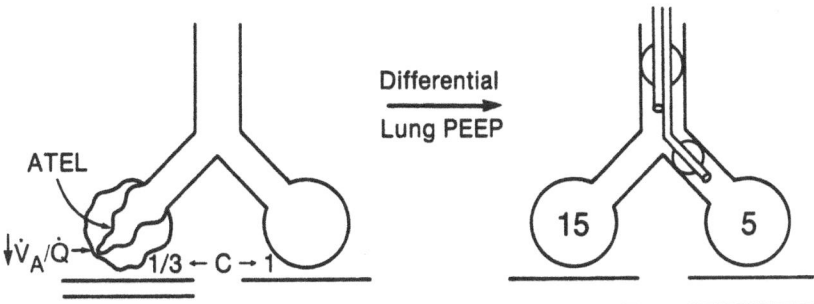

Figure 19–8. Differential lung PEEP applies PEEP to each of the two lungs in an amount that is inversely proportional to the compliance of each of the lungs. Differential lung PEEP must be applied via a double-lumen tube. In this example the diseased lung has one third the compliance of the more normal lung and, therefore, receives three times as much PEEP. (ATEL = atelectasis; $\downarrow \dot{V}_A/\dot{Q}$ = low ventilation-perfusion ratio.)

FIGURE 5. Reproduced with permission from Benumof JL: Anesthesia for Thoracic Surgery. Philadelphia, W.B. Saunders Co., 1987.

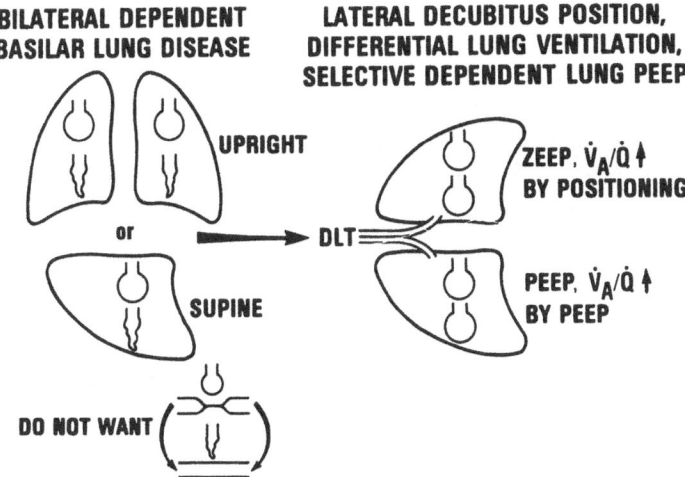

Figure 19–9. Schematic summarization of the results of the study in reference 57. Ventilation-perfusion ratios ($\dot{V}_A/\dot{Q}$) may be improved in patients with bilateral dependent basilar lung disease (viewed from either the upright or supine position) by turning the patient into the lateral decubitus position and ventilating the patient with differential lung ventilation via a double-lumen tube (DLT). The differential lung ventilation consists of zero end-expiratory pressure (ZEEP) to the nondependent lung and positive end-expiratory pressure (PEEP) to the dependent lung. The nondependent lung will improve its ventilation to perfusion relationship by virtue of being in a favorable nondependent position (see Figure 19–11), whereas the dependent lung will improve its ventilation to perfusion relationship by virtue of selectively receiving PEEP. This method avoids the problem of distension of the apical regions causing increased apical pulmonary vascular resistance resulting in blood flow diversion to basilar regions of the lung (see lower left-hand corner inset).

FIGURE 6. Reproduced with permission from Benumof JL: Anesthesia for Thoracic Surgery. Philadelphia, W.B. Saunders Co., 1987.

has most often resulted in equal functional residual capacities and blood flows to each lung. Poorer results have been obtained with ventilator settings resulting in equal end-tidal carbon dioxide concentrations or equal airway pressures. (8)

It was originally thought that the two lungs would have to be ventilated synchronously because asynchronous differential lung ventilation would cause mediastinal movements that would impair cardiovascular performance. However, experimental and clinical experience has not supported this hypothesis, and the two lungs do not have to be ventilated synchronously. (9,10)

In fact, some studies suggest that asynchronous or alternating differential lung ventilation actually improves compliance of each lung because one lung does not have to compete with the other during inspiration for space within the thorax. (9,10) When the two lungs have achieved an equal compliance and the chest roentgenogram has improved, the double-lumen tube should be switched to a single-lumen tube, and treatment should proceed to goals 2 and 3 below.

The specific management of differential lung ventilation and PEEP for the patient with bilateral lung disease is similar to that for the patient with unilateral lung disease, except for a few important differences. First, the nondependent lung should receive none or a relatively low level of PEEP, and the dependent lung should receive a relatively high level of PEEP (which is the opposite from differential lung ventilation of the patient with unilateral lung disease in the lateral decubitus position). Second, the tidal volume to each lung should be proportional to the assumed perfusion to each lung. (6) Third, the patient should be turned from side to side every 2 to 3 hours so that each lung may be in a nondependent position for a time. Fourth, the need for fiberoptic bronchoscopy to check the position of the double-lumen tube is increased because of the much more frequent patient movement.

REFERENCES

1. Benumof, J.L., Rogers, S.N., Moyce, P.R., et al. Anesthesiology 51:503-507, 1979.
2. Carlon, G.C., Kahn, R., Howland, W.S., et al. Crit Care Med 6:380-383, 1978.
3. Powers, S., Mannal, R., Neclerio, M., et al. Ann Surg 178:265-272, 1973.
4. Powers, S., Dutton, R.E. Crit Care Med 3:64-68, 1975.
5. Carlon, G.C., Ray, C. Jr., Klein, R., et al. Chest 74:501-507, 1978.
6. Hedenstierna, G., Baehrendtz, S., Frostell, C., et al. Bull Eur Physiopathol Respir 21:281-285, 1985.
7. Kanarek, D.J., Shannon, D.C. Am Rev Respir Dis 112:457-459, 1975.

8. East, T.D., Pace, N.L., Westenskow, D.R., et al. Acta Anaesthesiol
   Scand 27:356-360, 1983.
9. Muneyuki, M., Konishi, K., Horiguchi, R, et al. Anesthesiology
   58:353-356, 1983.
10. Hameroff, S.R., Caukins, J.M., Waterson, C.K., et al: Anesthesiology
    54:237-239, 1981

PHYSIOLOGIC EFFECTS OF RAISED AIRWAY PRESSURE

JOHN B. DOWNS, M.D.

Department of Anesthesiology, The University of South
Florida College of Medicine, Tampa, Florida 33612

INTRODUCTION

Clinicians frequently adopt an empirical approach
to the respiratory care of patients with pulmonary
failure. As a result, only the symptomatology is
treated, which often fails to restore normal pulmonary
function. Now, more than at any other time in the
past, it is possible to direct care towards specific
pulmonary derangements and accurately evaluate the
effects of therapy. The following pages will emphasize
a goal-oriented approach to the treatment of patients
requiring respiratory support, through appropriate
adjustment of mechanical ventilation, inspired oxygen
and airway pressure. Because therapeutic interventions
may have variable physiologic consequences and rational
application of therapies requires an understanding of
such effects, applied cardiopulmonary physiology also
will be reviewed.

PHYSIOLOGIC CONSIDERATIONS

Ventilation

Inspiration will occur whenever a pressure
differential is created between the upper airway and
the alveoli. During spontaneous inspiration,
diaphragmatic contraction occurs, thereby decreasing
intrapleural pressure and creating a pressure
differential. During mechanical ventilation,

173

T. H. Stanley and R. J. Sperry (eds.), Anesthesia and the Lung, 173–213.
© 1989 by Kluwer Academic Publishers.

inspiration occurs when positive pressure is applied to the distal airway, which produces the pressure differential. In either case, the distending, or transpulmonary, pressure (airway pressure [P_{aw}] minus intrapleural pressure [P_{pl}]) is increased. The magnitude of change in transpulmonary pressure and the time during which the change occurs determine both tidal volume and inspiratory gas flow.(5) For a given tidal volume (V_T), the required transpulmonary prepressure depends upon the resistance of the respiratory system to deformation which is determined by the intrinsic elasticity of the system and resistance of the airways to gas flow.

Resistance of the respiratory system to deformation can be quantified by determining compliance, which is the change in volume divided by the change in pressure. Individual lung (C_L) and thorax (C_T) compliances determine lung-thorax compliance (C_{LT}).(6) These relationships are expressed by the following equations:(7)

$$\frac{1}{C_{LT}} = \frac{1}{C_L} + \frac{1}{C_T} \quad \text{where:}$$

$$C_{LT} = \frac{V_T}{\Delta P_{aw}}$$

$$C_L = \frac{V_T}{P_L} = \frac{V_T}{\Delta P_{aw} - \Delta P_{pl}}$$

$$C_T = \frac{V_T}{\Delta P_{pl}}$$

An understanding of these equations is helpful in clinical practice. Lung-thorax compliance usually is decreased in patients who have acute lung injury. The decrease may result from a decremental change in lung and/or thorax compliance.

To determine the contribution of each would require measurement of intrapleural pressure, a difficult procedure clinically. Attempts to estimate intrapleural pressure by measuring esophageal pressure are very error-prone and, therefore, may not be useful in determining compliance. Resistance to gas flow increases when laminar flow becomes turbulent, or if airway diameter decreases.(8) For a given tidal volume, an increased flow resistance may require a greater change in transpulmonary pressure because gas flow is related to the product of resistance and transpulmonary pressure. Thus, if there is a decrease in intrinsic elasticity, as may occur following lung injury, or an increase in resistance to gas flow, or both, the change in transpulmonary pressure required for spontaneous breathing may become extreme. Since an increased change in transpulmonary pressure requires greater diaphragmatic contraction, the work of breathing also will increase. These considerations will be discussed later.

The change in transpulmonary pressure required to produce a given tidal volume is similar whether it is generated by spontaneous breathing or mechanical ventilation. However, the distribution of inspired gas varies. Bynum, Rehder, and their coworkers have shown that mechanical ventilation alters the anatomical distribution of inspired gas.[9,10] They found that gas is delivered preferentially to dependent lung regions during spontaneous ventilation. After mechanical ventilation is instituted, gas is distributed primarily to superior lung regions. This redistribution of inspired gas appears to be unrelated to the rate of gas flow.(11)

Froese and her colleagues offered an explanation for these observations.(12) With fluoroscopy, they observed that posterior regions of the diaphragm have the greatest motion during spontaneous breathing in supine individuals, presumably because of the smaller radius of curvature of that portion of the diaphragm. Hence, the distribution of inspired gas should be greatest to the posterior dependent lung fields. During mechanical ventilation, diaphragmatic motion is limited in the dependent regions and greatest superiorly. Therefore, gas distribution occurs preferentially in the superior lung regions. This anatomical alteration of gas distribution explains the previously observed increase in physiological dead-space volume during mechanical ventilation.

Physiological dead-space volume is the portion of each inhaled breath that does not participate in gas exchange. Both anatomical and alveolar compartments contribute to the total physiological dead space.(13) The calculated dead-space of patients requiring ventilatory support was found to decrease linearly when mechanical ventilator rates gradually were changed from 20 to 0 breaths per minute.(14,15) When patients began to breathe spontaneously, average dead-space decreased 50 percent, despite a ventilator rate between 9 and 6 breaths per minute. Physiological dead-space continued to decrease linearly as spontaneous ventilation became more effective and the ventilator rate was reduced to 0 breaths per minute. When patients breathed spontaneously without mechanical ventilation, dead-space volume returned to predicted normal values. To account for the increase in physiologic dead-space when spontaneous respiration ceases, a maldistribution of inspired gas, pulmonary perfusion, or both, must occur during mechanical ventilation. Thus, mechanical ventilation actually induces a mismatching of ventilation and perfusion.

Maintenance of normal alveolar minute ventilation may be difficult during mechanical ventilation and decreased $PaCO_2$ is common. During mechanical ventilation, normal alveolar minute ventilation and $PaCO_2$ usually can be achieved with a tidal volume of 12 to 15 ml/kg and a respiratory rate of 7.5 breaths/min.(16) With such settings, patients usually will attempt to breathe spontaneously, making control of ventilation difficult. To suppress such spontaneous efforts,

alveolar ventilation must be such that $PaCO_2$ is below the
apneic threshold, thereby abolishing the carbon dioxide
respiratory drive. This usually occurs when $PaCO_2$ is 30 to
32 torr, a level which may result in respiratory alkalemia
and associated undesirable side effects. To provide a more
normal alveolar ventilation and to avoid these effects in
patients receiving mechanical ventilation, the respiratory
response to carbon dioxide may be altered and the apneic
threshold increased with sedatives or narcotics.
Alternatively, some clinicians have administered muscle
relaxants. Attempts to achieve normal $PaCO_2$ by adding
mechanical dead-space or exogenous carbon dioxide are
successful only if the apneic threshold is elevated
sufficiently.

Assisted mechanical ventilation once was thought to
avoid such problems. However, if the ventilator is set to
cycle with minimal patient effort, mechanical cycling will
result whenever the patient attempts to breathe, which he
will do whenever the $PaCO_2$ exceeds the apneic threshold.
Therefore, it is not surprising that assisted ventilation
commonly produces respiratory alkalemia. This has been
confirmed by Llewellyn and Swyer[17] and Downs and
colleagues,[18] who found that controlled and properly
adjusted assisted mechanical ventilation produce equivalent
$PaCO_2$ values.

Intermittent mandatory ventilation, IMV, can avoid many
of these problems. Intermittent mandatory ventilation will
permit unrestricted, unassisted spontaneous ventilation to
occur between mechanical breaths which are applied at a rate
just sufficient to prevent respiratory acidemia. By
maintaining spontaneous ventilation, alterations in inspired
gas distribution and physiologic dead-space volume are
minimized. In addition, it is possible to maintain normal
alveolar minute ventilation without sedatives, muscle
relaxants, addition of dead space, carbon dioxide, or any
combination of these.[19] A person breathing spontaneously

will attempt to maintain normal ventilation by changes of
tidal volume and respiratory rate, depending upon respiratory
system compliance, airway resistance, $PaCO_2$, and carbon
dioxide production.(20,21) If a patient is unable to support
adequate ventilation, the IMV rate can be adjusted to deliver
the required amount of mechanical augmentation needed to
normalize alveolar ventilation. Thus, respiratory acidemia
and alkalemia can be minimized with IMV. As spontaneous
ventilation improves, IMV can be decreased progressively
until spontaneous breathing alone can maintain a normal
alveolar ventilation.

Recently, several manufacturers of mechanical
ventilators have offered an option described as a "pressure
assist" mode. An inspiratory effort by the patient will
initiate a variable flow of gas to cause a predetermined
airway pressure to be maintained throughout the patient's
effort. When inspiratory effort wanes, flow will decrease.
When the patient begins to exhale, pressure will decrease to
allow passive exhalation. Introduced in an effort to
decrease work of breathing with demand valve IMV systems,
pressure-support has been recognized as a true assist mode,
unlike patient-triggered mechanical ventilation mentioned
previously. The degree of assistance offered by pressure-
support depends on the level of airway pressure selected by
the clinician, but may vary from minimal to complete
ventilatory assistance.

Many criteria have been proposed to evaluate a patient's
ability and drive to breathe spontaneously.(22) Since
patients may require different levels of $PaCO_2$ to maintain
normal arterial pH, the latter usually is a superior
criterion of ventilatory adequacy. Therefore, this
measurement is used to evaluate the adequacy of mechanical
and spontaneous ventilation in patients receiving IMV.(19,22)

In summary, institution of mechanical ventilation and
loss of spontaneous efforts can alter normal respiratory
physiology. Changes include altered intrapulmonary gas

distribution, increased physiologic dead space, and difficulty in maintaining normal alveolar ventilation. IMV allows spontaneous breathing to persist during mechanical ventilation, which will assure more normal distribution of inspired gas, reduction of physiological dead-space and improved matching of ventilation and perfusion. In addition, a normal alveolar ventilation and arterial pH are more easily obtained.

Hemodynamic Responses

The respiratory system affects cardiovascular function primarily by variation in venous blood return and pulmonary vascular resistance. Return of venous blood to thoracic veins greatly depends upon the extrathoracic-intrathoracic intravascular pressure gradient. This gradient is determined largely by intrapleural pressure, which normally is subambient because of two opposing forces: lung recoil and retraction of the thorax.(6) Any change in these forces alters intrapleural pressure and the intravascular pressure gradient. Intrapleural pressure will increase following loss of spontaneous breathing, disruption of the chest wall, or application of positive airway pressure, thereby decreasing the extrathoracic-intrathoracic pressure gradient, venous inflow, and cardiac output. Intrapleural pressure is decreased by spontaneous inspiration, thereby increasing the pressure gradient, thoracic venous blood inflow and cardiac output.

The increase in intrapleural pressure following application of positive airway pressure depends upon how much of the airway pressure is transmitted to the intrapleural space. Transmission of airway pressure is determined by lung and thorax compliances and can be determined from the following equations:(7)

$$C_L = \frac{V_T}{\Delta P_L} = \frac{V_T}{\Delta P_{aw} - \Delta P_{pl}}$$

$$C_L = \frac{V_T}{\Delta P_{pl}}$$

Whenever lung volume changes, there must be an equivalent alteration in the volume of the thorax. Therefore:

$$V_T = C_L \ (\Delta P_{aw} - \Delta P_{pl}) = C_T \ \Delta P_{pl}$$

The fractional transmission of airway pressure to the intrapleural space (P_{pl}/ P_{aw}) can be determined:

$$C_L \ \Delta P_{aw} = (C_T + C_L) \ \Delta P_{pl}$$

$$\frac{\Delta P_{pl}}{\Delta P_{aw}} = \frac{C_L}{C_T + C_L}$$

When lung and thorax compliances are equal, 50 percent of a change in airway pressure is transmitted to the intrapleural space. If lung compliance decreases, fractional transmission is less than 50 percent. A decrease in thorax compliance increases pressure transmission. These relationships can explain some frequent clinical observations.

Patients with acute respiratory failure often tolerate high levels of positive end-expiratory pressure (PEEP) without deleterious cardiovascular consequences. This reflects decreased airway pressure transmission secondary to decreased lung compliance. Patients who have abdominal distention, or who have decreased lung volume following operative procedures, often have reduced thorax compliance and increased airway pressure transmission. Thorax compliance is decreased, and lung compliance is increased in patients with chronic obstructive lung disease. As we would predict on a basis of increased transmission of the positive airway pressure to the intrapleural space, such patients

often are intolerant of mechanical ventilation and PEEP,
which may cause significant decline in cardiac output.
Thus, many clinical conditions can affect transmission of
positive airway pressure and the resulting hemodynamic
responses. Such conditions should be considered when assessing the effects of ventilatory support on cardiopulmonary
function.

Measurements of thoracic vascular pressures frequently
are used to evaluate cardiac filling and function. When
airway pressure increases, all or part of the change in
intrapleural pressure will be transmitted to the lumen of the
intrathoracic vessels.(23) Thus, evaluation of cardiac
function may be difficult without accurate estimation of
true intravascular filling pressure.(23,24,25) Intravascular
filling pressure is determined by subtraction of the
intrapleural from the intravascular pressure. Therefore,
precise knowledge of the intrapleural pressure may be
valuable. At present, the measurement of intrapleural
pressure is difficult and requires the placement of a
catheter into the pleural space.(25) Attempts to estimate
intrapleural pressure with an esophageal balloon have been
made, but interpretation of esophageal pressure is difficult
because great pressure variations occur within the
esophagus.(26) In addition, when esophageal pressure
exceeds atmospheric pressure, compliance of the esophageal
balloon may limit accuracy of the measurement.(27) Such
inaccuracy may influence calculated filling pressures and
lead to significant error.

Expiratory intrapleural pressure varies little with
different respiratory patterns, as long as expiratory airway
pressure is similar. Therefore, the most important
determinant of mean airway, intrapleural and vascular filling
pressures is the inspiratory airway pressure pattern. During
mechanical inspiration, filling pressures will decrease,
since airway and intrapleural pressures are increased. When
filling pressure, or preload, is lowered, cardiac output

likely will decrease. This is not the case during
spontaneous breathing, even with PEEP. During spontaneous
exhalation, intrapleural and filling pressures are equivalent
to those recorded during mechanical ventilation with the same
PEEP level. However, during inspiration, intrapleural
pressure decreases, increasing cardiac filling. The effect
of spontaneous inspiration on filling pressure of the heart
and cardiac output depends on the change in airway pressure.
Continuous positive airway pressure (CPAP) is produced by gas
flowing through a circuit terminated by a threshold resistor
valve. Airway pressure is increased throughout the
spontaneous respiratory cycle and inspiratory airway pressure
should not decrease significantly.(28) If the airway is not
pressurized throughout the respiratory cycle, inspiratory
airway pressure will decrease toward ambient during breathing
with PEEP. The resultant higher mean airway and intrapleural
pressure with CPAP may decrease thoracic venous inflow of
blood and cardiac output. Weinstein and coworkers found no
difference between CPAP and spontaneous ventilation with
PEEP.(29) However, they insured that filling pressure was
normal, or elevated, during CPAP. Other studies have
reported that venous return is affected most by controlled
mechanical ventilation and PEEP, less by CPAP, and least by
spontaneous respiration with PEEP and ambient inspiratory
airway pressure.(24,28,30,31)

Principal respiratory factors affecting pulmonary
vascular resistance and pulmonary blood flow and its
distribution, are airway pressure and lung volume. When
expiratory lung volume, functional residual capacity (FRC),
is normal, pulmonary vascular resistance is minimal.(32)
Changes in lung volume above or below normal FRC increase
pulmonary vascular resistance. Therefore, normal FRC should
be maintained whenever possible. Even though FRC may be
independent of the inspiratory airway pressure pattern, the
mode of inspiration can affect pulmonary vascular
resistance.

During mechanical inspiration with large tidal volumes, pulmonary vascular resistance may increase as some alveoli become overdistended. Resistance may be increased further by PEEP since compliant lung areas are enlarged further. Increased pulmonary vascular resistance and decreased venous return from elevated intrapleural pressure additively can depress cardiac output. This may account for reports that mechanical ventilation with PEEP greater than 11 torr frequently depresses cardiac output. (33,34) In contrast, cardiac output is not adversely affected with 11 torr PEEP when spontaneous ventilation is maintained.(35) In fact, the cardiac output of patients treated for respiratory failure with IMV was unaffected by PEEP at an average level of 22 torr. (35) The deleterious effects of PEEP on venous return, cardiac output, and pulmonary vascular resistance appear to be minimized by maintaining spontaneous respiration and a lower mechanical cycling frequency.

It has been suggested that nonsynchronous application of mechanical ventilation to spontaneously breathing patients may cause cardiovascular depression.(36) Recently, IMV synchronized with spontaneous breaths (SIMV) and nonsynchronous IMV were compared.(37) Mean airway pressure was an average of 0.5 torr lower during SIMV, but there were no differences in intrapleural pressure, cardiac output, or stroke volume. From these results one can conclude that SIMV offers little advantage when compared to IMV, and may be a disadvantage due to the extra cost for that capability.

Application of positive airway pressure during spontaneous breathing may benefit some patients with compromised myocardial function. Patients who breathed spontaneously with 11 torr PEEP after operation for coronary revascularization had increased stroke index and cardiac output.(28) It is possible that PEEP may affect several of the determinants of cardiac output. Intrapleural pressure, increased by PEEP, could augment ventricular contraction during exhalation. The external compression may serve to "unload" the left ventricle. Because intrapleural pressure is lower during spontaneous inspiration, left ventricular filling pressure may increase.

Positive airway pressure has been reported to depress renal function, presumably secondary to decreased cardiac output(23) or elevated plasma levels of vasopressin.(38,39) Renal function was compared in swine receiving continuous positive pressure ventilation (CPPV) with 10 torr PEEP to that in others breathing spontaneously with 10 torr CPAP.(31) Animals receiving CPPV responded with increased plasma vasopressin and decreased cardiac output, urine flow, glomerular filtration rate, and sodium excretion. Animals that received CPAP had decreased urine flow and glomerular filtration, but cardiac output, plasma vasopressin, and excretion of sodium did not differ from control values. Since urine flow and glomerular filtration were similarly affected by CPPV and CPAP, these alterations could not have been secondary to changes in cardiac output or vasopressin alone, but may be related to elevated venous pressures. The preservation of pulsatile venous blood flow during spontaneous inspiration may account for the differences. Such flow would be decreased during mechanical inspiration because increased intrapleural pressure would further increase inferior vena cava and renal vein pressures. Thus, a decrease in inspiratory intrapleural pressure during spontaneous breathing minimizes some detrimental renal effects of positive pressure breathing.

In summary, spontaneous ventilation maintains lower airway and intrapleural pressures. This augments venous blood return and does not affect pulmonary vascular resistance adversely. Therefore, cardiac output, and pulmonary blood flow and distribution are better maintained. Presence of spontaneous ventilation is even more important after the application of positive airway pressure. If mechanical ventilation is required, it should be titrated to the level necessary to normalize alveolar ventilation, thereby minimizing deleterious effects.

Ventilation-Perfusion Relationships

As previously discussed, spontaneous inspiration directs the majority of ventilation toward dependent regions of the lung.(10,40) Gravitational effects insure a similar distribution of blood flow. Thus, the alveolar ventilation-to-perfusion ratio (V_A/Q) normally approaches unity in all lung regions. Significant ventilation-perfusion mismatching usually necessitates therapeutic intervention. Unfortunately, therapy to correct one extreme V_A/Q abnormality frequently induces the other. An increased V_A/Q may require mechanical ventilation, if spontaneous breathing cannot provide adequate alveolar ventilation for carbon dioxide elimination. During mechanical ventilation, the majority of ventilation is directed toward superior lung regions. Blood flow, however, is still greatest in dependent lung regions. As a result, mechanical ventilation increases V_A/Q in the superior lung regions, causing an increase in dead-space. Because dead-space volume increases during mechanical ventilation, an increased ventilator rate may result in a paradoxical increase in $PaCO_2$.

A decrease in V_A/Q results in impaired arterial oxygenation. Since the majority of gas exchange occurs during exhalation, improvement in overall V_A/Q must occur primarily during exhalation. Mechanical ventilation usually is not effective in improving such problems since the ratio will increase only during the inspiratory phase of the respiratory cycle. Additionally, Zarins and associates observed a lower PaO_2 in baboons receiving controlled mechanical ventilation than in those receiving IMV with the same level of PEEP.(41) This suggests that mechanical ventilation promoted decreased V_A/Q and increased venous admixture. Positive airway pressure applied during exhalation can improve low V_A/Q. However, PEEP may increase physiological dead-space and decrease effective alveolar ventilation, especially when applied with mechanical ventilation. Therefore, when ventilatory support is

instituted, the goal must be to minimize
ventilation-perfusion mismatching in all lung regions. This
is best accomplished when spontaneous ventilation is allowed
to persist and when mechanical ventilation is used just to
prevent acidemia.

Acute respiratory failure often is characterized by a
decrease in FRC and an increase in pulmonary venous
admixture. Therapy should include PEEP to increase FRC,
improve pulmonary gas exchange, increase arterial oxygen
tension and decrease pulmonary vascular resistance. It has
been recommended that the appropriate (optimal) level of PEEP
be determined by titrating PEEP to minimize venous
admixture.(33,35)

Minimizing venous admixture appears to be least
efficient when PEEP is applied during mechanical ventilation.
Venous admixture of patients with severe, acute respiratory
failure was found to be reduced from 50 to 32 percent by
controlled ventilation with an average of 10 torr PEEP.(33)
When PEEP was raised above this level, venous admixture
increased and PaO_2 decreased. Venous admixture was reduced
to an average of 14 percent by IMV and mean value of 22 torr
PEEP in a similar group of patients.(35) This difference
may be explained by the increased mean airway and
intrapleural pressure in patients receiving mechanical
ventilation with PEEP. The greater mean airway pressure may
overdistend compliant alveoli, increasing pulmonary vascular
resistance and redirecting blood flow to less well
ventilated areas, thus increasing venous admixture. In
contrast, spontaneous breathing during IMV maintains lower
mean airway and intrapleural pressure, and allows higher
PEEP levels to increase FRC with fewer deleterious
effects.(35)

During evaluation of pulmonary gas exchange, the effects
of inspired oxygen concentration on ventilation and perfusion
should be considered. In a normal lung, V_A/Q changes very
little from inspiration to expiration. However, this is not

true in respiratory failure. The expiratory V_A/Q is less
than the inspiratory V_A/Q and will be decreased further by
oxygen breathing because more alveolar oxygen is absorbed.
Eventually the rate of gas flow from an alveolus into the
blood will balance exactly the rate of delivery of gas to the
alveolus during inspiration. Such an alveolus will be
unstable and any subsequent decrease in inspiratory V_A/Q, or
increase in oxygen concentration will result in a net flow
of gas from the alveolus to the blood, further loss of
volume, and collapse. It has been suggested that lung units
with an inspiratory V_A/Q of less than 0.08 would be stable
only when breathing ambient air.(42-45) They have found
when oxygen was breathed, blood flow that had been
distributed to areas with low V_A/Q during ambient air
breathing, subsequently perfused areas with zero
ventilation. Thus, oxygen breathing induced atelectasis and
shunting.

Other investigators also have found that oxygen
breathing increases shunting. When patients with respiratory
failure breathe an increased concentration of inspired
oxygen, a uniform response occurs.(46-48) As the inspired
oxygen is increased to 40 percent, venous admixture
decreases and remains unchanged until the inspired oxygen
reaches 60 percent. Venous admixture then increases as
inspired oxygen approaches 100 percent. Increasing inspired
oxygen to 40 percent will minimize oxygen diffusion
abnormalities and mask the hypoxemia producing effect of
lung areas with low, but finite, V_A/Q, thereby accounting
for the observed decrease in venous admixture. The observed
increase in venous admixture caused by breathing high
concentrations of oxygen may result from atelectasis.
However, altered pulmonary perfusion may also contribute to
this effect.(47) In areas of the lung with low V_A/Q,
hypoxic pulmonary vasoconstriction is thought to limit
perfusion by shunting blood to areas with better
ventilation. When the inspired oxygen concentration is

increased, alveolar PO_2 rises, precapillary pulmonary vasoconstriction decreases, and perfusion to areas with decreased V_A/Q increases. Another possible explanation is that oxygen inhalation increases extra-alveolar shunting of venous blood.(49-51) Such right-to-left intrapulmonary shunting of blood can increase venous admixture. Recently, we observed a detrimental effect of short term exposure to 50% inspired O_2 in post operative patients. (52) Thus, detrimental consequences of oxygen breathing should be considered when evaluating lung function and when providing therapy.

In summary, although mechanical ventilation may be necessary for adequate carbon dioxide elimination, spontaneous ventilation insures better matching of ventilation and perfusion. Oxygen administration may be required to prevent hypoxemia, but minimal amounts are best to assure the least detriment to pulmonary function and provide for more precise evaluation of pulmonary dysfunction and therapy. It is apparent that respiratory therapy, based upon measurement of venous admixture during breathing of oxygen-enriched air, may not be directed at the patient's pathophysiology. Acute lung dysfunction often results in lung areas with low V_A/Q. Therapy should be directed to correct the dysfunction and improve V_A/Q. Therefore it is preferable for the inspired oxygen concentration to be at a level that will not mask the effects produced by areas of low V_A/Q. Such an inspired oxygen concentration will better allow evaluation of low V_A/Q and the effects of therapy.

Work of Breathing

If patients with respiratory failure are to have effective spontaneous breathing, the work of breathing must be maximally efficient. Few clinical studies have attempted to quantify the work of breathing in patients with respiratory failure, perhaps because quantification of work requires techniques which are not readily available.[53] For our discussion, only a graphical representation of the elastic work of inspiration will be considered. Any alteration in the pressure-volume relationship of the lung can alter the work of breathing. A normal pressure-volume curve for the lung-thorax system is shown in Fig. 1. As a result of a small pressure change, normal tidal breathing from FRC occurs along the pressure-volume curve as indicated by the arrow. The elastic work of inspiration can be estimated by the stippled areas under the curve.

In Fig. 2, the pressure-volume curves for normal lung, thorax, and lung-thorax are plotted. When the distending pressure of the lung-thorax is zero, which occurs when airway pressure is ambient, the lung volume at this point is the FRC. At FRC, the distending pressure of the lung is equal but opposite to that of the thorax. Any alteration in the pressure-volume relationships for the lung and/or thorax will alter the lung-thorax curve and affect FRC.

The effects of a change in the lung pressure-volume curve, which are likely to occur in patients with acute lung injury, are shown in Fig. 3. Because the pressure-volume relationships of the lung and thorax can be altered in an infinite number of ways during respiratory failure, a family of right-shifted lung-thorax curves can result. Each will have a new, but decrementally changed FRC (Fig. 4).

A shift in the pressure-volume curve not only decreases FRC, but can increase the work of breathing. When FRC is decreased, the required pressure change may be increased for the same tidal volume (Fig. 5). When the required pressure change is increased, the area under the curve representing work, also is increased. If this occurs, the patient will decrease tidal volume and increase respiratory rate in an effort to minimize work. Because of these changes, clinicians often have assumed the work of breathing for the patient by instituting mechanical ventilation. However, an increase in FRC and compliance also may decrease the patient's work of breathing.

Restoration of FRC can be accomplished by applying PEEP to increase distending pressure (Fig. 6). Each pressure-volume curve will require a different level of PEEP to restore FRC and minimize the work of breathing. Therefore, PEEP must be individualized, titrated for each patient, and reassessed frequently. If PEEP is applied to meet these goals, FRC will be increased and often will lie on a favorable portion of the pressure-volume curve, where the required change in pressure to produce a tidal volume will be less. Thus, compliance will be improved and work of breathing reduced.

Following application of PEEP to restore FRC, a reduction in the work of breathing will occur only if inspiratory drop in airway pressure is small. (54) Again, the spontaneous inspiratory airway-pressure change is of clinical significance.(28) During CPAP, gas must flow at a rate equalling or exceeding the inspiratory flow rate of the patient. Therefore, airway pressure changes little throughout the respiratory cycle. During spontaneous respiration with PEEP, gas flow occurs only when inspiratory airway pressure is below ambient pressure. The terms expiratory positive airway pressure (EPAP) and inspiratory pressure (IPAP) have been suggested to help define these respiratory patterns more precisely.(55) During CPAP, the expiratory and inspiratory pressures (EPAP and IPAP) are nearly equal. When airway pressure is elevated only during exhalation (EPAP), airway pressure change is greater than with CPAP. Intrapleural pressure change also is greater with EPAP, causing an increase in the work of breathing. As lung compliance decreases, intrapleural pressure change is greater because the stiff lung requires a greater intrapleural pressure change to accomplish tidal breathing, and a further increase in the work of breathing results. Since our goal must be to minimize the patient's work of breathing, CPAP

(EPAP and IPAP) should be applied to restore FRC.

In summary, the appropriate ventilatory pattern depends upon intravascular volume, cardiac output, lung volume, compliance and the patient's ability to breathe. Careful evaluation of airway and intrapleural pressure patterns becomes important in providing optimal therapy. Using the principles described, we can define optimal CPAP as the airway pressure that minimizes physiologic intrapulmonary shunting of blood and reduces the work of spontaneous breathing, without causing detrimental cardiovascular effects.

RESPIRATORY CARE
Oxygen Therapy

Patients often have arterial hypoxemia secondary to areas of lung with low, but finite, ventilation-to-perfusion ratio. Arterial hypoxemia produced by such areas is worsened by a low inspired oxygen concentration and usually can be alleviated when oxygen is added to the inspired gas. Another source of arterial hypoxemia is the impairment of oxygen diffusion from alveoli to pulmonary capillary blood. A "diffusion defect" rarely is the only cause of arterial hypoxemia, but may contribute when the inspired concentration is low. Right-to-left intrapulmonary shunting of blood, a third source of hypoxemia, will be unaffected, even during pure-oxygen breathing. Thus, oxygen therapy may improve arterial hypoxemia when it is secondary to two of three abnormalities.

When evaluating and treating arterial hypoxemia, variables which may contribute to the hypoxemia should be considered. Increased oxygen consumption resulting from an increased metabolic rate, or a decrease in cardiac output, will cause lower mixed venous blood lower oxygen tension. A low hemoglobin concentration also will result in a lower mixed venous blood oxygen tension. When mixed venous oxygen

tension is reduced, a lower arterial oxygen tension often
results. Such factors should be evaluated in patients with
arterial hypoxemia. This may require the measurement of
mixed venous oxygen saturation and calculation of
arterial-mixed venous oxygen content difference and venous
admixture.(56) Such efforts may prevent inappropriate
therapy.

Evaluation of hypoxemia is further complicated by the
effects of inspired oxygen concentration on pulmonary gas
exchange. Breathing an increased oxygen concentration may
lead to absorption atelectasis in areas of lung with low, but
finite, V_A/Q, as discussed previously. Only if the inspired
nitrogen concentration is increased can absorption
atelectasis and increased right-to-left intrapulmonary
shunting of blood be prevented. Even the application of PEEP
will not prevent absorption atelectasis.(47) Therefore,
administration of high inspired oxygen concentrations, even
if limited to 24 hrs, is undesirable. Also, prolonged
administration of 50 percent oxygen to patients can no longer
be considered therapeutic, rational, or safe.(52) Rather,
rapid reduction of inspired oxygen is the preferred
practice.

In spite of the frequency with which oxygen is used to
treat hypoxemia, discontinuation of such therapy has received
little attention. Evaluating pulmonary gas exchange in
patients with areas of lung with low V_A/Q when breathing
increased concentrations of oxygen might lead to incorrect
conclusions, because administration of as little as 30
percent oxygen may mask the hypoxemic-producing effect of
areas with low V_A/Q. This should be considered when oxygen
therapy is discontinued. For example, a patient breathing 40
percent oxygen with a PaO_2 of 70 torr might be thought to
have adequate pulmonary gas exchange. The clinician might
then decide to wean the patient from mechanical ventilation
and PEEP. However, ventilation and perfusion could be
mismatched to such a degree that breathing only 30 percent

oxygen might decrease PaO_2 to 50 torr. Were the clinician aware of this abnormality, it is likely that PEEP would be increased rather than decreased. Such evaluations of pulmonary gas exchange and the rational application of PEEP are possible only when the inspired oxygen concentration is low. Often evaluation of pulmonary gas exchange is best when patients breathe room air.

In summary, it is best to use the lowest possible inspired oxygen concentration to maintain an acceptable PaO_2. This practice maximizes alveolar nitrogen concentration, minimizes absorption atelectasis, minimizes right-to-left intrapulmonary shunting and may decrease the need for PEEP. Since the low, but finite, V_A/Q is more apparent when the inspired oxygen concentration is low, the clinician is better able to evaluate the resolution of lung dysfunction as therapy is applied and time progresses. Oxygen should be viewed as any other drug and should be given only when clinically indicated, only in the amount required, and reduced and removed as soon as feasible. During this period, the sources of hypoxemia should be clarified and specific therapy instituted.

CPAP Therapy

Spontaneous respiration with elevated airway pressure was recognized four decades ago to decrease pulmonary edema in patients with congestive heart failure.(57) A motor-driven blower provided an inspiratory gas source and airway pressure was elevated with a face mask and an expiratory valve for constant positive-pressure breathing (CPPB). Shortly thereafter, CPPB was used to treat pulmonary edema secondary to traumatic lung injury (58) and pulmonary contusion in patients with flail chest injuries.(59) Thus, there is ample historical precedent for applying elevated airway pressures to spontaneously breathing patients. Much later, mechanical ventilation was

emphasized for the treatment of lung injuries and
spontaneous breathing with CPPB was abandoned.(60)   Because
of the early emphasis on mechanical ventilation,
discontinuation of mechanical ventilatory support often is
attempted only after the need for PEEP has been alleviated.
This may not be the most rational approach.

Lung compliance and arterial oxygenation are decreased,
and work of breathing is increased in patients with acute
lung injury. In fact, it is often the increased work of
breathing that leads many clinicians to institute mechanical
ventilation. By application of CPAP, FRC and compliance can
be increased. The increase in FRC will improve V_A/Q and
arterial oxygenation. Increased compliance will decrease the
work of breathing. Thus, CPAP may reduce the requirement for
mechanical ventilation and inspired oxygen supplementation.
Since application of CPAP also may alleviate many problems
associated with the mechanical ventilator and oxygen, we
prefer to wean patients from mechanical ventilation and
oxygen before removing CPAP.

Application of CPAP, like oxygen therapy, has been
widely discussed for more than four decades. However, little
attention has been directed toward the mechanics of weaning
patients from CPAP. The clinician would like to insure that
a reduction in CPAP will not reduce FRC below normal. Such a
decrease in FRC may cause two aspects of pulmonary function
to deteriorate. In some regions of the lung V_A/Q
may decrease, causing arterial hypoxemia. In addition, lung
compliance may decrease. Each of these FRC-dependent effects
should be evaluated separately as CPAP is reduced. Because a
small reduction in CPAP can cause a large fall in FRC, CPAP
should be withdrawn in decrements of 2 cm H_2O.(61)

To evaluate V_A/Q, arterial blood oxygenation must be
examined. Alterations in FRC and oxygenation are nearly
complete within one minute following a change in CPAP.
Therefore, the effect of CPAP on oxygenation should be
evaluated within minutes of the addition or removal of

CPAP.(61) This often requires measurement, not only of
PaO$_2$, but also of the oxygen tension in mixed venous blood
and calculation of venous admixture. If a reduction in CPAP
causes a deterioration of these values, CPAP should be
increased immediately.

To assess change in lung compliance, respiratory
mechanics must be evaluated. A shift to the right of the
pressure-volume curve of the respiratory system may decrease
both FRC and compliance, causing a greater intrapleural
pressure change for tidal breathing and increased work of
breathing. The greater negativity of intrapleural pressure
may cause subcostal, suprasternal, or intercostal retractions
that can be observed clinically. To minimize the work of
breathing, the patient will inhale with a smaller tidal
volume and increase the respiratory rate in an effort to
maintain adequate alveolar ventilation. Thus, after a change
in CPAP, the respiratory rate, tidal volume, and physical
appearance of the patient should be observed closely.
Because change in V_A/Q and compliance may occur
independently, it is important that gas exchange and
mechanics be evaluated separately. Deterioration in either
should be considered a contraindication to further reduction
of CPAP and an indication for its return to a higher level.

Three additional considerations deserve mention. First,
blood-gas exchange must be evaluated when the inspired oxygen
concentration is low and constant, because venous admixture
varies at different concentrations of inspired oxygen.(47)
For example, a patient breathing 30 percent oxygen with a
calculated venous admixture of 25 percent may have only a 15
percent venous admixture breathing 40 percent oxygen. Were
CPAP reduced with the patient breathing 30 percent oxygen,
venous admixture could increase to 30 percent, indicating a
deterioration in pulmonary function. However, if CPAP were
decreased and the inspired oxygen simultaneously increased to
40 percent, venous admixture could be 20 percent. The
clinician erroneously might conclude that the reduction of

CPAP is well tolerated when, in fact, the patient's pulmonary status has deteriorated greatly. Thus, it is important to evaluate gas exchange while the concentration of inspired oxygen is constant.

Circuit resistance is the second consideration. In order to evaluate respiratory mechanics accurately, the clinician must be sure that external or mechanical resistance to respiration is minimal and that effective spontaneous respiration exists. Mechanical resistance is best minimized by assuring a continuous flow of gas, or by use of a sufficiently sensitive demand valve in the inspiratory circuit, by use of large-bore tubing and low-resistance valves, and avoidance of acute angles in the system. Such care will prevent inspiratory airway and intrapleural pressures from decreasing to levels which might erroneously suggest a deterioration in pulmonary function.

Currently, there are no commercially available demand valve systems with acceptable sensitivity and flow characteristics. Pressure-assist has greatly improved patient acceptance of such systems, but their complexity and expense seems unwarranted. Therefore, we still prefer continuous flow systems for IMV and CPAP. Care must be taken to insure low inspiratory circuit resistance for reasons mentioned above. In addition, exhalation valve resistance may create excessive inspiratory work of breathing. Where the high flow of gas exits such a valve an increase in airway pressure will result. When the patient inhales, the decrease in flow past the exhalation valve will decrease airway pressure and increase work of breathing. Therefore, low-flow resistance, threshold resistor type exhalation/CPAP valves should be used.

Adequacy of spontaneous respiration is the third consideration. To insure that spontaneous respiration is effective, weaning from CPAP should begin only when the mechanical ventilator rate is low and spontaneous respiration provides the majority of alveolar ventilation. In most instances, weaning from CPAP should not be attempted until the patient is breathing spontaneously and fewer than 2 mechanical breaths per minute are being provided.

In summary, by applying CPAP, the requirement for oxygen and mechanical ventilatory support may be reduced. IMV and CPAP may allow the patient to be weaned expediently from oxygen and mechanical ventilation.

Mechanical Ventilation

During the last few decades, there has been a trend toward using mechanical ventilation for patients with inadequate arterial oxygenation and increased work of breathing.(60) Infrequently, these patients have difficulty eliminating carbon dioxide while breathing spontaneously. Since mechanical ventilation alone usually does not reverse the factors responsible for hypoxemia, a need often exists for an increased concentration of inspired oxygen. Classic criteria for initiating mechanical ventilation based on respiratory strength and drive often are not applicable to such patients. Without specific guidelines for patients with acute respiratory failure, the decision to initiate and terminate mechanical ventilatory support often is subjective. Such difficulty can be avoided if mechanical ventilation is reserved only for patients unable to sustain adequate spontaneous ventilation.

When IMV is used, mechanical ventilation can be applied to prevent acidemia and CPAP can be optimally applied, thereby reducing the need for an increased inspired O_2 concentration and mechanical ventilation. Weaning may be accomplished by lowering the IMV rate in decrements. When mechanical ventilation has been completely discontinued and spontaneous respiration is adequate to prevent acidemia, the patient is considered weaned from mechanical ventilation. It is important to emphasize the difference between acidemia and respiratory acidosis.

Compensatory respiratory acidosis has been thought to occur only rarely in conscious patients. However, use of IMV has led us to observe some patients who decrease ventilation to maintain a normal arterial pH even though $PaCO_2$ may exceed 60 torr. If the patient has no history of lung disease or chronic carbon dioxide elevation, therapy aimed at correction of the coexisting metabolic alkalosis will result in prompt reduction of $PaCO_2$. Therefore, $PaCO_2$ may not be the best index of adequacy of spontaneous respiration, nor should it be a criterion for IMV rate reduction in many patients. Rather, arterial pH should be used as a guide and the rate of IMV should be reduced as long as arterial pH remains greater than 7.35. In this way, patients can be weaned rapidly and safely from mechanical ventilatory support, even when metabolic alkalosis is present.

By promoting spontaneous respiration and rapid termination of mechanical ventilation, IMV may avoid several problems observed during conventional therapy. Occasionally, during prolonged mechanical ventilatory support, patients develop a psychological dependence upon the ventilator that may cause weaning problems. It appears that those allowed to breathe spontaneously throughout the period of ventilatory support do not develop such dependence.(62) In addition, for reasons that are not clear, a pronounced neuromuscular discoordination of the respiratory muscles may occur in patients who have prolonged mechanical ventilatory support. Some reports have indicated that almost all patients requiring ventilatory support for more than 24 hours develop discoordination of abdominal and accessory muscles of respiration.(63) Such discoordination may be sufficient to prevent adequate spontaneous respiration and may prolong ventilator dependence. This discoordination does not occur in patients who maintain spontaneous breathing. Recently, Andersen and associates confirmed the absence of respiratory muscle discoordination in patients who received IMV.(64)

Initially, IMV was used on adult patients only as a weaning technique. Currently, we employ IMV as a ventilatory support mode to allow greater flexibility in oxygen therapy, CPAP, and mechanical ventilation. Each is applied and weaned separately to meet established goals. Controversy still exists whether IMV can speed the weaning process more than conventional techniques. A prospective investigation compared the efficacy of IMV criteria with traditional criteria for weaning patients from mechanical ventilatory support. The study concluded that IMV results in faster and safer weaning for a majority of patients.(22)

In summary, the advantages of IMV depend on the ability to apply therapy in a goal-oriented manner, rather than rapidity of weaning from mechanical ventilation. Only IMV allows oxygen therapy and mechanical ventilation to be reduced early in the therapy of patients with respiratory failure, through the use of optimal CPAP.

Current Practice

Ventilatory care of patients with acute respiratory failure often proceeds in the following fashion. Initially, oxygen is added to the inhaled gas to alleviate arterial hypoxemia. If a satisfactory arterial oxygen tension is not achieved, or maintained, the trachea is intubated and mechanical ventilation instituted. If an adequate PaO_2 still cannot be obtained with inspired oxygen concentration less than 60 percent, an arbitrary amount of PEEP is added. Weaning from ventilatory support proceeds in reverse fashion. PEEP is decreased in decrements, as long as PaO_2 remains satisfactory and inspired oxygen is "nontoxic". After successful removal of PEEP, mechanical ventilation is withdrawn and the patient breathes spontaneously from a T-piece for increasingly longer periods. Once totally spontaneous respiration is deemed to be satisfactory, patients are extubated and an elevated inspired oxygen

concentration administered to prevent arterial hypoxemia.
By using IMV we have developed a practice that proceeds in a
more objective and efficient fashion.

Patients suffering acute respiratory failure often
require oxygen therapy, mechanical ventilatory support, and
CPAP. In general, patients are orotracheally intubated.
Initially, mechanical ventilatory support is supplied to
normalize alveolar minute ventilation. To treat arterial
hypoxemia, an elevated inspired oxygen concentration is
administered. Pulmonary mechanics and gas exchange are
evaluated and CPAP titrated to minimize abnormalities. Once
optimal CPAP is obtained, mechanical ventilation is reduced,
as long as arterial pH remains greater than 7.35.
Simultaneously, the inspired oxygen concentration is reduced
decrementally to a level that will not mask the
hypoxemic-producing effect of areas of lung with low V_A/Q,
yet, that will maintain PaO_2 at an acceptable level. Often
this may be accomplished with 30 percent oxygen, or less.
Pulmonary gas exchange and mechanics are evaluated frequently
and when considered adequate, CPAP is reduced without
allowing detrimental change to occur. Finally, the patient
is extubated. It is important to note that patients are
weaned from mechanical ventilation and oxygen first and from
CPAP last. This order is the reverse of the standard mode of
therapy. Because this general approach may not apply to all
patients, specific therapy for those who have had a major
operation, acute respiratory failure, chest trauma or acute
exacerbation of chronic obstructive lung disease may vary.

Most patients who have undergone major operations have
little or no underlying lung disease. They may require
mechanical ventilation and oxygen therapy for a short time
because of the effects of anesthesia and operation.
Initially, we provide these patients with 100 ml/kg min of
total minute ventilation using a mechanical tidal volume of
12-15 ml/kg and a rate of 7.5 breaths/min.(16)   Because
they usually have no problem with arterial oxygenation, the

initial inspired oxygen is 30 percent. A PEEP of 5 cm H_2O is added to the expiratory limb of the ventilator circuit. Within 10 minutes of the time mechanical support is instituted, an arterial blood sample is analyzed and gas exchange is evaluated. The rate of mechanical ventilation is adjusted to the point that it just prevents acidemia. As the patient recovers from the sedatives, narcotics, and/or muscle relaxants used for anesthesia, the ventilator rate is reduced rapidly. When arterial oxygenation is adequate with 30 percent inspired oxygen and 5 cm H_2O PEEP, and arterial pH is greater than 7.35 without ventilatory assistance, the patient is extubated. As mentioned previously, the use of IMV for managing such patients has decreased the period of mechanical ventilatory support slightly and has made weaning safer. It is likely that pulse oximetry will become more popular, will decrease the requirement for frequent arterial blood analysis and will further speed the weaning process.(22)

Ventilatory management of patients with acute respiratory failure with decreased FRC and lung compliance is more difficult. Occasionally, lung compliance may deteriorate so that patients cannot support adequate respiration and must have mechanical ventilatory support. Even though mechanical support may be necessary at first, CPAP often lessens this need by increasing both FRC and lung compliance, thereby reducing the work of breathing. Thus, only a very short period of mechanical ventilatory support may be required.[65]   Thereafter, spontaneous respiration with CPAP and a slightly increased inspired oxygen concentration are usually the only required therapeutic adjuncts.

This approach is beneficial in several respects. Weaning from mechanical ventilatory support may occur within minutes or hours of the initiation of therapy.(67) Patients who require controlled mechanical ventilation with PEEP often need intravenous infusions of large amounts of fluids to stabilize cardiovascular function.(23) Such intravascular fluid loading may increase pulmonary capillary hydrostatic pressure and cause deterioration in pulmonary function secondary to increased lung water, when weaning from mechanical support is attempted. If spontaneous breathing is allowed to persist in the early phase of therapy and mechanical ventilatory support is discontinued as soon as possible, intravascular volume expansion often is unnecessary and CPAP and oxygen may be withdrawn more rapidly. Barotrauma probably is caused by increased airway pressure during mechanical inspiration. If patients are weaned rapidly from mechanical ventilation, exposure to elevated airway pressure and barotrauma may be reduced. Available evidence suggests that barotrauma is lessened when IMV is used.(65)

Controlled mechanical ventilation has long been the standard form of therapy for patients with lung contusion and flail chest.(66) However, the efficacy of such therapy has been questioned.(67) The treatment of patients with severe chest trauma should be similar to that just described. Patients with lung injury and flail chest often cannot breathe spontaneously with ambient airway pressure because of the reduction in lung compliance. Elevation of airway pressure with CPAP may increase FRC and lung compliance, so that mechanical ventilatory support is unnecessary.(68) In such cases, stabilization of the chest wall occurs without mechanical ventilation. However, if the chest wall is very unstable, mechanical ventilatory support should not be discontinued. Thus, the appropriate function of mechanical ventilation in the treatment of chest trauma should be to allow immobilization of the chest wall, but only until lung compliance improves enough that spontaneous respiration can occur without disruption of unstable segments. In many instances, mechanical ventilatory support can be discontinued within a matter of hours. Only in the rarest cases, when totally unstable chest wall segments make spontaneous respiration ineffectual, is mechanical

ventilatory support necessary for more than a week.(68)
These patients should be weaned from mechanical ventilation,
oxygen and CPAP according to evaluation of gas exchange an
pulmonary mechanics, as outlined previously.

Ventilatory support of patients with acute exacerbation
of chronic obstructive lung disease is difficult. These
patients have a high rate of mortality, and their clinical
course often is marked by extreme fluctuation in blood
pressure, barotrauma, electrolyte imbalance, and other
undesirable side effects of mechanical ventilatory
support.(69) Weaning them from mechanical support often is
hampered by respiratory and metabolic alkalosis,
malnutrition, and sedation. Although currently popular,
allowing patients to "rest" with mechanical ventilation may
not be therapeutic. The longer mechanical ventilation is
maintained, the smaller is the chance of survival. Within
24 to 48 hours, the cause of the acute respiratory failure
usually is resolving, so that such a rest is unnecessary.
Furthermore, controlling the patient's respiration and
administering sedatives often leads to problems with
weaning. Using IMV we have developed the following clinical
approach. A patient with chronic obstructive lung disease
often has a hypoxemic drive to breathe. Therefore, the
initial inspired oxygen concentration usually does not
exceed 30 percent. Spontaneous respiration is encouraged.
If mechanical ventilation is required, the initial
ventilator rate is low, in most cases no more than 2 or 3
breaths per minute, with a tidal volume of 10 ml/kg. This
amount of support usually results in a slow, but consistent
fall in $PaCO_2$ and an increase in arterial pH. In this
manner, rapid reduction in $PaCO_2$ and alkalosis may be
avoided.(70) Such patients usually have increased FRC and
lung compliance. Therefore, PEEP may not improve V_A/Q.
Once ventilatory support has been instituted, a vigorous
regimen of bronchodilation and tracheo-bronchial toilet is
initiated. As the patient improves, mechanical ventilation

can be withdrawn rapidly. When IMV has been reduced to zero, the patient should be extubated without a prolonged trial of spontaneous respiration.

SUMMARY

Respiratory therapy should be directed at underlying pathology, not symptomatology. Mechanical ventilation, oxygen, and CPAP therapy should be administered to patients in independently prescribed amounts. Removal should follow suit. The method of determining optimal mechanical ventilation, oxygen, and CPAP is not unlike that recommended for many other therapeutic modalities. Each should be applied to achieve a predetermined goal, each should be continually re-evaluated, and each should be withdrawn when no longer required. Optimal CPAP should be applied to improve matching of ventilation and perfusion and to assist lung mechanics so that the requirement of oxygen and mechanical ventilation is reduced. Reduced inspired oxygen may promote resistance to atelectasis and allow more rapid discontinuation of mechanical ventilation and CPAP. Minimal mechanical ventilatory support will eliminate iatrogenic respiratory alkalosis, and improve distribution of ventilation. This approach minimizes the detrimental effects of mechanical ventilation on acid-base balance and cardiovascular function, as well as decreasing the possibility of barotrauma. Sixteen years of prospective evaluation have demonstrated numerous clinical advantages of IMV. This approach has simplified the clinical management of patients with compromised respiratory function and has decreased morbidity and mortality.

1. Campbell EJM, Agostoni E, Davis JN. The Respiratory Muscles: Mechanical and Neural Control. 2nd ed., Philadelphia. WB Saunders, 1970.
2. Fenn WO, Rahn H (eds.). Handbook of Physiology, Section 3. Respiration, Vol. I. Washington, D.C. American Physiological Soc., 1959.
3. Nunn JF. Applied Respiratory Physiology. 2nd ed., London, Boston, Butterworth, 1977.
4. Shapiro BA. In: Critical Care: State of the Art, Vol. II. Shoemaker WC, Thompson WL (eds.) Fullerton, California. The Society of Critical Care Medicine, 1980, p. II(C):1-53.
5. Nunn JF. Applied Respiratory Physiology. 2nd ed., London, Boston, Butterworth, 1977; p. 112-43.
6. Nunn JF. Applied Respiratory Physiology. 2nd ed., London, Boston, Butterworth, 1977; p. 45-73.
7. Chapin JC, Downs JB, Douglas ME, Murphy EJ, Ruiz BC. Arch Surg 1979; 114:1193-97.
8. Nunn JF. Applied Respiratory Physiology. 2nd ed., London, Boston, Butterworth, 1977; p. 74-111.
9. Bynum LJ, Wilson JE III, Pierce AK. J Appl Physiol 41:341-347, 1976.
10. Rehder K, Sessler AD, Rodarte JR. J Appl Physiol 42:391-402, 1977.
11. Rehder K, Knopp TJ, Brusasco V, Didier EP. Am Rev Respir Dis 124:392-396, 1981.
12. Froese AB, Bryan AC. Anesthesiology 41:242-55, 1974.
13. Nunn JF. Applied Respiratory Physiology. 2nd Ed., London, Boston, Butterworth, 1977; p. 177-208.
14. Downs JB, Mitchell LA. Crit Care Med 4:295-300, 1976.
15. Downs JB, Douglas ME. In: Intermittent Mandatory Ventilation. Kirby RR, Graybar GB (eds.). Int Anesthesiol Clin 18(2):81-95, 1980.
16. Downs JB, Marston AW. Crit Care Med 5:112-14, 1977.
17. Llewellyn MA, Swyer PR. Br J Anaesth 43:926-31, 1971.
18. Downs JB, Douglas ME, Ruiz BC, Miller NL. Crit Care Med 7:5-8, 1979.
19. Downs JB, Perkins HM, Modell JL. Arch Surg 109:519-23, 1974.
20. Campbell EJM, Agostoni E, Davis JN. The Respiratory Muscles: Mechanics and Neural Control. 2nd Ed., Philadelphia. WB Saunders, 1970; p. 115-142.
21. Nunn JF. Applied Respiratory Physiology. 2nd Ed., London, Boston, Butterworth, 1977; p. 144-176.
22. Millbern SM, Downs JB, Jumper LC, Modell JH. Arch Surg 113:1441-43, 1978.
23. Qvist J, Pontoppidan H, Wilson RS, Lowenstein E, Laver MB. Anesthesiology 42:45-55, 1975.
24. Downs JB, Douglas ME, Sanfellippo PM, Stanford W, Hodges MR. Anesth Analg 56:88-96, 1977.
25. Downs JB. Crit Care Med 4:207-10, 1976.
26. Mead J, Gaensler EA. J Appl Physiol 14:81-3, 1959.

206

27. Milic-Emili J, Mead J, Turner JM, Galuser EM. J Appl Physiol 19:207-11, 1964.
28. Sturgeon CL Jr, Douglas ME, Downs JB, Dannemiller FJ. Anesth Analg 56:633-41.
29. Weinstein ME, Rice CL, Peters RM, Virgilio RW. J Trauma 18: 231-35, 1978.
30. Kirby RR, Perry JC, Calderwood HW, Ruiz BC, Lederman DS. Anesthesiology 43:533-39, 1975.
31. Marquez JM, Douglas ME, Downs JB, Wu WH, Mantini EL, Kuck EJ, Calderwood HW. Anesthesiology 50:393-98, 1979.
32. Nunn JF. Applied Respiratory Physiology. 2nd Ed., London, Boston, Butterworth; 1977 p. 209-31.
33. Downs JB, Klein EF Jr, Modell JH. Anesth Analg 52:210-15, 1973.
34. Suter PM, Fairley HB, Isenberg MD. N Engl J Med 292:284-89, 1975.
35. Kirby RR, Downs JB, Civetta JM, Modell JH, Dannemiller FJ, Klein EF Jr, Hodges M. Chest 67:156-63, 1975.
36. Shapiro BA, Harrison RA, Walton JR, Davison R. Respir Care 21:521-25, 1976.
37. Heenan TJ, Downs JB, Douglas ME, Ruiz BC, et al. Chest 77:598-602, 1978.
38. Baratz RA, Philbin DM, Patterson RW. Anesthesiology 34:510-13, 1971.
39. Kumar A, Pontoppidan H, Baratz RA, Laver MB. Anesthesiology 40:215-21, 1974.
40. Landmark SJ, Knopp TJ, Rehder K, Sessler AD. J Appl Physiol 43:993-1000, 1977.
41. Zarins CK, Bayne CG, Rice Cl, et al. J Surg Res 22 (3):299-304, 1977.
42. Briscoe WA, Cree EM, Filler J, Houssax HEJ, Cournand A. J Appl Physiol 15:785-95, 1960.
43. Wagner PD. In: Anesthesia and Respiratory Function. Kafer ER (ed.) Int Anesthesiol Clin 15(2):81-111, 1977.
44. West JB. Anesthesiology 41:124-38, 1974.
45. West JB. Anesth Analg 54:409-18, 1975.
46. Suter PM, Fairley HB, Schlobohm RM. Anesthesiology 43:617-27, 1975.
47. Douglas ME, Downs JB, Dannemiller FJ, Hodges MR, Munson ES. Anesth Analg 55:688-95, 1976.
48. Barany JS, Saltzman AR, Locke RA. Chest 74-34-38, 1978.
49. Strauss HW, Hurley PJ, Rhodes BA, Wagner HN Jr. J Lab Clin Med 74:597-607, 1969.
50. Tobin CE. Thorax 21:197-204, 1966.
51. Balchum OJ, Jung RC, Turner AF, et al. In: Proceedings of the Ninth Annual Aspen Emphysema Conference, Aspen, Colorado, 223-38, 1968.
52. Register SD, Downs JB, Stock, MC, Kirby RR. Crit Care Med 15:598-601, 1987.
53. Gherini S, Peters RM, Virgilio RW. Chest 76:251-6, 1979.

54. Douglas ME, Downs JB. Anesth Analg 57:347-50, 1978.
55. Greenbaum DM, Miller JE, Eross B, Snyder JV, Grenvik A, Safar P. Chest 69:615-20, 1976.
56. Mitchell LA, Downs JB, Dannemiller FJ. Anesthesiology 43:583-6, 1975.
57. Barach Al, Martin J, Eckman M. Ann Intern Med 12:754-95, 1988.
58. Burford TH, Burbank B. J Thorac Surg 14:415-24, 1945.
59. Jensen NK. Dis Chest 22:319-46, 1952.
60. Ashbaugh DG, Petty TL, Bigelow DG, et al. J Thorac Cardiovasc Surg 57:31-41, 1969.
61. Rose DM, Downs JB, Hennan TJ. Crit Care Med (9): 79-82, 1981.
62. Downs JB, Klein EF Jr., Desautels D, Modell JH, Kirby RR. Chest 64:331-5, 1973.
63. Chiang H, Pontoppidan H, Wilson RS, et al. In: Abstracts of the 1973 Annual Meeting of the American Society of Anesthesiologists. San Francisco, California, p. 211-212, 1973.
64. Andersen JB, Kann T, Rasmussen JP, et al. Am Rev Respir Dis Annual Meeting Supplement. (Abstract) 117(4): 89-90, 1978.
65. Douglas ME, Downs JB. Chest 71:18-23, 1977.
66. Avery EE, Morch ET, Benson DW. J Thorac Surg 32:291-309, 1956.
67. Trinkle JK, Richardson JD, Franz JL, Grover FL, Aron KV, Holmstrom FMG. Ann Thorac Surg 19:355-63, 1975.
68. Downs JB (commentor), Parham AM, Yarbrough DR III, Redding JS. Editorial comment. Arch Surg 113:903, 1978.
69. Kilburn KH. Ann Intern Med 65:977-84, 1966.
70. Downs JB, Block AJ, Vennum KB. Anesth Analg 53:437-41, 1974.

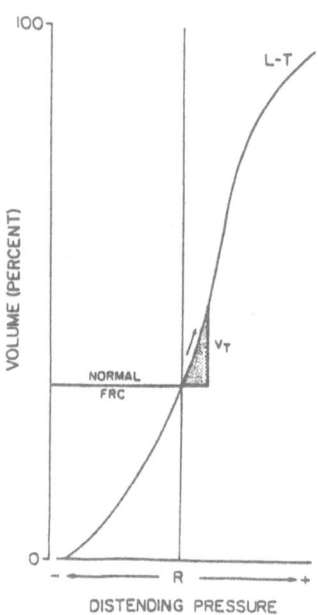

FIG. 1. Normal pressure-volume curve of the lung-thorax (L-T). Volume as a percent of total lung capacity, is plotted as a function of distending pressure. Pressure R corresponds to ambient airway pressure. During inspiration, distending pressure. Pressure R corresponds to ambient airway pressure. During inspiration, distending pressure is increased and lung volume (VT) increases from normal functional residual capacity (FRC).

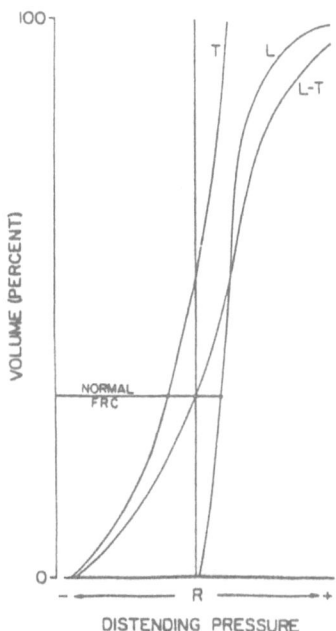

FIG. 2. Normal pressure-volume curve of the thorax (T),
lung (L), and lung-thorax (L-T). Volume, as a percent of
total lung capacity, is plotted as a function of distending
pressure. Distending pressure R occurs when airway pressure
is ambient. When the distending pressure of the lung-thorax
is zero, the distending pressure of the lung is equal, but
opposite, to that of the thorax. These equal counterforces
are responsible for determining and maintaining FRC.

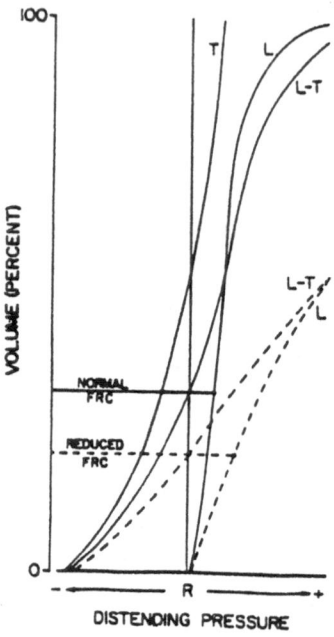

FIG 3. Normal pressure-volume curve of the thorax (T),
lung (L), and lung-thorax (L-T) (solid lines). Abnormal
pressure-volume curves of the lung (L) and lung-thorax (L-T)
(dotted lines). Distending pressure R occurs when airway
pressure is ambient. The abnormally right-shifted
pressure-volume curve of the lung results in a new
pressure-volume curve for the lung-thorax, and reduction in
functional residual capacity (FRC).

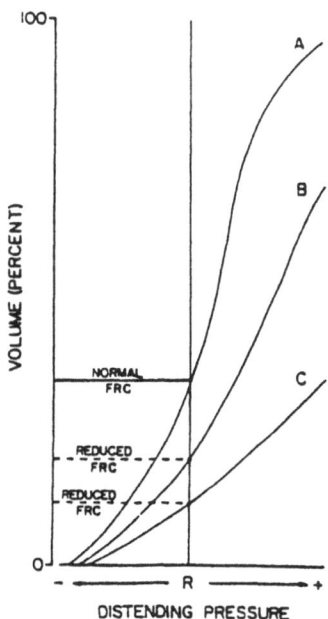

FIG 4. Pressure-volume curves of the lung-thorax. Volume,
as a percent of total lung capacity, is plotted as a
function of distending pressure. Distending pressure R
occurs when airway pressure is ambient. Curve A represents
a normal pressure-volume relationship for the lung-thorax.
Curves B and C are shifted to the right. It should be noted
that each curve results in a reduced functional residual
capacity (FRC).

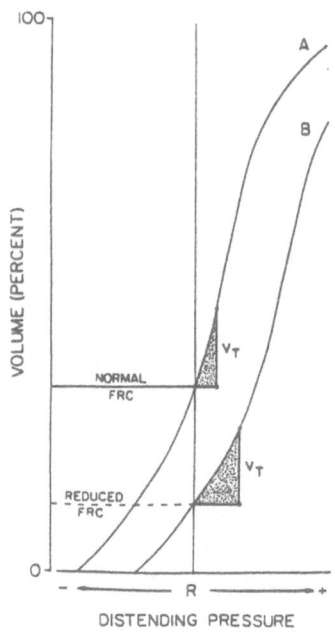

<u>**FIG 5.**</u> Pressure-volume curves of the lung-thorax. Volume, as a percent of total lung capacity, is plotted as a function of distending pressure. Distending pressure R occurs when airway pressure is ambient. Curve A represents a normal pressure-volume relationship and B represents a right-shifted curve.

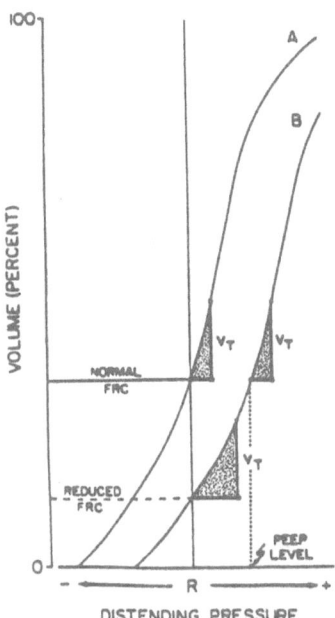

FIG 6. Pressure-volume curves of the lung-thorax. These curves are equivalent to those illustrated in Fig 5. When distending pressure is increased by application of positive airway pressure (PEEP), FRC can be normalized. When FRC is increased, the expenditure of work for tidal breathing may be reduced to a value which is nearly normal.

HFJV, PS, IRV, MMV, APRV, "NEW" VENTILATORY MODES

STEVEN J. ALLEN

Department of Anesthesiology, Center for Microvascular and
Lymphatic Studies, The University of Texas Medical School at
Houston, 6431 Fannin, Houston, Texas

INTRODUCTION

Positive pressure ventilation has been a mainstay in the
treatment of respiratory failure since the 1950's. However, conventional mechanical ventilation has been associated with a number of
problems including cardiovascular depression, barotrauma, increased
work of breathing, inadequate gas exchange and interference with
weaning. A number of investigators have attempted to develop new
forms of mechanical ventilation that address these problems. In
this review we will briefly discuss the progress of four modes of
mechanical ventilation.

MANDATORY MINUTE VENTILATION

Intermittent mandatory ventilation (IMV) and t-tube trials are
common methods for the weaning of patients from mechanical ventilatory support. Both techniques involve a time interval of
ventilatory support reduction followed by some type of evaluation
by a health care provider as to whether the wean should continue.
Mandatory minute ventilation (MMV) has been advocated as a better
technique for weaning patients. Essentially, a minimum amount of
minute ventilation is set on an appropriately equipped ventilator.
The machine then monitors the spontaneous tidal volume and
respiratory rate of the patient. If the patient fails to breathe
sufficiently to meet the set minute ventilation, the ventilator
provides breaths. During a successful wean, the ventilator reduces
support as the patient assumes more of his own ventilation, with

T. H. Stanley and R. J. Sperry (eds.), Anesthesia and the Lung, 215–219.
© 1989 by Kluwer Academic Publishers.

the result of an automatic wean. A potential problem may arise in the patient who is breathing rapidly with shallow breaths, thus generating an "adequate" minute ventilation despite persistence of respiratory failure. Although initially suggested in 1977 (1), no clinical trials have yet demonstrated the superiority of MMV (or for that matter any other wean technique) over IMV.

PRESSURE SUPPORT

Both IMV and assist-control ventilation have been shown to increase the patient's work of breathing (WOB). Ventilator imposed work may impair a patient's ability to wean. The development of pressure support (PS) has been aimed at compensating for the increased WOB due to 1) flow resistance in ventilator tubing and endotracheal tube, 2) opening the demand valve, and 3) compensating for the inadequate flow rates after the demand valve opens. PS is a form of pressure limited assisted ventilation. When the patient begins a spontaneous breath while on CPAP or IMV, he reduces the airway pressure. The reduction in airway pressure either opens a demand valve or diverts a continuous flow of gas. Without PS, the tidal volume depends on maintenance of the reduced airway pressure. When PS is instituted, the drop in airway pressure also triggers a flow of gas sufficient to increase the airway pressure to a preset level, typically +10 to +20 cm H_2O. This results in an increase in tidal volume related to the level of PS. When the flow of gas increases below some set amount, signaling end inspiration, the pressure assist ends. Patients on IMV reported being more comfortable when PS was added (2). As expected with the institution of partial ventilatory assist, studies have documented a decrease in WOB in postoperative and ICU patients (3).

The main difficulty of PS and any form of ventilatory assist is how much assist to administer. Ideally, we want to compensate for mechanically induced WOB but we still have the patient assume as much of his ventilatory needs as is reasonable. If PS is set too high, the technique becomes pressure limited assisted ventilation, and the patient is essentially completely supported. On the other hand, if PS is set too low, respiratory fatigue may develop. Much work needs to be done to determine when and to what degree PS is appropriate.

AIRWAY PRESSURE RELEASE VENTILATION

Patients with severe respiratory failure are traditionally treated with PEEP and tidal volumes of 10-15 ml/kg, which may result in markedly elevated airway pressures in low compliant lungs. Airway pressure elevations are thought to be the cause of cardiovascular depression and barotrauma. Airway pressure release ventilation (APRV) has been developed in an attempt to maintain gas exchange with lower airway pressures. Similar to conventional ventilator management, some level of positive airway pressure is maintained between breaths. Spontaneous breaths by the patient are similar to those in a CPAP circuit. However, with APRV, regular and transient decrease in the CPAP level occur, resulting in temporary lung deflation. Thus, the periodic lung deflations provide for CO_2 removal and the positive airway pressure between airway pressure releases maintains FRC and PaO_2. This technique results in a lower peak airway pressure compared with traditional ventilator management (3).

Only preliminary data is currently available concerning the efficacy of APRV. Experimentally, APRV is associated with improved gas exchange when compared to IPPV with similar mean airway pressure, respiratory frequency, and tidal volume (4). Patient studies have documented the ability of APRV to adequately ventilate postoperative patients (5).

INVERSE RATIO VENTILATION (PRESSURE CONTROL)

The term inverse ratio ventilation (IRV) describes a type of mechanical ventilation where the inspiratory time is 3-4 times the expiratory time. This is done by a combination of prolonging the inspiratory time and adding an inspiratory hold. IRV appears to maintain oxygenation by maintaining FRC during inspiration rather than during expiration. The effect of this manipulation of ventilatory pattern is to avoid the markedly elevated peak inspiratory pressures often seen with traditional ventilatory management. The airway pressure contour of IRV is similar to APRV in that, between machine "breaths," the airway pressure is held at some elevated level which is transiently decreased by the machine at set intervals. However, IRV does not allow the patient to breathe spontaneously. Thus, IRV is to APRV as assist-control ventilation is to IMV.

Clinical studies have not shown an overwhelming benefit of IRV when compared to IPPV. Cole, et. al. (6) found that an I:E of 4:1 resulted in a reduction in pulmonary shunt similar to that produced with a mean PEEP of about 13 cm H2O in patients with acute respiratory failure. However, oxygen delivery was decreased by both of these interventions. They found that an I:E of 1.1:1 or 1.7:1 produced an overall increases in oxygen delivery largely due to improved oxygenation and negligible cardiovascular effects.

HIGH FREQUENCY VENTILATION

The term high frequency ventilation (HFV) covers an ever increasing number of ventilator designs that deliver low tidal volumes at supraphysiologic rates. Similar to other new forms of mechanical ventilation, investigators have sought to find some form of HFV that provides adequate gas exchange but does not induce cardiovascular depression or barotrauma.

High Frequency Positive Pressure Ventilation (HFPPV) was developed by Sjostrand in the later 1960's. It is a volume preset ventilator that has negligible dead space and internal compliance. Thus, the machine generated tidal volume is not lost in the ventilator or circuit. Limited studies in patients have been performed with little evidence to show superiority of HFPPV over conventional ventilation.

High Frequency Jet Ventilation (HFJV) has been used extensively in this country for a variety of indications. The technique involves the injection of gas at 10 to 40 psi into a 14 gauge needle placed at the elbow connector of an IMV ventilator circuit. The passage of gas through the needle results in a marked decrease in pressure but a tremendous increase in gas velocity.

The action of this high speed gas is to draw additional gas from the IMV circuit. This additional gas may constitute the majority of the tidal volume.

Although HFJV has been suggested as being beneficial in a number of clinical situations, such as pulmonary edema, thoracic surgery, neurosurgery, increased intracranial pressure, upper airway surgery, bronchoscopy, ARDS, and tracheomalacia, the FDA has approved HFJV only for the treatment of airway disruption. Disadvantages of HFJV include tracheal mucosal damage if humidification of the injected gas is not optimal and the variable tidal volume that results when lung compliance changes.

High Frequency Oscillation (HFO) is delivered by a piston moving back and forth within a cylinder. As opposed to HFPPV and HFJV, both inspiration and expiration are active. Also unlike the other forms of HFV, the tidal volumes generated by HFO are typically below that of the dead space. Nonetheless, adequate gas exchange can be maintained in normal individuals as well as in a number of disease states. Whether HFO offers improvement to patients over conventional ventilation has yet to be determined.

REFERENCES

1. Hewlett, A.M., Platt, A.S. and Terry, V.G. Anaesthesia 32:163, 1977.
2. MacIntyre, N.R. Chest 89:677-683, 1986.
3. Viale, J.P., Annat, G.J., Bouffard, Y.M,. Delafosse, B.X., Bertrand, O.M. and Motin, J.P. Chest 93:506-509, 1988.
4. Stock, M.C., Downs, J.B. and Frolicher, D.A. Crit. Care Med. 15:462-466, 1987.
5. Stock (Personal Communication).
6. Cole, A.G.H., Weller, S.F. and Sykes, M.K. Int. Care Med. 10:227-232, 1984.

ADULT RESPIRATORY DISTRESS SYNDROME

Roger C. Bone, M.D.

The adult respiratory distress syndrome (ARDS) was described as a clinical entity in 1967.[1] The mortality in early reports was as high as 70%. This was disappointing since the entity was shown to be common (estimated as high as 150,000) per year in the United States), and potentially reversible.

Positive End Expiratory Pressure

The application of Positive End Expiratory Pressure has been an integral component in the treatment of adult respiratory failure. Ashbaugh and Petty popularized its use in the management of adult patients with diffuse lung injury (ARDS) over 15 years ago.[2] PEEP is still a mainstay in the treatment of diffuse lung processes since it supports the PaO_2 and allows reduction in the FIO_2. There are excellent comprehensive reviews on the use of PEEP to which the interested reader is referred for a more detailed discussion.[3-14]

Positive End Expiratory Pressure produces an increase in the alveolar and airway pressure at the end of expiration to levels greater than the atmospheric pressure. Thus, a continuous positive distending pressure is produced across the alveolar and airway walls. This results in the maintenance of patency in many closed or atelectactic gas exchange units through the process of recruitment.[4-6] Areas of shunt and ventilation/perfusion mismatch may be improved resulting in improved oxygenation.[4-6] Fluid filled alveoli may also be stabilized by allowing the fluid to occupy a relatively flat layer on the alveolar wall and, thus, would permit improved gas exchange.[4] The use of PEEP does not decrease the amount of extravascular lung water and, in fact, lung water may actually increase at high lung volumes.[4,15]

T. H. Stanley and R. J. Sperry (eds.), Anesthesia and the Lung, 221–232.

The beneficial effects of PEEP therapy (Table 1) include an increase in functional residual capacity, an increase in pulmonary compliance, a decreased shunt fraction (Qs/Qt), an increased PaO_2 for a given FIO_2, and possibly conservation of alveolar surfactant and the reduction of alveolar surface tension.[34,4] There may be a decrease in intrapulmonary shunting associated with the decreased cardiac output produced by high levels of PEEP.[4] These attributes of PEEP therapy have made it a standard in the treatment of respiratory failure secondary to diffuse parenchymal lung disease. PEEP therapy helps to improve several of the physiologic alterations associated with diffuse lung injury, but there are no data to substantiate that PEEP is anything more than supportive therapy. Despite this aggressive supportive therapy, there has been no appreciable change in survival over the past 17 years in the management of ARDS. Positive End Expiratory Pressure has been advocated in the treatment of flail chest and mechanical dysfunction of the chest, the Infant Respiratory Distress Syndrome, during the post-operative period to improve oxygenation, and in the treatment of obstructive sleep apnea.[3] Several reports have suggested that the early use of PEEP might protect a susceptible patient from developing ARDS.[35-37,16,17] This has been the topic of much controversy and will be a difficult issue to resolve because of the heterogeneity of the ARDS syndrome. In an attempt to answer the question, Pepe and co-workers randomized 92 mechanically ventilated patients at risk to develop ARDS to receive either no PEEP (control group) or cmH$_2$0 PEEP).[17] No effect on the incidence of ARDS or other associated complications were noted between the two study groups. Thus, the value of prophylactic PEEP in patients at high risk for the development of ARDS remains to be proven.

Another controversial issue in PEEP therapy has been the proper level of PEEP to administer.[18-20] Most would agree that PEEP should be increased or decreased in small increments and that the patient's cardiac output and tissue oxygen delivery need to be monitored during this therapy.[34] If the cardiac output falls, it must be supported with volume infusions and inotropic agents.[8] Suter defined "optimal PEEP" as the level of PEEP that produced the maximal pulmonary compliance.[18] Gallagher and associates described the "best PEEP" as that amount of PEEP that reduces the intrapulmonary shunt fraction to less than 15 percent of the cardiac output.[19] Kirby defined the "optimum PEEP" as the highest level of PEEP that produces a maximum decrease in shunt without a detrimental effect on the cardiac output.[20] Considering these recommendations, the ideal level of PEEP appears to be that amount that allows the inspired oxygen concentration to be reduced to less toxic ranges and still maintain adequate tissue oxygen delivery.[34]

Unfortunately, the use of positive end expiratory pressure also has some undesirable effects. Intra-alveolar pressure may exceed intracapillary pressure and result in an increase in VD/VT (dead space ventilation). There may also be a decrease in cardiac output and organ perfusion. While the use of PEEP is usually associated with an increase in the PaO_2, there may be a fall in the PaO_2 as a result of the decrease in cardiac output, alveolar overdistention, or an increase in pulmonary arterial resistance and decreased pulmonary capillary size.[3,4,8,21,22] Blood may also be diverted from the well preserved and ventilated lung unit to poorly ventilated units resulting in an increased shunt. PEEP may elevate cerebral venous pressure and intra-cranial pressure, both of which may produce cerebral dysfunction.[4] As previously stated PEEP does not decrease extravascular lung water, but it can signifi-cantly decrease intravascular pulmonary fluid volume as a consequence of the reduction in cardiac output.[23,24] The PEEP related reduction in cardiac output is primarily on the basis of a decrease in venous return caused by the elevation in intrathoracic pressure.[25] Other hemodynamic effects of PEEP include an increase in pulmonary vascular resistance, a decrease in left ventricular afterload, decreased myocardial blood flow, and altered geometry and compliance of the right and left ventricles.[25-30] High levels of PEEP we found to gradually increase the radius of septal curvature and progressively decrease the dimensions of the left ventricle at both end-diastole and end-systole.[30] Equalization of the right and left ventricular transmural end-diastolic pressures were also noted.[30] The reduction in cardiac output with PEEP therapy subsequently leads to a decrease in hepatic, adrenal, bronchial, fundal mucosa, hepatic, renal, coronary, and subendocardial arterial blood flow.[31,32] The renal blood flow was found to decrease 32% in one study of PEEP and renal function.[33] Coupled with this decrease in glomerular filtration rate, a 33% decrease in sodium excretion, and a 26% decrease in potassium excretion.[33] All of these changes returned to baseline levels when PEEP was stopped. There was an ADH like effect associated with PEEP therapy.[33] Initially the water was retained on the basis of the hemodynamic impairment of renal function, which eventually led to an increase in plasma renin, aldosterone, and ADH secretion.[33]

The use of PEEP may predispose the patient to pulmonary barotruma (Table 40, especially when large tidal volumes are used.[25] The physician needs to be

aware of this potential complication and realize that a
tension Pneumothorax may develop quite rapidly in a
patient ventilated with PEEP. Despite the potential for
PEEP to reduce cardiac output and produce pulmonary
barotrauma, PEEP therapy does have a beneficial role in
the management of respiratory failure secondary to
diffuse parenchymal lung disease. When using PEEP
attention must be directed to the maintenance of organ
perfusion and function. At present there is no evidence
that PEEP decreases extravascular lung water or prevents
the development of ARDS in susceptible patients. The
primary goal of PEEP therapy is, therefore, to obtain an
adequate arterial oxygen saturation on a nontoxic
FIO_2, while maintaining cardiac output and tissue
oxygen delivery.

Differential Lung Ventilation

When gas is administered under positive pressure it
tends to follow the path of least resistance or toward
areas of greater compliance. When dealing with diffuse
lung processes this does not present a problem; however,
in the case of unilateral lung disease where there is a
great disparity between the compliance of the two lungs,
a problem with oxygenation may result. The pathophysiologic mechanism for the oxygenation defect is the
creation of a larger West Zone I in the more compliant
lung. The more compliant lung will receive the larger
volume of the tidal volume and the greater pressure from
the ventilator breath. The resultant increase in
alveolar pressure may lead to a West Zone I formation,
where the alveolar pressure (PA) exceeds both the
arterial (Pa) and the venous (Pv) pressures. The
resultant ventilation-perfusion imbalance may also be
accompanied by areas of shunting as the blood flow is
divered toward the less ventilated lung. This process
is amplified when high inflation pressures of PEEP are
used since the gradient between the compliance of the
two lungs is further increased.

To overcome the difficulties of ventilating
patients with unilateral lung disease the technique of
differential lung ventilation was developed. Differential lung ventilation is not required in the treatment
of all patients with unilateral lung disease who require
mechanical ventilation, but it is a resource for chose
patients who have compromised oxygenation on the basis
of the pressure changes described above. The technique
was introduced in a synchronized fashion in 1950 by
Bjork and Carlens for use with operative patients.[10]
Since that report there have been a number of case
reports detailing the use of differential lung ventilation in either a synchronized or an asynchronized
mode.[11-14]

When using differential lung ventilation a double lumen endotracheal tube is required. Each lung is then connected to a separate ventilator which may then be synchronized to administer the inspiratory and expiratory cycles together or they may act independently (asynchronously). Differential lung ventilation has been suggested to be of value in maintaining adequate gas exchange in patients with broncho-pleural fistulae,[14] in the reexpansion of an atelectatic lung,[12] and in the treatment of unilateral pneumonia, pulmonary edema, pulmonary hemorrhage, or aspiration pneumonitis.[11,13] Theoretically, cardiac output may be worse with the use of asynchronous ventilation. However, Hillman found no problem with cardiac output in four patients treated with asynchronous lung ventilation and three of the four improved.[13] The use of asynchronous lung ventilation may also interfere with the interpretation of pulmonary artery catheter pressures.[13]

High Frequency Ventilation

A relatively new ventilatory technique involves the use of smaller than usual tidal volumes and faster rates to accomplish mechanical ventilation. The rate used is usually more than four times the normal ventilatory rate for the individual and in adults the rate may vary from 1-100 Hz (60-6000 breaths per minute). The usual principle of mechanical ventilation is to use a volume of air that is greater than the dead space and a rate that approximates the normal resting respiratory rate so that normal ventilation is achieved. In high frequency ventilation the tidal volumes are usually much smaller than the dead space volume and much faster rates are utilized. There are three basic types of high frequency ventilation in use today; high frequency positive pressure ventilation (rates of 60-120 bpm), high frequency jet ventilation (rates up to 600 bpm), and high frequency oscillation (rates up to 6000 bpm).[15]

The development of high frequency ventilation dates back to 1959 when Emerson suggested that high frequency oscillation could improve gas mixing.[16] In 1967 Oberg and Sjostrand developed high frequency positive pressure ventilation while investigating carotid reflexes.[36] There have been a vast number of subsequent studies of each of the various types of high frequency ventilation in a wide range of clinical and research trials which have confirmed the ability to achieve adequate ventilation with these techniques.[15-30] A review of these studies is beyond the scope of this discussion. Some generalities into basic mechanisms of gas exchange and the clinical uses for high frequency ventilation will follow.

Conventional ventilation is based on the delivery of a volume of gas greater than dead space volume into the tracheo-bronchial tree.[15] The gas is transported by convective flow in the larger airways and gas transport occurs through molecular diffusion in the smaller airways and the alveoli. This gas transport is somewhat enhanced by the process of cardiogenic mixing in these areas.[15] Differences in the regional compliance-resistance times constants of the lung direct the distribution and flow of the inspired gas.[15] In high frequency ventilation, a small volume of gas under high pressure is delivered to the proximal trachea. There is rapid deceleration of the pressurized gas as it mixes with gas already present in the airway and effective ventilation is accomplished through a process of augmented or enhance diffusion.[16] Effective ventilation takes place at lower peak and mean airway pressure.[17] This serves to minimize the pressure gradients through bronchopleural fistulae or major airway disruptions and, hence, maintain adequate alveolar ventilation since there will be less gas loss through the fistulous tract as compared to conventional ventilation.[17]

The ability to achieve adequate alveolar ventilation using lower airway pressures and the finding that spontaneous ventilatory efforts cease in some patients ventilated with high frequency ventilation has lead to its use in a variety of clinical situations (Table 20. High frequency positive pressure ventilation was initially utilized to facilitate the performance of direct laryngoscopy and rigid bronchoscopy.[18] High frequency ventilation may allow for the removal of the endotracheal tube from the operative field and help thoracic surgical procedures since there is cessation of respiratory motion. In patients whose respiratory drive ceases with the use of high frequency ventilation, prevention of asynchrony between the patient and the ventilator may be achieved without the use of sedative or paralyzing agents.

Pulmonary barotrauma (see ahead - Complications of mechanical ventilation) has been estimated to occur in 5-20% of mechanically ventilated patients.[43] High peak inspiratory pressures and changes in lung compliance are two of the factors implicated in the production of pulmonary barotrauma.[31] The use of high frequency ventilation is associated with a decrease in mean and peak inspiratory pressure and, thus, may be advantageous in the prevention of pulmonary barotrauma.[31] The decreased inspiratory pressures have been shown by several studies to be useful in the treatment of patients with broncho-pleural fistulae, tracheoesophageal fistulae, and major airway disruption.[16,17,21] It

may be difficult to achieve adequate alveolar ventilation in these patients using conventional ventilatory
techniques because of the loss of inspired gas through
the fistulous tract. This gas loss through the fistulous tract may also delay the closure of the fistula.
Elevated airway pressures are also transmitted, at least
to some extent, to the intrapleural space and the chest
cavity. Elevations in intrathoracic pressure can result
in impaired venous return and a subsequent decrease in
cardiac output. The lower airway and intrathoracic
pressure produced with high frequency ventilation will
produce less effect on the venous return and cardiac
output. This same reasoning may be advantageous in
patients with head injuries where it is important to
avoid elevating the intracranial pressure.

Use of high frequency ventilation requires the
expertise of experienced personnel. There are no
uniform guidelines regarding initial ventilator settings
for a given ventilator or type of patient and there may
be a protracted period of stabilizing the patient. Some
of the ventilator's lack the sophisticated alarms and
monitoring devices that we have come to rely on in the
use of conventional ventilators. There is also the
potential to develop very high working pressures in some
of the systems which is a potential danger to the
patient in the event of a malfunction.

The role of the high frequency ventilator must
still be regarded as a research tool at this point in
time. There are still some fine points of operation and
monitoring of ventilator and patient function that need
to be worked out prior to its incorporation in routine
ventilatory management. The technique does have its
current place in clinical ventilatory management in the
treatment of bronchopleural fistulae, major airway
disruption and other clinical situations in which
adequate alveolar ventilation cannot be achieved with
conventional mechanical ventilation.[15] [21] [27] [29]

Extracorporeal Membrane Oxygenation

The National Institutes of Health sponsored a
randomized multicenter trial of extracorporal membrane
oxygenation (ECMO) in the hope that this advanced
technology might improve survival. The results were
discourging; survival was not improved.[45] This negative
study was an important contribution to the literature
since if the ECMO study has been positive, every center
treating these patients would be using this costly and

labor-intensive therapy. A negative study thus introduced phase 2, the study of basic mechanisms of lung injury in this condition and experimentation in animals. Phase 3 is now underway, the application of findings in experimental animals in controlled clinical trials in humans.

Recently, forty-three patients with ARDS were treated with extracorporeal membrane lung support.[46] The methods differed from those of the ECMO study in that a low flow venous bypass was used with low frequency ventilation. The hope was that this technique would prevent damage to diseased lungs by reducing their motion. Survival was 48.8%

Other problems with this technique of therapy are its cost and its invasiveness. Most intensive care units in the United States are in smaller hospitals which, in most circumstances, do not have the capability of ECMO. The nurse/patient ratio was 1:1 and a physician or technician with expertise in ECMO was always present.[46] The daily cost of patient care was twice that of a severely ill patient requiring standard care with mechanical ventilation. As these authors indicate, the most we can expect from the "best" respiratory treatment is to support gas exchange without further damage to the lungs.[46]

REFERENCES

1. Ashbaugh DG, Bigelow DB, Petty TL, et al.: Acute respiratory distress in adults. Lancet 2:319, 1967.

2. Ashbaugh, D.G., Bigelow, D.B., Petty, T.L., et al. Acute respiratory distress in adults. Lancet 2:319, 1967.

3. Tyler, D.C. Positive end-expiratory pressure: a review. Crit Care Med 11:300-308, 1983.

4. Gong, H. Positive-pressure ventilation in the adult respiratory distress syndrome. Clin Chest Med 3:69-88, 1982.

5. Weisman, I.M., Rinaldo, J.E., Rogers, R.M. Current concepts: positive end-expiratory pressure in adult respiratory failure. NEJM 307:1381-1384, 1982.

6. Powers, S.R., Mannal, R., Neclerio, M., et al.
    Physiologic consequences of positive end-expiratory
    pressure (PEEP) ventilation. Ann Surg 178:265-272,
    1973.

7. Wayne, K.S. Positive end-expiratory pressure
    (PEEP) ventilation: A review of mechanisms and
    actions. JAMA 236:1394-1396, 1976.

8. Shapiro, B.A., Cane, R.D., Harrison, R.A. Positive
    end-expiratory pressure therapy in adults with
    special reference to acute lung injury: A review of
    the literature and suggested clinical correlations.
    Crit Care Med 12:127-141, 1984.

9. Shelhamer, J.H., Natanson, C., Parrello, J.E.
    Positive end-expiratory pressure in adults. JAMA
    251:2692-2695, 1984.

10. Simmons, D.H. Therapy of ARDS: positive end-
    expiratory pressure. Western J Med 130:229-235,
    1979.

11. Pontoppidan, H., Geffin, B., Lowenstein, E. Acute
    respiratory failure in the adult (Part 2). NEJM
    287:743-752, 1972.

12. Pontoppidan, H., Geffin, B., Lowenstein, E. Acute
    respiratory failure in the adult (Part 3). NEJM
    287:799-806, 1972.

13. Kuckelt, W., Scharfenberg, J., Mrochen, H., et al.
    Effect of PEEP on gas exchange, pulmonary mechanics
    and hemodynamics in adult respiratory distress
    syndrome (ARDS). Intensive Care Med 7:177-185,
    1981.

14. Cassan, S.M. PEEP and barotrauma. Western J Med
    131:47-48, 1979.

15. Russell, J.A., Hoeffel, J., Murray, J.F. Effect of
    different levels of positive end expiratory
    pressure on lung water content. J Appl Physiol
    53:9-15, 1982.

16. Wright, J.A., Mitchell, R.A., Snyder, W.H., III.
    Early positive end-expiratory pressure in the adult
    respiratory distress syndrome. Arch Surg
    114:497-501, 1979.

17. Pepe, P.E., Hudson, L.D., Carrico, C.J. Early
    application of positive end-expiratory pressure in
    patients at risk for the adult respiratory distress
    syndrome. NEJM 311:281-325, 1984.

18. Suter, P.M., Fairly, H.B., Isenberg, M.D. Optimum end-expiratory airway pressure in patients with acute pulmonary failure. NEJM 292:284-289, 1975.

19. Gallagher, T.J., Civetta, J.M., Kirby, R.R. Terminology update: Optimal PEEP. Crit Care Med 6:323-326, 1978.

20. Kirby, R.R., Downs, J.B., Civetta, J.M., Modell, J.H., Dannamiller, F.J., Klein, E.F., and Hodges, M. High level positive end-expiratory pressure (PEEP) in acute respiratory insufficiency. Chest 67:156-163, 1975.

21. Pesenti, A., Riboni, A., Marcolin, R., Sattinoni, L. Venous admixture (Qau/Q) and true shunt (Qs/Qt) in ARF patients: effects of PEEP at constant F_IO_2. Int Care Med 9:307-311, 1983.

22. Holzapfel, L., Robert, D., Perrin, F., Blanc, P.L., Palmier, B., Guerin, C. Static pressure-volume curves and effect of positive end expiratory pressure on gas exchange in adult respiratory distress syndrome. Crit Care Med 11:591-597, 1983.

23. Slutsky, R.A. Reduction in pulmonary blood volume during positive end-expiratory pressure. J Surg Res 35:181-187, 1983.

24. Helbert, C., Paskanik, A., Bredenberg, C.E. Effect of positive end-expiratory pressure on lung water in pulmonary edema caused by increased membrane permeability. Annals Thoracic Surg 36:42-48, 1983.

25. Bone, R.C. complications of mechanical ventilation and positive end-expiratory pressure. Resp Care 27:402-407, 1982.

26. Brown, D.R., Bazaral, M.G., Nath, P.H., et al. Canine left ventricular volume response to mechanical ventilation with PEEP. Anesthesiology 54:409-412, 1981.

27. Laver, M.B., Strass, H.W., Pohost, G.M. Right and left ventricular geometry: adjustments during acute respiratory failure. Crit Care Med 7:509-519, 1979.

28. Jacobs, H.K., Venus, B. Left ventricular regional myocardial blood flows during controlled positive pressure ventilation and positive end-expiratory pressure in dogs. Crit Care Med 11:872-875, 1983.

29. Marini, J.J., Culver, B.H., Bulter, J. Effect of positive end-expiratory pressure on canine ventricular function curves. J Appl Physiol 51:1367-1374, 1981.

30. Jardin, F., Farcot, J.C., Boisante, L., Curien, N., Margairaz, A., Bourdarias, J.P. Influence of positive end-expiratory pressure on left ventricular performance. NEJM 304:387-392, 1981.

31. Bonnet, F., Richard, C., Glaser, P., et al. Changes in hepatic flow induced by continuous positive pressure ventilation in critically ill patients. Crit Care Med 10:703-705, 1982.

32. Bredenberg, C.E., Paskanik, A.M. Relation of portal hemodynamics to cardiac output during mechanical ventilation with PEEP. Ann Surg 198:218-222, 1983.

33. Annat, G., Viale, J.P., Xuan, B.B., Aissa, O.H., Benzoni, D., Vincent, M., Gharib, C., Motin, J. Effect of PEEP ventilation on renal function, plasma renin, aldosterone, neurophysins, and pituatary ADH, and prostaglandins. Anesthesiology 58:136-141, 1983.

34. Bone, R.C. and Balk, R. Mechanical ventilation in current pulmonology. Vol. 5, Ed., Simmons, D.H. John Wiley & Sons, Inc. 201-228, 1984.

35. Valdes, M.E., Powers, S.R., JR., Shah, D.M., et al. Continuous positive airway pressure in prophylaxis of the adult respiratory distress syndrome in trauma patients. Surg Forum 29:187-198, 1978.

36. Schmidt, G.B., O'Neill, W.W., Kith, K., et al. Continuous positive airway pressure in the prophylaxis of the adult respiratory distress syndrome. Surg Gyn Obstet 143:613-618, 1976.

37. Hagyo, T., Hialt, I.M. The effect of continuous positive airway pressure on the course of respiratory distress syndrome: the benefits of early initiation. Crit Care Med 9:38-41, 1981.

38. Gedeon, A., Mebius, C. The hygroscopic condensor humidifier. Anesthesia 34:1043-1047, 1979.

39. Bone, R.C. Assisted ventilation in oxygen transport to human tissues, edited by Loeppky, J.A., Reidesel, M.L. Elsevier North Holand, Inc., 345-555, 1982.

40. Downs, J.B., Klein, E.F., Desautels, D., et al. Intermittent mandatory ventilation: a new approach to weaning patients from mechanical ventilators. Chest 64:331-335, 1973.

41. Luce, J.M., Pierson, D.J., Hudson, L.D. Intermittent mandatory ventilation. Chest 79:678-685, 1981.

42. Schachter, E.N., Tucker, D., Beck, G.J. Does intermittent mandatory ventilation accelerate weaning. JAMA 246:1210-1214, 1981.

43. McPherson, S.P. Respiratory therapy equipment. St. Louis, MO, C.V. Mosby Co., 1977.

44. Bone RC. Treatment of adult respiratory distress syndrome. A need for comparative studies. Arch Int Med 138:908, 1978.

45. Gattinoni L, Pesenti A, Mascheroni L, et al.: Low frequency positive pressure ventilation with extracorporeal CO_2 removal in acute respiratory failure:Clinical results. JAMA (this issue).

46. Zapol WM, Snider MT, Dill JD, et al.: Extra-corporeal membrane oxygenation in severe acute respiratory failure. JAMA 242:2193-2196, 1979.

HEMODYNAMICS AND THERAPY IN ARDS

WARREN M. ZAPOL, M.D.

Department of Anesthesia, Massachusetts General Hospital,
Boston, MA 02114

The pulmonary artery pressure (PAP) and vascular
resistance (PVR) are elevated in moderate and severe ARDS of
diverse etiology (1,2). This occurs despite a normal PaO_2 and
can occur within a few hours after acute lung injury. We
remain uncertain as to the precise cause of the increased PVR
but its effect, pulmonary hypertension, places a severe load
on the lung which exchanges fluid in the face of both an
increased microvascular permeability and an increased
hydrostatic pressure. Late in ARDS the PVR cannot be reduced
by infusing vasodilators (nitroprusside, phentolamine,
ibuprofen). However, early in ARDS, Snider et al. reported
that infusing nitroprusside reduced the PAP and pulmonary
capillary wedge pressure (PCWP), while increasing cardiac
output, thus vasodilation or vascular recruitment occurred
(2,3). During ARDS there was no effect on the elevated PVR of
altering PvO_2 or pH_v over a wide range of partial venoarterial
bypass flow rates using ECMO.

What is the structural basis of the elevated PVR in ARDS?
Two techniques have provided information on pulmonary vascular
alterations in ARDS. Balloon occlusion pulmonary
arteriography was employed by Greene et al. to study the
pulmonary vasculature in over 220 patients with ARDS. He
learned that 80 of the patients had multiple PA filling
defects (PAFD). These filling defects were associated with
DIC, an elevated PVR, increasing severity of ARDS, and death
of the patients (approximately 85% died). On the other hand,
ARDS patients without PAFD often survived their illness (4).

These angiographic studies were correlated with
morphologic examinations of post mortem and lung biopsy
specimens. K. Kobayashi et al. used silicone rubber
perfusions to demonstrate widespread arterial occlusions of
ARDS lungs. Greene et al. reported that most patients with
PAFD had pulmonary artery thromboembolism at autopsy. We were
surprised by the large number of PA vascular occlusions in
ARDS lungs. Jones et al. (5) and Tomashefski et al. (6)
subsequently reported that 21 of 22 ARDS lungs cast with
gelatin-barium at autopsy had thromboemboli. In addition,
Tomashefski et al. described major remodelling of the
pulmonary arteries with marked medial muscular thickening and
growth of smooth muscle into distal regions of the pulmonary

T. H. Stanley and R. J. Sperry (eds.), Anesthesia and the Lung, 233–238.
© 1989 by Kluwer Academic Publishers.

artery where muscle is not normally present. Muscle may encroach upon the lumen and increase the PVR in later stages of ARDS.

The right ventricle faces an increased afterload in ARDS. As the PAP increases this thin-walled muscular cavity must eject blood into the pulmonary artery at higher pressures. There is a general finding that in ARDS as PAP increases the right ventricular ejection fraction (RVEF) decreases. This has been confirmed by gated (7) and first pass (8,9) radionuclide studies as well as thermodilution measurements of RVEF. In late stage ARDS with the PAP greater than 40 mm Hg the patient can exhibit a low cardiac output, high PCWP and RVEDP and an enlarged poorly contracting right ventricle with a small, hyperdynamic left ventricle. Strategies to improve survival require increasing RV contractility (e.g. inotropic agent infusion) and possibly efforts to reduce the elevated PVR (e.g. thrombolytic therapy with streptokinase infusions in selected patients). Greene et al. have reported a pilot trial of streptokinase infusions in ARDS patients (10). Such supportive maneuvers may be required to buy time to allow pulmonary healing.

Two randomized prospective studies have been completed to examine if drugs can inhibit the progression of ARDS once it has developed. Bernard et al. completed a study of corticosteroid therapy in established ARDS in 99 patients, the majority with sepsis and pneumonia (control vs treated with high dose methylprednisolone) (11). There was no difference in the survival rates between the groups. A prospective study of the effects of infusing PGE_1 (30 ng/kg min) for a week was reported by Holcroft et al. (12) in patients with ARDS (mechanical ventilation with FIO_2 0.4, PEEP > 5 cm H_2O, and effective compliance < 50 ml/cm H_2O). At thirty days after the end of the infusion 15 of 21 PGE_1 patients (71%) were alive, compared with 7 of 20 placebo patients (35%), although the overall survival rate in PGE_1 patients was not statistically greater than control patients. This study of PGE_1 infusion has been repeated by a number of collaborating investigators in several countries to learn if PGE_1 is a useful therapy for ARDS. A randomized trial is purported to show no significant differences but results are not yet published. Shoemaker et al. (13) reported PGE_1 lowered the PAP and PVR in doses up to 30 ng/kg min while PaO_2 tended to increase, suggesting PGE_1 acts as an unusual pulmonary vasodilator without increasing the shunt fraction. This may be one salutary mechanism of PGE_1, as well as acting to suppress pulmonary inflammation.

Interstitial fibrosis is often progressive in ARDS. To inhibit fibrosis for periods of up to 21 days, we infused L-3,4-dehydroproline. This agent is a proline analog which reduces fibrous tissue synthesis (14). In 12 severe ARDS patients we infused L-3,4-dehydroproline 30-50 mg/kg day for

periods lasting up to three weeks, eight patients survived
(15). This drug shows promise for inhibiting interstitial
fibrosis during ARDS and may increase the survival rate.

TNF$_\alpha$

Tumor necrosis factor alpha, also known as cachectin, is
a macrophage and monocyte produced polypeptide hormone with a
sub-unit of approximately 17 kilodaltons. Recent studies
increasingly implicate TNF$_\alpha$ as a key agonist producing shock
and death following endotoxemia (16). Animal research shows
TNF$_\alpha$ appears in the circulation within minutes after endotoxin
is injected and peaks at blood levels near 0.3 μM. Of
singular significance is the finding that mice passively
immunized against this hormone are protected against the
lethal effects of endotoxin injection. Researchers are hoping
to determine whether this effect can be exploited to man's
benefit, a task made possible largely because rapid advances
in molecular biologic engineering have yielded ample amounts
of highly purified recombinant human TNF$_\alpha$ (rh-TNF$_\alpha$).
Researchers are now able to examine in vivo the effects of
infusing this hormone.

It has been determined that TNF$_\alpha$, infused intravenously
into rats and dogs in quantities similar to those produced
endogenously after endotoxin injection, causes hypotension,
metabolic acidosis, hemoconcentration and death within a few
hours (16,17). Autopsy reveals diffuse pulmonary inflammation
and hemorrhage. The similarity of these effects of cachectin
to the acute lung injury which occurs when ARDS arises in the
context of bacterial sepsis gives added importance to the
study of this hormone. Focusing on its pulmonary and systemic
effects in larger animals, we have found that infusing human
recombinant TNF$_\alpha$ (25-150 μg/kg) into sheep with a lung lymph
fistula produces immediate neutropenia and progressive
hypotension with hemoconcentration. A major fluid infusion is
required to replace the intravascular fluid loss. Progressive
increase of lung lymph flow rate occurs at an unchanged L/P
ratio. This demonstrates that rh-TNF$_\alpha$ can increase lung
permeability. A recent study suggests passive immunization to
TNF$_\alpha$ in monkeys 1-2 hours before i.v. gram negative bacterial
challenge protects against septic hypotension and death (18).
Whether treatment of humans with antibodies to TNF$_\alpha$ can
prevent septic shock or ARDS from occurring is unknown but of
great interest.

Endotoxin Neutralization by Antibodies. Gram negative
endotoxin releases mediators which cause acute lung injury,
pulmonary hypertension and increase lung microvascular
permeability. In order to fortify cells against such an
attack, we begin with the known fact that immunity to specific
bacterial types protects many animals against challenge by the
homologous bacterial species.

Ziegler et al. (19) have found that transfusion of polyclonal anti E.coli J5 human sera reversed clinical gram negative endotoxin shock. Teng et al. (20,21) recently produced a human monoclonal antibody to J5 strain E.coli. This monoclonal antibody protects rabbits from the lethal effects of many gram negative endotoxins and shields mice from gram negative bacterial infections.

A recent report by Feeley et al. (21) has shown that pretreating rats with 0.6 mg/kg of this human anti-endotoxin MAb 15 mins before infusing i.v. 3 mg/kg endotoxin prevented increased ^{99m}Tc DTPA clearance from lung into blood at 24 hours as well as the increase of serum lipid peroxidation products but did not prevent neutrophil accumulation in the lung. At present 30 major centers are assessing this human monoclonal antibody raised against J5 in a double-blind, prospective and randomized multicenter study of patients with a known source of sepsis, fever and evidence of the early onset of single organ failure. Such therapy given early during a gram negative infection may prevent the subsequent release of noxious mediators and thereby prevent ARDS (or other organ failure).

This study is sponsored by Centocor (Malvern, PA) and is also analyzing the effects of this MAb on the incidence and progression of ARDS. Another ongoing prospective randomized study of a murine MAb against E.coli J5 is being sponsored by Xoma Corp (Berkeley, CA). It is eventually hoped that neutralizing gram negative endotoxins with antibodies will prevent ARDS.

References

1. Zapol WM, and Snider MT: Pulmonary hypertension in severe acute respiratory failure. N. Engl. J. Med. 296:476-480, 1977.

2. Zapol WM, Snider MT, Rie M, Frikker M, and Quinn D: Pulmonary circulation during ARDS. In: WM Zapol and K Falke eds., Acute Respiratory Failure, in the series Lung Biology in Health and Disease. New York: Marcel Dekker, 1985, pp 241-273.

3. Snider MT, Rie MA, Lauer J, and Zapol WM: Normoxic pulmonary vasoconstriction in ARDS: detection by sodium nitroprusside (N) and isoproterenol (I) infusions. Am. Rev. Respir. Dis. 121:191, 1980 (Abstract).

4. Greene R, Boggis CRM, and Jantsch HS: Radiography and angiography of the pulmonary circulation in ARDS. In: WM Zapol and K Falke eds., Acute Respiratory Failure, in the series Lung Biology in Health and Disease. New York: Marcel Dekker, 1985, pp 275-302.

5. Jones R, Reid LM, Zapol WM, Tomashefski JF, Kirton OC, and
    Kobayashi K: Pulmonary vascular pathology: human and
    experimental studies. In: WM Zapol and K Falke eds.,
    Acute Respiratory Failure, in the series Lung Biology in
    Health and Disease. New York: Marcel Dekker, 1985, pp 23-
    160.

6. Tomashefski JF, Zapol WM, and Reid LM: The pulmonary
    vascular lesions of the adult respiratory distress
    syndrome. Am. J. Pathol. 112:112-126, 1983.

7. Laver MB, Strauss WA, and Pohost GM: Right and left
    ventricular geometry: adjustments during acute
    respiratory failure. Crit. Care Med. 7:509-519, 1979.

8. Rajagopalan B, Lowenstein E, and Zapol WM: Cardiac
    function in the adult respiratory distress syndrome. In:
    WM Zapol and K Falke eds., Acute Respiratory Failure, in
    the series Lung Biology in Health and Disease. New York:
    Marcel Dekker, 1985, pp 555-576.

9. Sibbald WJ, Driedger AA, Myers ML, Short AIK, Wells GA:
    Biventricular function in the adult respiratory distress
    syndrome. Chest 84(2): 126-134, 1983.

10. Greene R, Lind S, Jantsch H, Wilson R, Lynch K, Jones R,
    Carvalho A, Reid L, Waltman AC, Zapol W: Pulmonary
    vascular obstruction in severe ARDS: angiographic
    alterations after i.v. fibrinolytic therapy. Am. J.
    Roentgenol. 148:501-508, 1987.

11. Bernard GR, Luce JM, Sprung CL, Rinaldo JE, Tate RM,
    Sibbald WJ, Kariman K, Higgins S, Bradley R, Metz CA,
    Harris TR, Brigham KL: High-dose corticosteroids in
    patients with the adult respiratory distress syndrome. N.
    Engl. J. Med. 317:1565-1570, 1987.

12. Holcroft JW, Vassar MJ, and Weber CJ: PGE_1 and survival
    in patients with the Adult Respiratory Distress Syndrome.
    Ann. Surg. 203:371-378, 1986.

13. Shoemaker WC and Appel PL. Effects of prostaglandin E_1 in
    Adult Respiratory Distress Syndrome. Surgery 99:275-282,
    1986.

14. Salvador RA, Fiedler-Nagy C, and Coffey JW: Biochemical
    basis for drug therapy to prevent pulmonary fibrosis in
    ARDS. In: Acute Respiratory Failure, in the series Lung
    Biology in Health and Disease. New York: Marcel Dekker,
    1985, pp 477-506.

15. Zapol WM, Quinn D, Coffey J, and Salvador RA: L-3,4-dehydroproline suppression of fibrosis in ARDS: early clinical results. Am. Rev. Respir. Dis. 129:102, 1984 (Abstract).

16. Beutler B, Cerami A: Cachectin: more than a tumor necrosis factor. N. Engl. J. Med. 316:319, 1987.

17. Tracey K, Lowry SF, Fahey III TJ, Albert JD, Fond Y, Hesse D, Beutler B, Manogue KR, Calvano S, Wei H, Cerami A, Shires GT: S. Gyn. and Obst. 164:415-422, 1987.

18. Tracey KJ, Fong Y, Hesse DG, Manogue KR, Lee AT, Kuo GC, Lowry SF, Cerami A: Anti-cachectin/TNF monoclonal antibodies prevent septic shock during lethal bacteraemia. Nature 330:662-664, 1987.

19. Ziegler EJ, McCutchan A, Fierer J, Glauser MP, Sadoff JC, Douglas H, Braude AI. Treatment of gram-negative bacteremia and shock with a human antiserum to a mutant Escherichia coli. N. Engl. J. Med. 307:1225-1230, 1982.

20. Teng NN, Kaplan HS, Hebert JM, Moore C, Douglas H, Wunderlich A, Braude AI: Protection against gram-negative bacteremia and endotoxemia with human monoclonal IgM antibodies. Proc. Natl. Acad. Sci. 82:1790-1794, 1985.

21. Feeley TW, Minty BD, Scudder CM, Garet Jones J, Royston D, Teng NN: The effect of human anti-endotoxin monoclonal antibodies on endotoxin induced lung injury in the rat. Am. Rev. Respir. Dis. 135:665-670, 1987.

Septic Shock

Roger C. Bone, M.D.

Abstract

The Septic Syndrome can be defined as hypothermia (T < 96°F rectal) or hyperthermia (T > 101°F rectal), tachycardia (> 90 bpm), tachypnea (> 20 bpm), a presumed site of infection, and evidence of inadequate perfusion as evidenced by either poor or altered cerebral function, arterial hypoxia (PaO_2 < 75 mm Hg) elevated plasma lactate level, or urine output less than 0.5 ml/kg body weight/hr without corrective therapy. Thirty-six patients with the Septic Syndrome were prospectively evaluated and found to have a 39% mortality rate. Forty-seven percent of the patients were found to be bacteremic and 64% manifested at least one episode of shock (systolic blood pressure < 90 mmHg or a decrease in systolic blood pressure > 40 mmHg that is sustained for at least one hour) during their hospitalization.

Survivors had a significantly lower mean age (48.8 ± 16.3 yrs vs. 59.8 ± 7.6 yrs X ± S.D.; p < 0.02) than the nonsurvivors. There was no significant difference in the incidence of bacteremia between survivors and nonsurvivors. Shock was present twice as often in nonsurvivors as in survivors (93% vs. 45%). Nonsurvivors had a higher initial plasma lactate level, and a greater degree of multi- organ

239

T. H. Stanley and R. J. Sperry (eds.), Anesthesia and the Lung, 239–251.
© 1989 by Kluwer Academic Publishers.

failure as evidenced by an increased APACHE score (Acute Physiology and Chronic Health Evaluation) and an increased mean organ system dysfunction index.

These results indicate that the Septic Syndrome is associated with a significant mortality rate and the survival rates were not related to the presence or absence of bacteremia. The presence of shock and increased age were both associated with decreased survival rates. Nonsurvivors also exhibited a greater degree of multiorgan system dysfunction. The identification of the Septic Syndrome may allow for earlier treatment of patients with sepsis and potentially result in improved survival through prevention of shock and multiple organ system dysfunction.

Key words: Sepsis, Septic Syndrome, Septic Shock.

Sepsis is most often defined in terms of hemodynamic alterations associated with bacteremia. When shock accompanies sepsis it is referred to as septic shock. Although the exact incidence is not known, 70,000-300,000 cases of sepsis are estimated to occur in the United States each year.[1] Shock is present in approximately 40% of these patients and adversely affects survival.[2] Some authors postulate that a number of recent innovations in medical practice may have increased the likelihood of sepsis and septic shock.[1] These innovations include: aggressive oncologic chemotherapy, corticosteroid or immunosuppressive therapy for organ transplantation or inflammatory diseases,

increasing survival of patients predisposed to sepsis, and
more frequent use of invasive medical devices.(1,3)

A review of gram-negative bacteremia in 612 patients
found early institution of appropriate antibiotic treatment
reduced the fatality rate and the frequency of shock in
septic patients by approximately one-half.(2) Thus, it is
essential to recognize these severely ill patients early in
an attempt to improve overall survival. This study defines
the Septic Syndrome and prospectively evaluated patients
with the Septic Syndrome in comparison to the bacteremic
group of patients (the more classical definition of
sepsis).

Methods

This study was conducted under the guidance and
approval of the Human Research Investigations Committee of
the University of Arkansas and the Little Rock Veterans
Administration Medical Center and was part of a multi-
centered study evaluating the role of corticosteroids in,
septic shock. Patients between the age of 18 and 75 years
admitted to either the University of Arkansas for Medical
Sciences Hospital or the Little Rock Veterans Administration Medical Center from November, 1982 through June, 1984
were prospectively studied. The study population consisted
of patients who fulfilled the criteria of Septic Syndrome
and were evaluated within 4 hours of the onset of the Septic
Syndrome.

The Septic Syndrome was defined as the presence of
hypothermia (T < 96°F) or hyperthermia (T > 101°F) measured

rectally, tachycardia (> 90 bpm), tachypnea (> 20 bpm), a presummed site of infection, and evidence of inadequate perfusion as evidenced by either poor or altered cerebral function, arterial hypoxia (PaO_2 < 75 mmHg) elevated plasma lactate level, or urine output less than 30 ml/hr (< 1/2 ml/kg body weight/hr) without corrective therapy.

All of the patients were treated in the usual and customary fashion using state of the art technologic and pharmacologic interventions. The patients were followed for fourteen days unless they died or were discharged from the hospital prior to the fourteenth day. Patients who survived fourteen days or were discharged from the hospital after a full recovery prior to the fourteenth day were considered to be survivors. The various parameters monitored throughout the evaluation period included: age, presence of shock, survival, blood culture and other culture results, white blood cell count, plasma lactate, PaO_2, pH, development of the Adult Respiratory Distress syndrome (ARDS), presummed site of infection, transfusion requirement, need for Dopamine or other pressors, hemoglobin (Hg), hematocrit (Hct), platelet count, prothrombin time, partial thrombo-plastin time, temperature, serum albumin, Apache score (Acute physiology and chronic health evaluation (4)), and an organ system dysfunction score. The organ system dysfunction score was used as an index of multiple organ system disease and reflected abnormalities of liver function tests, abnormal pulmonary, renal, cardiovascular, gastrointestinal, and neurologic function. If the function was

abnormal, a score of 1 was given for that organ system, if
the function was normal, a score of 0 was given. The organ
dysfunction range was 0 to 6, with 6 reflecting multiple
organ system dysfunction.

Shock was defined as a sustained drop of at least one
hour duration of the systolic blood pressure of greater than
or equal to 40 mmHg or a resultant systolic blood pressure
less than or equal to 90 mmHg within 24 hours of the
presumptive diagnosis of severe sepsis. The hypotension was
noted in the absence of antihypertensive therapy and in the
presence of an adequate fluid challenge. The definition of
ARDS reflected the development of bilateral diffuse alveolar
infiltrates with a normal cardiac silhouette. A pulmonary
capillary wedge pressure (PCWP) less than or equal to 18
mmHg, hypoxemia ($PaO_2 < 60$ mmHg) despite high FIO_2 ($> 50\%$),
and the absence of pre-existing severe cardiopulmonary
disease resulting in the hypoxemia.

Data Analysis:

The descriptive variables were analyzed using student's
T-test and the non-descriptive variables were analyzed using
Chi-Square. The data are presented in percentage form or as
the mean plus or minus the standard deviation. Statistical
significance was defined as a $p < 0.05$.

Results:

Thirty-six patients, 29 males and 7 females, with the
septic syndrome were studied. The age range was from 21-75
years with a mean age of 53.1 ± 14.3 (X $\pm$ S.D.). Twenty-two
of the 36 patients (61%) survived. Shock was noted in 64%

(23 of 36) and 47% of the patients had at least one positive
blood culture (17 of 36). The mean initial blood chemistries
and blood gases are listed in Table 1.

Forty-seven percent of the patients were bacteremic and
would fit the more traditional definition of sepsis (Table
2). There was no significant difference between the mean age
of the bacteremic group 51.1 ± 14.6 years and the nonbacteremic group 55.0 ± 13.8 years. As a group, the bacteremic
patients tended to have a greater incidence of shock, 82%
(14/17) versus 47% (9/19), and a lower survival rate, 53%
(9/17) versus 68% (13/19), in comparison to the nonbacteremic
group.

ARDS was found in 6% (1/17) of the bacteremic patients
and 16% (3/19) of the nonbacteremic patients. Shock was
noted in all of these patients. Overall there was a 50%
mortality rate in patients with ARDS. All of the initial
platelet counts were above 150,000 (Table 3).

There were 22 survivors (16 male and 6 female) and 14
nonsurvivors (13 male and 1 female) of the 36 patients
identified to have the Septic Syndrome. The demographic data
for the survivors and nonsurvivors are presented in Tables 4
and 5. Survivors had a significantly lower mean age than the
nonsurvivors (48.8 ± 16.3 yrs vs. 59.8 ± 7.6 yrs; p < 0.02).
Forty-one percent (9/22) of the survivors had at least one
positive blood culture compared to 57% (8/14) of the nonsurvivors (p > 0.05). Shock was present twice as often in
nonsurvivors compared to survivors [93% (13/14) vs. 45%
(10/22)]. The initial white blood cell and platelet counts

were not significantly different between the survivors and nonsurvivors (15,500 $\pm$ 10,500 cells/mm^3 vs. 12,700 $\pm$ 8,000 cells/mm^3 and 187,200 $\pm$ 122,000 cells/mm^3 vs. 236,000 $\pm$ 86,000 cells/mm^3). The initial PaO$_2$ was also similar between the two groups. Nonsurvivors had a higher initial plasma lactate level (7.8 vs. 1.6 mg/dl).

A greater degree of multiorgan failure as measured by both the Organ System Dysfunction index and the Apache score was noted in the nonsurivors. The nonsurvivors had a mean organ system dysfunction index of 4.5 $\pm$ 1.5 vs. 2.68 $\pm$ 1.39 for the survivors (p $<$ 0.001) and nonsurvivors had an Apache score of 30.8 $\pm$ 7.7 vs. 20.7 $\pm$ 7.7 for the survivors. The mean Apache score for all patients enrolled in the study was 24.8 $\pm$ 9.2. Among the survivors, 36% had abnormal liver function tests, 64% had abnormal pulmonary function, 50% had abnormal renal function, 32% had abnormal cardiovascular function, 73% had abnormal neurologic function, and 14% had abnormal gastrointestinal function. In the nonsurvivors, 86% had abnormal liver function tests, 93% had abnormal pulmonary function, 86% had abnormal renal function, 50% had abnormal cardiovascular function, 71% had abnormal neurologic function, and 64% had abnormal gastrointestinal function.

Discussion:

The Septic Syndrome can be defined as the systemic manifestations of presumed sepsis. The criteria for diagnosis include the presence of hypo- or hyperthermia, tachycardia, tachypnea, a presumed site of infection, and evidence of inadequate perfusion; manifested by either poor or altered

cerebral function, arterial hypoxia, elevated plasma lactate
level, or a urine output less than 0.5 ml/kg body weight/hr
without corrective therapy. The Septic Syndrome does -7- not
require the presence of documented bacteremia, or shock which
are integral to the diagnosis of sepsis and septic shock,
respectively. Previous reports have noted the presence of
shock in approximately 40% of septic patients and have noted
a 40-90% mortality rate in patients with septic shock.(1-3,5)

In hopes of detecting the systemic response to sepsis
prior to the documentation of bacteremia or septic shock, the
guidelines for the septic syndrome were used to evaluate
patients in a prospective fashion. Thirty-six patients were
identified who fulfilled the criteria of the Septic Syndrome.
Forty-seven percent of these patients were subsequently found
to be bacteremic and 64% eventually developed shock. As a
group, these 36 patients with the Septic Syndrome had a 39%
mortality rate.

The presence or absence of bacteremia did not significantly influence survival [53% (9/17) vs. 68% (13/19)
bacteremic vs. nonbacteremic]. Shock was more prevalent in
the bacteremic group (82% - 14/17) as compared to the nonbacteremic group (47% - 9/19). The presence of advanced
age, shock, increased plasma lactate, and evidence of
multiple organ system dysfunction were all associated with a
decreased survival rate. Shock was found twice as often in
nonsurvivors and the altered organ perfusion associated with
the shock state may have been at least partially responsible
for the higher incidence of multiple organ system failure.

Our prospective results in patients with the septic syndrome are similar to the findings of a large retrospective review of bacteremia.(2,5) Kreger and McCabe found that 44% of their bacteremic patients experienced shock and the presence of shock increased the mortality rate from 7% to 47%.(2) Other factors which adversely affected survival were the prior use of corticosteroids, age greater than 60 years, underlying host disease, granulocytopenia, congestive heart failure and antecedent treatment with antibiotics, corticosteroids, or antimetabolites.(2) Appropriate antibiotic therapy was found to decrease the frequency of shock and the mortality by approximately 50%.(2) The mortality rate ascribed to septic shock ranges from 40-90% in most reviews.(1-3,5,6) The importance of early recognition of the signs and symptoms of circulatory embarrassment in patients with presumed sepsis is crucial and may allow for improved survival (7). Early death is related to inadequate cardiac performance and decreased intravascular volume status.(8) The importance of effective blood flow and organ perfusion has been stressed.(9,10) This is not gauged soley by an adequate cardiac output. Excess lactate production, presumably from anaerobic metabolism of underperfused tissues indicates inadequate tissue perfusion. Plasma lactates in excess of 4 mMoles/liter have been shown to prognosticate poor survival.(10) Nonsurvivors in our study were found to have elevated plasma lactate levels in comparison to survivors. Abraham and associates evaluated sequential cardiorespiratory patterns in patients with septic shock. (11,12) The 19 survivors were found to have significantly greater cardiac index, oxygen delivery, oxygen consumption, and left cardiac work index during the 24 hour period before the hypotensive crisis as compared to the 14 nonsurvivors. The authors suggested that survival patterns are determined even before the onset of the hypotensive crisis.(11,12)

Even among our surviving patients evidence of organ system dysfunction was common with a mean organ system dysfunction index approaching 3 (2.68 $\pm$ 1.39). The nonsurvivors averaged over 4 on their organ system dysfunction index and 93% of the patients had abnormal pulmonary function. Pulmonary injury is a common result of the systemic manifestations of sepsis and may take a variety of forms.(13) One of the most devastating is the Adult Respiratory Distress Syndrome (ARDS) which has been reported to have a mortality rate up to 90% when related to gram negative sepsis.(14) Fein and coworkers evaluated 116 consecutive septic patients over a 9 month period and found 21 (18%) episodes of ARDS.(15) It was noted that shock preceded all cases of ARDS while occurring in only 15% of the septic population. Thrombocytopenia was also significantly more common in the ARDS group as compared with the non-ARDS group. The ARDS group had a significantly decreased survival (19% vs. 65%). The presence of multiple organ system failure and bacteremia without a clinically identified site of infection have both been associated with increased mortality.(16)

Four of the 36 (11%) patients in our study were found

to have ARDS. All of these patients were noted to have shock preceding the development of the ARDS. In contrast to Fein's results, our patients all had initial platelet counts greater than 150,000 cells/mm^3. The 50% survival rate is somewhat greater than the 19% noted by Fein and coworkers and may reflect the smaller population size in the current study. Nonetheless, ARDS still represents a significant risk factor for death.

We have shown that patients with a systemic response to sepsis, septic syndrome, have similar risks for morbidity and mortality as do patients with septic shock. The septic syndrome is associated with a 39% mortality rate and there was an 11% incidence of ARDS. Multiorgan system dysfunction is commonly encountered. The presence of advanced age, shock, multiple organ system dysfunction, and elevated plasma lactate levels are all associated with an increased mortality rate. It is hoped that through earlier identification of patients with the systemic response to sepsis that appropriate therapy can be initiated and lead to improved survival.

Table 1

Mean Data in 36 Patients With the Septic Syndrome

Age - 53.1 + 14.3 years[1]
Shock present in 23/36 (64%)
Positive Blood Cultures in 17/36 (47%)
Survival 22/36 (61%)
Initial·White Blood Cell Count 14,400 + 9,700 cells/mm^3
Initial Plasma Lactate 3.9 + 14.0 mg/dl
Initial Hemoglobin 11.3 + 2.9 gms/dl
Initial Platelet Count 213,000 + 107,500 cells/mm^3
Initial Prothrombin Time 14.7 + 10.3 sec
Initial Partial Thromboplastin Time 39.5 + 21.7 sec
Initial PaO$_2$ 61.4 + 19.7 mmHg
Temperature 101.3 + 2.9°F
Heart Rate 125.7 + 18.7 beats/minute
Systolic Blood Pressure 106.8 + 29.7 mmHg
Diastolic Blood Pressure 62.3 + 22.7 mmHg
Mean Blood Pressure 77.1 + 23.8 mmHg
Apache Index 24.8 + 9.2
ARDS developed in 4/36 (11%)
Dopamine Treatment used in 15/36 (42%)
Abnormal Liver Function Tests 20/36 (56%)
Abnormal Pulmonary Function 27/36 (75%)
Abnormal Renal Function 23/36 (64%)
Abnormal Cardiovascular Function 14/36 (39%)
Abnormal Neurologic Function 26/36 (72%)
Abnormal Gastrointestinal Function 12/136 (33%)
Initial pH 7.4 + 0.1
Initial PaCO$_2$ 36.1 + 10.1 mmHg
Initial Albumin 2.7 + 0.8 gm/ds
Initial Glucose 197 + 120.3 mg/dl
BUN 35.7 + 28.1 mg/dl
Creatinine 2.3 + 1.7 mg/dl
Total Protein 5.9 + 1.4 gm/dl
Total Bilirubin 3.7 + 6.0 mg/dl
SGOT 94.3 + 209.5 mU/ml
Alkaline Phosphatase 185 + 313 mU/ml
HCO$_3^-$ 21.6 + 6.9 mEq/L
K$^+$ 3.9 + 0.8 mEq/L
Na$^+$ 136 + 11.4 mEq/L
Cl$^-$ 101 + 11.5 mEq/L
[1] X + SD

REFERENCES

1. Parker, M.M., Parrillo, J.E. Septic Shock: Hemodynamics and Pathogenesis. JAMA 250:3324-3327, 1983.
2. Kreger, B.E., Craven, D.E., McCabe, W.R. Gram Negative Bacteremia IV. Re-evaluation of Clinical Features and Treatment in 612 Patients. Am J of Med 68:344-355, 1980.
3. Shubin, H., Weil, M.H. Bacterial Shock. JAMA 235:421-424, 1976.
4. Knaus, W.A., Zimmerman, J.E., Wagner, D.P., Draper, E.A., Laurence, D.E. APACHE - Acute Physiology and Chronic Health Evaluation: A Physiologically Based Classification System. Crit Care Med 9:591-597, 1981.
5. Kreger, B.E., Craven, D.E., Carling, P.C., McCabe, W.R. Gram Negative Bacteremia III. Reassessment of Etiology, Epidemiology and Ecology in 612 Patients. Am J of Med 63:332-343, 1980.
6. Pollack, M.M., Fields, A.I., Ruttimann, U.E. Distributions of Cardiopulmonary Variables in Pediatric Survivors and Nonsurvivors of Septic Shock. Crit Care Med 13:454-459, 1985.
7. Christy, J.H. Treatment of Gram-Negative Shock. Am J of Med 50:77-87, 1971.
8. MacLean, L.D., Mulligan, W.G., McLean, A.P.H., Duff, J.H. Patterns of Septic Shock in Man, a Detailed Study of 56 Patients. Ann Surg 166:554-563, 1967.
9. Hinshaw, L.B., Beller-Todd, B.K., Archer, L.T. Review Update: Current Management of the Septic Shock Patient: Experimental Basis for Treatment Circulatory Shock. 9:543-553, 1982.
10. Udhoji, V.N., Weil, M.H. Hemodynamic and Metabolic Studies on Shock Associated with Bacteremia. Annals of Int Med 62:766-798, 1965.
11. Abraham, E., Shoemaker, W.C., Bland, R.D., Cobo, J.C. Sequential Cardiorespiratory Patterns in Septic Shock. Crit Care Med 11:799-803, 1983.
12. Abraham, E., Bland, R.D., Cobo, J.C., Shoemaker, W.C. Sequential Cardiorespiratory Patterns Associated with Outcome in Septic Shock. Chest 85:75-80, 1984.
13. Clowes, G.H.A., Jr. Pulmonary Abnormalities in Sepsis. Surg Clinics of N.A. 54:993-1013, 1974.
14. Kaplan, R.L., Sahn, S.A., Petty, T.K. Incidence and Outcome of the Respiratory Distress Syndrome in Gram-Negative Sepsis. Arch Intern Med 139:867-869, 1979.
15. Fein, AM, Lippman, M., Holtzman, H., Eliraz, A., Goldberg, S.K. The Risk Factors, Incidence, and Prognosis of ARDS Following Septicemia. Chest 83:40-42, 1983.
16. Bell, R.C., Coalson, J.J., Smith, J.D., Johanson, W.G., Jr. Multiple Organ System Failure and Infection in Adult Respiratory Distress Syndrome. Ann Int Med 99:293-298, 1983.

RESPIRATORY MECHANICS IN ICU PATIENTS

J. Milic-Emili and A. Rossi

Meakins-Christie Laboratories, McGill University, Montreal, Quebec,
H3A 2B4, Canada

Measurements of respiratory mechanics in patients mechanically
ventilated for acute respiratory failure are not performed routinely.
This reflects the general notion that in the intensive care setting
(ICU) results of respiratory mechanics are difficult to obtain (1). As
a matter of fact, however, in mechanically ventilated patients a
detailed analysis of respiratory mechanics can readily be performed with
simple and commonly available equipment, namely a pneumotachograph to
measure flow (V), an integrator to obtain   volume changes (ΔV) from
the flow signal and a transducer to measure the pressure at the airway
opening (Pao). Here it should be noted that some commercial ventilators
allow direct measurement of these variables (e.g., Siemens Servo 900C).
With the above equipment it is possible to determine noninvasively the
static and dynamic compliance of the total respiratory system (2-4), the
frequency-dependence of respiratory flow resistance (5,6) and to
establish if respiration is limited by dynamic compression of the
intrathoracic airways (2).

In this article we first describe a simple, noninvasive method for
measurement of respiratory mechanics which has been adapted to
mechanically ventilated patients, and next we present results obtained
in patients with adult respiratory distress syndrome (ARDS) and with
chronic airway obstruction (CAO).

OCCLUSION TECHNIQUE

Static compliance

The static compliance of the total respiratory system (Cst,rs) is
conventionally obtained by dividing the inflation volume (ΔV) by the
difference between the plateau pressure measured at the airway opening
(tracheal pressure) during end-inspiratory airway occlusion (breathhold

253

T. H. Stanley and R. J. Sperry (eds.), Anesthesia and the Lung, 253–260.
© 1989 by Kluwer Academic Publishers.

for 2 to 4 sec) and the PEEP set by the ventilator. Such measurements
are correct provided that at end-expiration the elastic recoil pressure
of the respiratory system (Pel,rs) is zero, i.e., that no further
pressure is available to produce expiratory flow. This was the case for
the ARDS patient in Fig. 1 in whom the expiratory flow prior to lung
inflation became nil (expiratory pause) indicating that during
expiration the respiratory system had time to reach its elastic
equilibration point (Pel,rs=0). In most ICU patients, however, Pel,rs
does not become zero during expiration, the end-expiratory Pel,rs being
termed "auto" (7) or "intrinsic" PEEP (PEEPi) (8). When present, PEEPi
needs to be subtracted from the end-inspiratory plateau pressure, to
obtain the correct value of Cst,rs (8):

$$Cst,rs = \frac{\Delta V}{\text{end-inspiratory plateau Pel,rs - PEEP - PEEPi}} \tag{1}$$

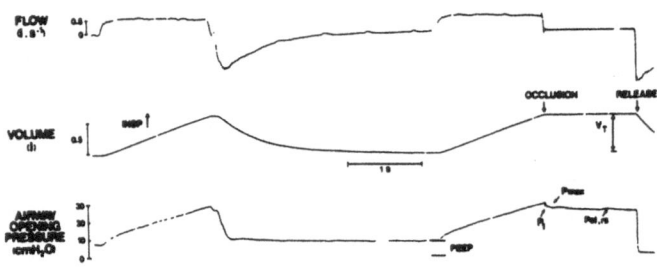

Fig. 1. Tracings of flow, volume, and pressure at the airway opening in
a mechanically ventilated patient with ARDS, with PEEP of 8.5 cm water.
Airway occlusion at end-inspiration was performed at point indicated by
the first arrow. This results in an immediate drop of pressure from a
peak value (Pmax) to P1, thereafter decreasing gradually to a "plateau"
value representing the end-inspiratory elastic recoil pressure of the
total respiratory system (Pel,rs). In this subject, expiratory flow
became nil before the end of expiration, and inspiratory flow started
synchronously with the onset of positive pressure inflation, indicating
that the end-expiratory Pel,rs relative to PEEP is zero. (Modified from
Ref. 8).

PEEPi can be readily measured with ventilators (e.g., the Siemens Servo 900C) provided with an end-expiratory occlusion hold which allows measurement of the end-expiratory plateau pressure (i.e. PEEPi). Most ventilators, however, do not have this option, and hence assessment of PEEPi is more problematic. A discussion of the different ways to assess PEEPi and of the factors determining its magnitude, as well of its implications in terms of cardiovascular function and weaning, can be found elsewhere (4,7).

Respiratory resistance

The end-inspiratory occlusion technique also allows to determine the flow-resistive properties of the respiratory system. In fact two types of resistance can be obtained from records such as that shown in Fig. 1. Both of these resistance measurements were introduced in 1927 by von Neergaard and Wirz (9,10), but paradoxically never applied simultaneously by these authors. The first resistance measurement is based on the interrupter method which consists in rapid airway occlusion at some point during inspiration or expiration (10). As shown in Fig. 1, sudden end-inspiratory airway occlusion during constant flow inflation is associated with an immediate drop in airway opening pressure from a maximal value (Pmax) to P1. Dividing Pmax - P1 by the flow ($\dot{V}$) immediately preceding the occlusion yields a resistance which has been termed minimum resistance (Rmin) (5,6):

$$Rmin = \frac{Pmax - P1}{\dot{V}} \qquad (2)$$

The significance of Rmin has been recently clarified by Bates et al (5). It represents a "true" or "ohmic" resistance. In humans, it mainly reflects airway resistance.

The second method proposed by von Neergaard and Wirz (9) to determine resistance is known as the elastic subtraction method. When applied to mechanically ventilated patients, this method consists of subtracting the static elastic recoil pressure (Pel,rs) from the total pressure applied by the ventilator in order to obtain the dynamic component of the driving pressure (Pdyn), and dividing Pdyn by the corresponding $\dot{V}$. In Fig. 1, Pdyn following end-inspiratory airway occlusion is equal to Pmax-Pel,rs. If the flow preceding the occlusion is constant, as in the case in Fig. 1, the "resistance" measured in this way is called Rmax (5,6):

$$Rmax = \frac{Pmax-Pel,rs}{\dot{V}} \qquad (3)$$

Rmax is always greater than Rmin. In fact, as shown in Fig. 1, the airway opening pressure does not reach a plateau value immediately after the occlusion; instead it exhibits a gradual drop from P1 to its plateau values (=Pel,rs). The pressure drop from P1 to Pel,rs reflects two phenomena: (a) "Pendelluft" resulting from unequal time constants within the lung and chest wall (11,12); and (b) stress relaxation due to viscoelastic behaviour of the respiratory system (13,14). Both of these phenomena involve non-ohmic behaviour, and hence the difference between Rmax and Rmin [= (P1-Pel,rs)/$\dot{V}$] does not represent a "true" resistance. Nevertheless, P1 - Pel,rs reflects dynamic pressure losses which involve dynamic work. Accordingly, Rmax [= Rmin + (P1-Pel,rs)/$\dot{V}$] is of considerable clinical interest. In this connection it should be noted that Rmax corresponds to the effective resistance at zero respiratory frequency while Rmin is resistance at high frequency (5,6). Thus, the difference between Rmax and Rmin is a measure of the frequency-dependence of resistance, an index of considerable clinical importance (12,15). In fact, in patients with severe chronic airway obstruction, there is an increase of time constant inhomogeneities within the lungs which results in an increased difference between Rmax and Rmin (5,6).

RESPIRATORY MECHANICS IN PATIENTS WITH ARDS AND CAO
"Intrinsic" PEEP

It has been shown that, in mechanically ventilated patients, alveolar pressure can remain positive throughout expiration, even when PEEP is not intentionally applied by the ventilator (7,8). This occurs when the time required for passive expiration to proceed to completion is disproportionately increased relative to the expiratory duration set by the ventilator (8). In patients with acute exacerbation of chronic airway obstruction, the rate of lung emptying is unduly slowed by high expiratory resistance and expiratory flow limitation (3-4) and, by necessity, it is interrupted by the next mechanical inflation (8). Therefore the end-expiratory volume during mechanical ventilation will exceed the relaxation volume of the total respiratory system, and hence alveolar pressure will be positive at the end of the expiration, i.e., PEEPi will be present. PEEPi has been consistently observed in mechanically ventilated patients with CAO (8), reaching values up to 22 cmH_2O (Rossi et al., unpublished observations).

In patients with ARDS, in whom the lungs are stiffer (see below), the rate of lung emptying should be faster and expiration should be completed before the onset of the next mechanical inflation. This is the case for the patient in Fig. 1. However, PEEPi was present in 8 out of 12 consecutive, unselected patients with ARDS, examined on the first day of mechanical ventilation and in the absence of any PEEP applied by the ventilator. In four of these patients PEEPi ranged between 5 and 8 cm water (Rossi et al., unpublished observations). The presence of PEEPi in ARDS patients should reflect an increased expiratory resistance, reflecting in part that of the endotracheal tubes.

Static respiratory compliance

In ICU patients with CAO, the static compliance of the respiratory system is almost invariably increased, reflecting dynamic pulmonary hyperinflation, i.e., the presence of PEEPi (3,6,8).

In patients with ARDS, the static compliance of the respiratory system decreases with progression from interstitial to alveolar edema, and loss of ventilating units, due to air space flooding by a protein rich fluid (16). Cst,rs is therefore generally accepted as a good indicator of the amount of fluid in the alveoli and has become the most widely used physiologic variable to assess the status and progress of the respiratory function in patients with ARDS (1). In 12 patients with ARDS, examined in the first day of mechanical ventilation, Cst,rs averaged 0.037 ± 0.007 (SEM) L/cmH_2O, which is about one third of the normal value (17). In this connection it should be noted that in these patients Cst,rs was corrected for PEEPi. This was not the case for previous values of compliance in ARDS patients reported in the literature. In ARDS patients, the percent difference between the corrected and uncorrected values of Cst,rs can amount to as much as 30%.

Respiratory resistance

Measurement of respiratory resistance is not common in patients with ARDS because these patients are generally thought to have a "compliance disease". In fact, no systematic investigation of respiratory resistance in ARDS patients has as yet been reported in the literature. Fig. 2 depicts data of respiratory resistance in ARDS patients (Rossi et al., unpublished observations). Average results (SEM) for both minimum (Rrs,min) and maximum (Rrs,max) resistance of the total respiratory system (after subtraction of equipment and endotracheal tube resistance) for 12 patients are shown together with similar values obtained in 10 mechanically ventilated patients with acute exacerbation of CAO.

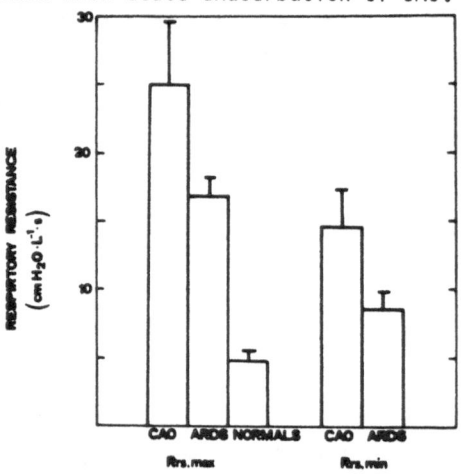

Fig. 2. Average values (SEM) of maximum (Rrs,max) and minimum (Rrs,min) respiratory resistance (after subtraction of resistance of endotracheal tube and equipment) in 10 mechanically ventilated patients with acute exacerbation of chronic airway obstruction (CAO), and 12 patients with ARDS; normal values are from Ref. 18.

To our knowledge, Rrs,min has as yet not been measured in normal subjects. However, using a technique similar to ours, Don and Robson (18) have measured Rrs,max in normal anesthetized subjects and found a mean value of 4.8 cm water/L/s. In both CAO and ARDS patients, Rrs,max was higher than in normals, the difference being somewhat greater for CAO. Rrs,min was higher in CAO than in ARDS. In both groups of patients it exceeded the normal value of Rrs,max, indicating an increase of the "true" resistance of the respiratory system, probably reflecting a reduction in bronchial caliber caused by fluid in the airways, reflex bronchoconstriction, reduced lung volume, etc. In both CAO and ARDS patients, Rrs,max was considerably greater than Rrs,min, suggesting the presence of substantial frequency-dependence of resistance, probably due to time constant inequalities within the lung. This is a well-known phenomenon in patients with CAO, both in stable condition (15) and in acute respiratory failure (6), but has not been previously reported for patients with ARDS. The results in Fig. 2 suggest that ARDS is not only a "compliance" but also a "resistance" disease, with an important peripheral component, as reflected by the difference between Rrs,max and Rrs,min.

SUMMARY

The airway occlusion method during constant flow inflation for determination of the mechanical properties of the respiratory system has been reviewed. This method can provide valuable on-line information in patients mechanically ventilated in the intensive care unit setting. More extensive use of this method should provide a better understanding of the pathophysiologic processes and the adaptative mechanisms in ARDS and CAO patients.

REFERENCES
1. Suter, P.M. In: "Acute respiratory failure" (Eds. Z.M. Zapol, K.J. Falke), Lung Biology in Health and Disease, No. 24, New York, 1985, pp. 507-519.
2. Gottfried, S.B., Higgs, B.D., Rossi, A., Carli, F., Mengeot, P.M., Calverley, P.M.A., Zocchi, L., and Milic-Emili J. J. Appl. Physiol. 59: 647-652, 1985.
3. Gottfried, S.B., Rossi, A., Higgs, B.D., Calverley, P.M.A., Zocchi, L., Bozic, C., and Milic-Emili, J. Am. Rev. Respir. Dis. 131: 414-420, 1985.
4. Gottfried, S.B., Rossi, A., and Milic-Emili, J. Int. Crit. Care Digest 5: 30-33, 1986.
5. Bates, J.H.T., Rossi, A., and Milic-Emili, J. J. Appl. Physiol. 58: 1840-1848, 1985.
6. Rossi, A., Gottfried, S.B., Zocchi, L., Grassino, A., and Milic-Emili, J. J. Appl. Physiol. 58: 1849-1858, 1985.
7. Pepe, P.E., and Marini, J.J. Am. Rev. Respir. Dis. 126: 166-170, 1982.
8. Rossi, A., Gottfried, S.B., Zocchi, L., Higgs, B.D., Lennox, S., Calverley, P.M.A., Begin, P., Grassino, A., and Milic-Emili, J. Am. Rev. Respir. Dis. 131: 672-678, 1985.
9. Neergaard von, K., and Wirz, K. Z. Klin. Med. 105: 51-82, 1927.

10. Neergaard von, K., and Wirz, K. Z. Klin. Med. <u>105</u>: 35-50, 1927.
11. Barnas, G., Katsuki, Y., Loring, S.H., and Mead, J. J. Appl. Physiol. <u>62</u>: 71-81, 1987.
12. Otis, A.B., McKerrow, C.B., Bartlett, R.A., Mead, J., McIlroy, M.B., Selverstone, N.J., and Radford E.P. J. Appl. Physiol. 8: 427-433, 1956.
13. Hildebrandt, J. J. Appl. Physiol. <u>27</u>: 246-250, 1969.
14. Hildebrandt, J. J. Appl. Physiol. <u>28</u>: 365-372, 1969.
15. Grimby, G., Takishima, T., Graham, W., Macklem, P.T., and Mead, J. J. Clin. Invest. 47: 1455-1465, 1968.
16. Staub, N.C. Physiol. Rev. <u>54</u>: 678-811, 1974.
17. Agostoni, E., and Mead, J. In: Handbook of Physiology, Respiration, Washington, DC, Am. Physiol. Soc., Sec. 3, Vol. I, Chap. 13, 1964, pp. 387-409.
18. Don, H.F, Robson, JC: Anesthesiology <u>26</u>: 168-178.

DYNAMIC HYPERINFLATION: INTRINSIC PEEP AND ITS RAMIFICATIONS IN PATIENTS
WITH RESPIRATORY FAILURE

J. Milic-Emili, S.B. Gottfried, and A. Rossi

Meakins-Christie Laboratories, McGill University, Montreal, Quebec,
H3A 2B4, Canada

Pulmonary hyperinflation, namely a consistent increase in the
end-expiratory lung volume above the predicted functional residual
capacity (FRC), is a characteristic abnormality in patients with acute
or chronic airways obstruction (1). While this may be the result of
loss of lung elastic recoil (e.g. pulmonary emphysema), dynamic factors
may also be responsible. For example, when there is a significant
increase in airway resistance, the rate of lung emptying is unduly
slowed and, by necessity, is interrupted by the next inspiratory
effort. When the breathing frequency increases, as in exercise or
when the ventilatory demands are increased for other reasons, the
expiratory time shortens and hence the end-expiratory lung volume may
increase above the relaxed FRC position (elastic equilibrium volume).
This is referred to as <u>dynamic hyperinflation</u>. Expiratory flow may also
be reduced by other mechanisms. These include activity of the
inspiratory muscles during expiration (post-inspiration inspiratory
activity) as well as activation of laryngeal adductor muscles with
expiratory narrowing of the glottic aperture (2-5).

Dynamic hyperinflation is often present during passive mechanical
ventilation (6-10). Indeed, the end-expiratory volume during mechanical
ventilation will exceed the elastic equilibrium volume of the
respiratory system whenever the time required for passive expiration to
proceed to completion is disproportionately increased relative to the
expiratory duration imposed by the chosen ventilator settings (7-10).
In the absence of respiratory muscle activity, the rate of passive lung
deflation is determined by the balance between the elastic recoil stored
during the preceeding lung inflation and the opposing total
flow-resistance offerred by the respiratory system (including
endotracheal tube, ventilator and additional equipment). Accordingly,

261

T. H. Stanley and R. J. Sperry (eds.), Anesthesia and the Lung, 261–268.
© 1989 by Kluwer Academic Publishers.

the stiffer the respiratory system (i.e. decreased compliance) the
quicker will be the rate of lung emptying; conversely, increased
flow-resistance impedes the rate of lung deflation. Thus, as a general
rule, the magnitude of dynamic hyperinflation will be proportional to
the tidal volume and the mechanical time constant of the respiratory
system (i.e. the product of total respiratory resistance and compliance)
and inversely related to expiratory duration (11,12).

In patients with chronic obstructive pulmonary diseases (COPD),
mechanically ventilated for management of acute respiratory failure,
dynamic hyperinflation is almost invariably present because the
time-course of passive expiration is prolonged by increased respiratory
resistance (7,9,10). Thus, when airway obstruction worsens or
expiratory time decreases with increased ventilatory demands, the
dynamically determined FRC will rise. It should be noted, however, that
dynamic hyperinflation is not restricted to patients with endstage COPD
and expiratory airflow limitation. Respiratory resistance may be
increased by a number of reasons in critically ill, intubated and
mechanically ventilated patients (13,14). For example, the added
flow-resistance due to a narrow bore endotracheal tube can be
substantial (7,15); and can be very effective in retarding expiratory
flow and thereby contributing to dynamic hyperinflation. Tachypnea with
a concomitant reduction in expiratory duration will also have a similar
effect (7,9,10).

The presence of dynamic hyperinflation implies that the alveolar
pressure remains positive throughout the expiratory time. This is
equivalent to the deliberate use of PEEP and has been referred to as
"intrinsic" or "auto" PEEP (7,9,10). In contrast with positive
end-expiratory pressure set by the ventilator, however, intrinsic PEEP
(PEEPi) is not recorded by the ventilator pressure manometer. As a
result, PEEPi is frequently not recognized and this has led to use of
the term "occult" PEEP (9). This is not surprising in that the
ventilator manometer measures the pressure at the airway opening (Pao)
relative to atmosphere - and not alveolar pressure. To the extent that
end-expiratory lung volume is increased and results in continued
expiratory flow, then alveolar pressure must exceed the measured airway
pressure. This is in contrast with mechanical PEEP devices which in
general provide a constant applied pressure at the airway opening

independent of expiratory flow. This problem is perhaps best illustrated in patients with advanced COPD and dynamic airway compression, where the ventilator manometer is downstream from the site of flow limitation and gives no indication of the existing upstream alveolar pressure proximal to the point of flow limitation (9).

In clinical practice, PEEPi should be suspected whenever one notices that the ventilator spirometer fills throughout expiration with an abrupt interruption at the onset of the next ventilator breath. As suggested by Pepe and Marini (9), the presence of PEEPi can be confirmed and its magnitude directly measured by simply occluding the airway opening at end-expiration immediately prior to the onset of the subsequent mechanical inflation. Under these conditions, i.e. in absence of expiratory flow with the airway occluded, alveolar pressure will be transmitted to the airway opening and PEEPi will be accurately recorded by the ventilator manometer (9,10).

PEEPi has several clinical implications in the mechanically ventilated patient. Static compliance of the total respiratory system (Crs) is frequently measured in the ICU in order to assess respiratory mechanical function and aid in clinical decision making (16,17). This is conventionally determined from single measurements of volume and pressure during airway occlusions performed at end inflation. Crs is then computed by dividing the tidal volume (V_T) by the difference between the "plateau" in airway pressure during end-inspiratory airway occlusion (Pplateau) plus the level of PEEP set by the ventilator (if any), i.e. $Crs = V_T/(Pplateau + PEEP)$. This approach assumes that the end-expiratory lung volume during mechanical ventilation corresponds to the relaxed FRC position of the respiratory system, or that it is increased by a predicted amout with applied PEEP. In the presence of dynamic hyperinflation and PEEPi, clearly this assumption is false and will result in a systematic underestimation of Crs. Taking PEEPi into account, Rossi et al. (10) have found underestimations of Crs of up to 48%. In fact, such errors were not uncommon and occurred in 10 of 14 patients studied. This problem can be easily overcome by routinely performing airway occlusions both at the end of passive expiration and at end-inflation. The airway pressure recorded during end-expiratory "cclusion will indicate the true magnitude of positive end-expiratory pressure, whether set by the ventilator or by PEEPi resulting from dynamic hyperinflation. Crs may then be accurately determined as the tidal volume divided by the difference in airway pressure between end-inspiratory and end-expiratory occlusions. Clearly, commercial ventilators should be provided not only with the capability of performing automatic end-inspiratory airway occlusions, as is presently the case, but also automatic end-expiratory occlusions.

It is generally assumed that patient effort is minimal during "assisted" mechanical ventilation and, as a result, the work of breathing is largely assumed by the ventilator (18). This assumption is true provided that only a modest inspiratory effort is needed to "trigger" assisted ventilator breaths. Under usual conditions this requires the ventilated patient to reduce airway pressure below the chosen "sensitivity" level, generally set 1-5 cmH_2O below the prevailing end-expiratory pressure. In the presence of PEEPi, however, the patient must generate a negative inspiratory pressure equivalent in magnitude to the opposing elastic recoil pressure plus the triggering pressure before an assisted ventilator breath can be initiated. Clearly, the inspiratory efforts performed by the patient during "assisted" mechanical ventilation cannot be assumed to be negligible in the presence of PEEPi. In fact, we have seen patients who had to generate active inspiratory pressures greater than 20 cmH_2O. This has great importance in the management of ICU patients because the large inspiratory efforts due to PEEPi, associated with decreased inspiratory muscle strength (implicit with hyperinflation), can lead to inspiratory muscle fatigue.

Pepe and Marini (9) have recognized and discussed the hemodynamic consequences of PEEPi in mechanically ventilated patients. No different from externally applied PEEP set on the ventilator, the increased intrathoracic pressure present with significant levels of PEEPi will impede venous return, reduce cardiac output, and to some extent be transmitted to the intrathoracic vasculature. This will introduce errors in the measurement and interpretation of central hemodynamic pressure recordings. Failure to recognize the presence of PEEPi in this setting may result in inappropriate fluid restriction and unnecessary vasopressor therapy (9,10). Moreover, the adverse hemodynamic effects of PEEPi may in fact be greater than comparable amounts of externally applied PEEP in patients with severe COPD. First, a given amount of

end-expiratory pressure will most likely be associated with a higher
mean intrathoracic pressure averaged over the course of expiration
(20). Second, unlike patients with acute respiratory distress syndrome
in whom PEEP therapy is most frequently utilized, increased compliance
in patients with pulmonary emphysema will permit a relatively greater
fraction of alveolar pressure to be transmitted to the intrathoracic
vasculature (9).

While the presence of dynamic hyperinflation and PEEPi has
significant implications for the management of the mechanically
ventilated patient, it is also of considerable importance when weaning
from ventilatory support is being attempted. Patients with acute
respiratory failure almost invariably exhibit rapid, shallow
breathing during periods of spontaneous ventilation (21,22). To the
extent that respiratory frequency increases, and hence expiratory time
is decreased, this will result in the development of dynamic
hyperinflation and increasing PEEPi. In fact, in a study on 14
spontaneously breathing patients with COPD in acute respiratory failure,
PEEPi was found in each individual and averaged approximately 9 cmH_2O
(21,22). The presence of PEEPi in the spontaneously breathing patient
implies that, in addition to the pressure needed to produce the actual
breathing movements, the inspiratory muscles are required to generate
sufficient inspiratory force in order to overcome the opposing positive
recoil pressure (i.e., PEEPi) before inspiratory airflow will begin. In
this respect, PEEPi represents an inspiratory threshold load (23). This
additional pressure requirement places a significant burden on the
inspiratory muscles, whose performance as pressure generators is already
impaired because of pulmonary hyperinflation and other factors (24,25).
As a maximum inspiratory pressure of 20-30 cmH_2O is generally taken as
indicating sufficient respiratory muscle strength to enable spontaneous
ventilation in such patients (26,27), the additional mechanical load
which PEEPi imposes upon the inspiratory muscles is indeed
considerable. This is particularly important when considering that the
increased end-expiratory lung volume will necessarily reduce the
inspiratory muscle strength, increase the mechanical work and oxygen
cost of breathing, and decrease the respiratory muscle blood flow and
energy supply. This should also predispose to inspiratory muscle
fatigue (19,25). Clearly, the presence of high levels of PEEPi should

herald difficulty in weaning the patient from mechanical ventilation.

As mentioned above, maximum inspiratory pressure is commonly used as a criterion for weaning (26,27). In the presence of dynamic hyperinflation, maximum inspiratory pressure will decrease in a predictable fashion with increasing lung volume, related in part to the force-length properties of the inspiratory muscles. Under these conditions, however, maximum inspiratory pressure does not represent the total pressure actually developed by the inspiratory muscles but is underestimated because of the opposing positive elastic recoil pressure present at lung volumes above the relaxed FRC, i.e. PEEPi. Nevertheless, the maximum inspiratory pressure measured in this fashion is clinically relevant to the extent that it does in fact represent the net pressure available to produce respiratory movements and airflow. While changes in maximum inspiratory pressure may be due to alterations in lung volume rather than intrinsic respiratory muscle function, it accurately reflects the extent of the reduction in effective ventilatory capacity of the inspiratory muscles. In this regard, with extreme hyperinflation, mechanical ventilation may be achieved at lung volumes exceeding the voluntary total lung capacity (8,28). This condition, which perhaps is not uncommon, indicates inability to generate sufficient net inspiratory muscle force to provide for spontaneous respiration and hence complete ventilator dependence must ensue. It is apparent that mechanical ventilation cannot be discontinued until lung volume sufficiently decreases (because of reduced airways obstruction, alveolar dead space, or minute ventilation) or intrinsic inspiratory muscle function itself improves significantly for other reasons.

Fundamental in the approach to the mechanically ventilated patient in whom dynamic hyperinflation and PEEPi occur is to recognize if PEEPi is in fact present. Indeed, we believe that measurement of PEEPi should become a part of routine ventilator monitoring in mechanically ventilated patients, particularly those with airways obstruction. This will allow for reliable measurement and interpretation of other frequently determined cardiopulmonary variables, such as respiratory system compliance, pulmonary capillary wedge pressure, and maximum inspiratory pressure. The potential adverse effects of PEEPi require that, in addition, management should be specifically directed towards those factors contributing to the development of PEEPi. This includes medical therapy aimed at reducing the severity of airflow obstruction as well as excessive minute ventilation (due to fever, metabolic acidosis, inadequate pain relief, etc.). The inspiratory flow setting should be adjusted to maximize the time provided for passive expiration to occur. While in theory a reduction in tidal volume should be beneficial, for a given minute ventilation this would require an increased respiratory frequency (and therefore a decreased expiratory time) so that it is unlikely that the level of PEEPi will be appreciably altered (10).

REFERENCES
1. Bates, D.V., Macklem, P.T. and Christie, R.V. (Eds), WB Saunders Company, Philadelphia PA, 1971.
2. Collett, P.W., Brancatisano, T. and Engel, L.A. Am. Rev. Respir. Dis. 128: 719-723, 1983.
3. Martin, J., Powell, E., Shore, S., Emrich, J. and Engel, L.A. Am. Rev. Respir. Dis. 123: 441-447, 1980.
4. Mortola, J.P., Milic-Emili, J., Noworaj, A., Smith, B., Fox, G. and Weeks, S. Am. Rev. Respir. Dis. 129: 49-53, 1984.
5. Muller, N., Bryan, A.C. and Zamel, N. J. Appl. Physiol. 49: 869-874, 1980.
6. Bergman, N.A. Anesthesiology 37: 626-633, 1972.
7. Gottfried, S.B., Rossi, A., Higgs, B.D., Calverley, P.M.A., Zocchi, L., Bozic, C. and Milic-Emili, J. Am. Rev. Respir. Dis. 131: 414-420, 1985.
8. Kimball, W.R., Leith, D.E. and Robins, A.G. Am. Rev. Respir. Dis. 126: 991-995, 1982.
9. Pepe, P.E. and Marini, J.J. Am. Rev. Respir. Dis. 126: 166-170, 1982.
10. Rossi, A., Gottfried, S.B., Zocchi, L., Higgs, B.D., Lennox, S., Calverley, P.M.A., Begin, P., Grassino, A. and Milic-Emili, J. Am. Rev. Respir. Dis. 131: 672-677, 1985.
11. LeSouef, P.N., England, S.J. and Bryan, A.C. Am. Rev. Respir. Dis. 129: 552-556, 1984.
12. Vinegar, Sinnett, E.E., Leith, D.E. J. Appl. Physiol. 46: 867-871, 1979.
13. Lavietes, M.H. and Rochester, D.F. Lung 159: 219-229, 1981.
14. Sybrecht, G.W., Taubner, E.M., Bohm, M.M. and Fabel, H. Lung 156: 49-56, 1979.
15. Behrakis, P.K., Higgs, B.D., Baydur, A., Zin, W.A. and Milic-Emili, J. J. Appl. Physiol. 55: 1085-1092, 1983.
16. Bone, R.C. Chest 70: 740-746, 1976.
17. Suter, P.M., Fairley, H.B. and Isenberg, M.D. N. Engl. J. Med. 292: 284-289, 1975.
18. Marini, J.J., Capps, J.S. and Culver, B.H. Chest 87: 612-18, 1985.
19. Bellemare, F. and Grassino, A. J. Appl. Physiol. 55: 8-15, 1983.
20. Colgan, F.J., Barrow, R.E. and Fanning, G.L. Anesthesiology 34: 145-151, 1971.
21. Fleury, B., Murciano, D., Talamo, C., Aubier, M., Pariente, R. and Milic-Emili, J. Am. Rev. Respir. Dis. 131: 822-827, 1985.

22. Murciano, D., Aubier, M., Bussi, S., Derenné, J-Ph., Pariente, R. and Milic-Emili, J. Am. Rev. Respir. Dis. 126: 837-841, 1982.
23. Mead, J. Bull. Eur. Physiopath. Respir. 15: 61-71, 1979.
24. Kelly, S.M., Rosa, A., Field, S., Coughlin, M., Shizgal, H.M. and Macklem,P.T. Am. Rev. Respir. Dis. 130: 33-37, 1984.
25. Rochester, D.J. and Arora, N.S. Med. Clin. N. Amer. 67: 573-597, 1983.
26. Feeley, T.W. and Hedley-White, J. New. Engl. J. Med. 292: 903-906, 1975.
27. Sahn, S.A. and Lakshminarayan, S. Chest 63: 1002-1005, 1973.
28. Sharp, J.T., van Lith, P., Nuchprayoon, C.V., Briney, R. and Johnson, F.N. Am. J. Med. 44: 39-46, 1968.
29. Martin, J.G., Shore, S. and Engel, L.A. 126: 812-817, 1982.

WHY INTERMITTENT MANDATORY VENTILATION (IMV) FAILS?

JOHN B. DOWNS, M.D.

Department of Anesthesiology, University of South Florida
College of Medicine, Tampa, Florida, 33612

Since the introduction of intermittent mandatory
ventilation (IMV) to adult medical practice in 1973, the
technique has been fraught with numerous difficulties.(1)
Initially, IMV was felt to be purely a weaning tool.
Subsequently, as clinicians at the University of Florida
began treating patients with severe respiratory failure
with IMV, many other clinicians felt that
the technique was being used to prematurely discontinue
mechanical ventilatory support of critically ill
patients.(2,3) Subsequent publications from the University
of Florida, the University of Miami, Lackland Air Force Base
and other institutions, attempted to support the physiologic
basis for allowing spontaneous respiration to persist during
mechanical ventilatory support. Initially, the technique
did not enjoy wide-spread acceptance. As time as passed,
the reasons for this lack of acceptance have become obvious
and, in spite of continued controversy, the technique now is
applied world-wide.(4,5)

Failure of a patient to adequately support spontaneous
respiration may result from three major deficiencies.
Often, patients have inadequate respiratory muscle strength
to support spontaneous respiration. Others may have marked
decrease in lung compliance and/or increase in airways
resistance, such that work of breathing is so great that
spontaneous respiration can be maintained for only a limited
time. Finally, some patients suffer from decreased
respiratory drive and even in the face of normal

269

T. H. Stanley and R. J. Sperry (eds.), Anesthesia and the Lung, 269–276.
© 1989 by Kluwer Academic Publishers.

respiratory mechanics, hypoventilation may occur. Failure of the clinician to properly assess a patient's ability and drive to breath has led to "failure of IMV", which in reality is a failure of appropriate patient selection and/or application of the technique.

Some patients require total ventilatory support. For example, patients who have residual muscle paralysis following an operative procedure, cannot support spontaneous respiration. Clearly, such patients require ventilatory support until adequate reversal of muscle relaxation has occurred. Not surprisingly, when such patients receive inadequate ventilatory support with IMV, they fare poorly. Similarly, patients with decreased respiratory drive, for example, those who have received large doses of narcotics, will not respond to low-rate IMV with an appropriate degree of spontaneous respiratory activity. In both of these examples, use of IMV may result in an untoward result which represents failure of appropriate patient selection, rather than failure of the technique.

Often times, patients with marked decrease in lung compliance secondary to decreased expiratory lung volume have marked increase in their work of breathing, represented by tachypnea and shallow respiration. Such patients often will respond to application of continuous positive airway pressure (CPAP) with increased functional residual capacity (FRC), increased lung compliance, decreased work of breathing, increased tidal volume, and decreased respiratory rate. Such patients often receive mechanical ventilatory support, often without positive end-expiratory pressure (PEEP). In such patients, application of IMV, without application of PEEP or CPAP, will result in a tachypneac patient, who often resists ventilatory support. In such patients, application of CPAP during IMV results in a more comfortable ventilatory pattern and improvement in arterial blood oxygenation. Furthermore, such patients often

tolerate rapid reduction in IMV rate, and total weaning from
ventilatory support. Again, failure of patients to tolerate
mechanical ventilation with IMV does not represent failure
of the technique. Rather, it presents inappropriate
application of the technique. Most often, weaning from IMV
is accomplished by linear decrements in mechanical
ventilator rate. Thus, the patient receiving twelve IMV
breaths each minute (bpm) is likely to have ventilator rate
reduced to 10,8,6 bpm, and so forth, over a period of time.
Frequently, such patients seem to tolerate the weaning
process well, until 4 to 6 bpm is reached. Then, they seem
to fail. Such failure often is attributed to "fatigue".
However, more likely, such failure is predictable, and
represents ventilator dependance from the outset. When
ventilator rate is lowered in such a linear fashion, the
time between breaths is increased at a non-linear rate. For
example, 12 bpm represents a respiratory cycle time of 5
sec. A linear decrement in respiratory rate, as mentioned
previously, would cause an increase in cycle time from 5 sec
to 6 sec, to 7.5 sec, to 10 sec, to 15 sec to 30 sec, to
infinity. In other words, the patient would seem to
tolerate an increase in cycle time of 1 sec, then 1.5 sec,
and even 2.5 seconds, but would fail to tolerate increases
of 5 sec, 15 sec, and total discontinuation of ventilatory
support. Clearly, the marked increase in time between
ventilator breaths is responsible for intolerance of
weaning, rather than sudden onset of respiratory muscle
fatigue. Weaning from ventilatory support should proceed by
increasing respiratory cycle time in a linear fashion. This
will avoid the rapid imposition of an intolerable
respiratory load on the ventilator dependent patient. I
recommend that cycle time be increased in 2 sec intervals
for difficult to wean patients. Thus decrements in
ventilatior rate would procede as follows:

```
Cycle time     :  4  6  8  10 12  14  .. 20  ....  30     60
Ventilator rate: 15 10 7.5  6  5  4.3 ..  3  ....   2      1
```

It should be stressed that such a weaning regime is rarely necessary, since most patients tolerate rapid discontinuation of mechanical ventilation when the etiology of their ventilator dependance has resolved.

Most frequently, IMV has been unsuccessful because of an unacceptable increase in work of breathing imposed by the IMV circuit. The work created by each breath is dependent upon the volume of gas taken into the lung and the pressure gradient responsible for generation of that breath. Total work of breathing also is dependent on respiratory rate. Clearly, patients with a minimal decrease in lung or thoracic compliance can tolerate an increase in the extrinsic work of breathing. However, most patients with acute lung injury and respiratory failure, of either the obstructive or restrictive type, cannot tolerate a significant increase in work of breathing imposed by a breathing circuit. It is not surprising that the early circuitry described for IMV was successful. Such equipment most often was used to wean patients from mechanical ventilatory support who were quite able to tolerate a significant increase in their work of breathing. In addition, such patients frequently were required to breathe through the IMV circuitry for only a few hours. However, as IMV became more popular and was used for patients who required long-term ventilatory support, the significance of circuit resistance in increased work of breathing, became apparent.

Any resistance to gas flow will increase inspiratory and/or expiratory work of breathing. There are numerous sources of increased resistance within a breathing circuit, including valves, humidifying devices, and the inspiratory gas flow source, itself. Inspiratory circuit flow resistance has received the greatest attention during the last decade. Any decrease in airway pressure during the inspiratory phase of the respiratory cycle will increase work of breathing. The greater the change in inspiratory airway pressure, the greater the work of breathing. Such a decrease in airway pressure may result from a variety of circuit deficiencies. One-way valves, acute angles, narrow bore tubing, etc. all will increase resistance to gas flow and create undesirable fluctuation in airway pressure during inspiration. Since most ventilator circuits include a humidifier, strict attention must be given to this source of resistance. Many humidifiers are designed to create turbulent gas flow and air is forced through a fine mesh screen in order to increase surface area and improve efficiency of humidification. Such humidifiers are acceptable when the increase in work of breathing is performed by a mechanical ventilator. However, they are unacceptable for use during spontaneous respiration. Currently, "wick-type" humidifiers are preferable. They are efficient and have little, or no, flow resistance. In addition, they are capable of humidifying very large volumes of gas at rapid flow rates.(6)

Less attention has been given to expiratory circuit resistance characteristics, in terms of inspiratory work of breathing. Whenever a rapid flow of gas is forced by a resistance, an increase in airway pressure will result. A decrease in flow then will cause a decrease in airway pressure. Thus, during spontaneous inspiration gas is diverted from the expiratory valve to the patient causing a decrease in CPAP level. Therefore, an increase in work of breathing will occur, secondary to expiratory circuit resistance. For this reason, only exhalation-PEEP valves with low flow resistance should be utilized. Unfortunately, most such valves have a high flow resistance and may result in an unacceptable work of breathing for the patient.(7)

The final consideration for IMV circuitry requires some historical perspective. Initially, IMV was introduced as a weaning technique.(1) Therefore, the original IMV circuit resulted from a circuit conversion using a mechanical ventilator circuit and T-Piece apparatus. A one-way valve

was used to connect the two circuits, such that spontaneous
inspiratory efforts by the patient opened a one-way valve
and generated a flow of gas from the T-Piece to the patient.
Thus, the mechanical ventilator and the weaning circuit were
joined. However, such a circuit should not be utilized when
PEEP is applied. In order for the patient to inhale, a
significant decrease in airway pressure must result in order
to open the one-way valve connected to the T-Piece. The
work of breathing is unacceptable whenever PEEP excedes 5 cm
H_2O. In order to decrease the work of breathing created
with the initial circuitry, a continuous flow of gas was
directed through the one-way valve, past the patient's
trachael tube and past the PEEP valve. As long as the
continuous flow of gas exceeded the patient's peak
inspiratory flow rate at all times, it was felt that there
would little or no decrease in inspiratory airway pressure.
However, because of expiratory flow resistance, it soon was
realized that even extremely high continuous flow rates
would not prevent significant decrease in inspiratory airway
pressure. In addition, various elastic reservoirs were
added to the inspiratory circuit, to decrease the need for
high continuous flows of gas. Currently, Venturi devices
have been utilized to prevent excessive use of compressed
gas and to decrease the need for an inspiratory gas
reservoir. When combined with a threshold resistor CPAP
valve, such circuits create minimal increase in work of
breathing.

Demand valves have been used for years in respiratory
care devices. For the last ten years, manufacturers have
attempted to utilize demand valves to provide gas flow
during spontaneous inspiration with IMV. Unfortunately,
these valves have sufficient insensitivity and inertia to
create an undesirable increase in the inspiratory work of
breathing. Many such devices have inadequate peak flow.
Therefore, patients have a sense of flow restriction
during inspiration and may become agitated and tachypneac.

Clearly, this represents an equipment failure, not failure
of the technique. Hopefully, manufacturers will respond to
these deficiencies and create appropriate equipment in the
future.(8)

IMV is a controversial ventilatory technique. However,
much of the controversy has resulted from lack of
understanding of the equipment and the physiologic basis for
its' application. When properly applied, with appropriate
equipment, to the appropriate patients, in the appropriate
clinical setting, IMV has increased the safety and efficacy
of respiratory therapy.

1. Downs JB, Klein EF Jr, Desautels D, Modell JH, Kirby RR: Intermittent mandatory ventilation: A new approach to weaning patients from mechanical ventilators. Chest 64:331-335, 1973.

2. Kirby RR, Downs JB, Civetta JM, Modell JH, Dannemiller FJ, Klein EF, Hodges M: High level positive end-expiratory pressure (PEEP) in acute respiratory insufficiency. Chest 67:156-163, 1975.

3. Petty TL: IMV vs. IMC. Chest 67:630, 1975.

4. Downs JB: Inappropriate applications of IMV, letter to the editor. Chest 78:897, 1980.

5. Venus B, Smith RA, Mathru M: National Survey of Methods and Criteria Used for Weaning From Mechanical Ventilation. Crit Care Med 15:530-533, 1987.

6. Poulton TJ, Downs JB: Humidification of rapidly flowing gas. Crit Care Med 9:59-63, 1981.

7. Banner MJ, Downs JB, Kirby RR, Smith RA, Boysen PG, Lampotang S: Effects of Expiratory Flow Resistance on Inspiratory Work of Breathing. Chest 93: p. 795-797, 1988.

8. Downs JB: Inappropriate applications of IMV, letter to the editor. Chest 78:897, 1980.

WEANING FROM VENTILATORY SUPPORT

JOHN B. DOWNS, M.D.

Department of Anesthesiology, The University of South
Florida College of Medicine, Tampa, Florida 33612

Weaning from various forms of respiratory support
usually is a technically simple task. However, occasionally
a patient may appear resistant to attempts to discontinue
mechanical ventilation, or continuous positive airway
pressure (CPAP), and may become persistently hypoxemic when
the fractional concentration of inspired oxygen (FIO_2) is
reduced. Unfortunately, conventional methods for
discontinuing respiratory support often have not provided a
methodical means of weaning patients and rarely were
conventional methods based on sound physiologic principles.
Therefore, weaning is often a subjective process which may
compromise patient care. The following approach represents
one way that successful discontinuation of respiratory
support may be systematically approached.

Oxygen

An increased FIO_2 is usually delivered to relieve
arterial hypoxemia. Most commonly, patients have arterial
hypoxemia secondary to low, but finite,
ventilation/perfusion ratios (V_A/Q) in some areas of the
lung. The arterial hypoxemia produced by low V_A/Q is
worsened by a low FIO_2 and is usually alleviated when oxygen
is added to the inspired gas. Diffusion of oxygen from
alveoli to pulmonary capillary blood also may be impaired.
Such a "diffusion defect" is rarely the only cause of
arterial hypoxemia, but may contribute to it, especially
when FIO_2 is low. Right-to-left intrapulmonary shunting of

277

T. H. Stanley and R. J. Sperry (eds.), Anesthesia and the Lung, 277–293.
© *1989 by Kluwer Academic Publishers.*

blood will decrease oxygen tension, even when the FIO_2 is elevated. Therefore, oxygen therapy is of little value in treating this condition, but it may be beneficial in treating hypoxemia when it is secondary to the other abnormalities.

In spite of the frequency with which oxygen is used to treat hypoxemia, methods to discontinue such therapy have received little attention. Recent evidence suggests that rapid discontinuation of oxygen may be indicated not only to prevent pulmonary toxicity but also to improve the pulmonary function of gas exchange. West(26) suggested that areas of the lung with very low V_A/Q may collapse when the FIO_2 is increased, even to levels as low as 0.30. Suter,(24) Douglas,(9) and their colleagues have demonstrated that intrapulmonary shunting of blood increases when the FIO_2 exceeds 0.6 for more than a few minutes; therefore, rapid reduction of FIO_2 appears to be desirable to improve pulmonary function. Certainly we can no longer consider it therapeutic or safe to give up to 50 percent oxygen to patients for weeks at a time.

Oxygen administration also can impair the evaluation of pulmonary function. Often patients who have arterial hypoxemia when breathing room air have areas of lung with low but finite V_A/Q. Evaluating pulmonary function in such patients when they are receiving an elevated FIO_2 might lead to incorrect conclusions since administration of as little as 30 percent oxygen may mask the hypoxemia-producing effect of low V_A/Q areas. For example, a patient with a PaO_2 of 70 torr and an FIO_2 of 0.4 may be considered adequately oxygenated. The clinician might then decide to wean the patient from mechanical ventilation and positive end-expiratory pressure (PEEP). However V_A/Q could be mismatched to such a degree that an FIO_2 decreased to 0.3 might cause the PaO_2 to fall below 50 torr. Were the clinician aware of this abnormality, he or she would probably increase PEEP rather than decrease it, to achieve early weaning. Such evaluations are possible only when FIO_2 is low.

For these reasons, it is best to use the lowest possible FIO_2 to maintain the PaO_2 between 60 and 80 torr. This practice maximizes inspired and alveolar nitrogen concentrations. An elevated nitrogen concentration in the alveoli minimizes absorption atelectasis and may decrease the need for PEEP. A decrease in FIO_2 also may increase hypoxic pulmonary vasoconstriction, thus promoting better matching of VA and Q. In addition, since the hypoxemia-producing effect of low, but finite, V_A/Q is more apparent when FIO_2 is decreased, the clinician is better able to evaluate the resolution of pathological conditions producing such effects.

CPAP

Four decades ago, Barach and associates (4) recognized that respiration with an elevated airway pressure often was therapeutic. They elevated airway pressure with a motor-driven blower and an expiratory valve, both of which were connected to the patient's airway with a face mask. This technique, continuous positive pressure breathing (CPPB), was found to decrease pulmonary edema in congestive heart failure. In 1945, Burford and Burbank(5) recommended that CPPB be used to treat pulmonary edema secondary to traumatic lung injury. In 1952, Jensen(17) used CPPB to treat pulmonary contusion in patients with flail chest injuries. Thus, there was ample historical precedent for applying elevated airway pressures to patients breathing spontaneously. However, treatment of lung injuries with mechanical ventilation in the early 1960's and emphasis on controlled mechanical ventilation (CMV) by Ashbaugh, Petty and Bigelow(2) effectively discredited CPPB as a useful form of therapy. Because of the emphasis on mechanical ventilation, most of the literature during the last decade has recommended that mechanical ventilatory support be discontinued only after the need for PEEP has been alleviated. Thus, weaning patients from PEEP has come to depend on the discontinuation of mechanical ventilatory support. However, this dependence may be inappropriate in some patients. In patients with acute respiratory failure, functional residual capacity (FRC), lung compliance, and arterial oxygenation frequently fall. Work-of-breathing, which largely depends on lung compliance, usually increases in patients with acute respiratory failure. In fact, this increase in work-of-breathing led many clinicians to believe that CMV should be instituted. However, we have taken a different approach to this problem. CPAP can increase FRC and lung compliance. Therefore, CPAP applied during spontaneous respiration can decrease work-of-breathing in some patients with acute respiratory failure.(8) The increase in FRC also may improve V_A/Q and arterial oxygenation, which will reduce the requirement for increased FIO_2. Therefore, CPAP may reduce the requirements for mechanical ventilatory support and increased FIO_2. For these reasons we prefer to wean patients from mechanical ventilation and oxygen, before removing CPAP.

Even though the application of PEEP, like oxygen therapy, has been widely discussed for more than four decades, relatively.little attention has been directed toward the mechanics of weaning patients from PEEP. For this reason, much of the following discussion is based on theory and preliminary data.

The clinician would like to insure that a reduction in PEEP will not cause FRC to fall below normal. A decline in FRC may decrease V_A/Q in some regions of the lung and cause arterial oxygenation to deteriorate. Since lung compliance is volume dependent, it likely will decrease if FRC decreases, thereby altering respiratory mechanics. Each of these effects should be evaluated separately. A small reduction in PEEP could cause a large fall in FRC and deterioration of blood-gas exchange, with or without a change in compliance. The changes in FRC and PaO_2 are probably completed within one or two minutes after a change in PEEP. Therefore, PEEP should be withdrawn in decrements of 2 cm H_2O and the effect of PEEP on gas exchange evaluated within minutes of the addition or removal of PEEP.(22) Significant deterioration in lung mechanics or gas exchange indicates that CPAP should be restored to the previous level.

The effect on respiratory mechanics of discontinuing PEEP may best be evaluated when the patient is breathing spontaneously. By multiplying lung-thorax compliance by the amount that PEEP was altered, the clinician can roughly estimate the change in FRC after a reduction in PEEP. However, when PEEP is reduced, the pressure-volume curve of the respiratory system may shift to the right, decreasing lung-thorax compliance thereby invalidating the estimate of change in FRC. When lung compliance decreases, a lower intrapleural pressure is needed for tidal breathing. Thus, the decreased lung compliance increases the work-of-breathing, and the greater negativity of intrapleural pressure may cause subcostal, suprasternal, or intercostal retractions that can be observed clinically. To minimize the work-of-breathing, the patient will inhale with a smaller tidal volume (V_T) and will increase the respiratory rate in an effort to maintain adequate alveolar ventilation. Thus, after a change in CPAP, the respiratory rate, V_T, and physical appearance of the patient should be observed closely. Since pulmonary mechanics may be altered without a change in blood-gas exchange, and vice versa, both aspects of pulmonary function should be evaluated separately. Deterioration in mechanics or gas exchange should be considered a contraindication to further reduction of PEEP.

There are two technical problems in weaning patients from PEEP that deserve attention. It is imperative that blood-gas exchange be evaluated when FIO_2 is constant because calculated physiological shunt fractions vary at different concentrations of inspired oxygen.(9) Fractional concentrations of oxygen of less than 0.4 tend to unmask the hypoxemia-producing effect of low but finite V_A/Q in the lung.

An FIO_2 of 0.4 usually minimizes venous admixture, but when the FIO_2 is greater than 0.4, venous admixture may increase. This FIO_2 dependent variability of venous admixture must be considered during weaning. For example, assume that a patient has a calculated venous admixture of 25 percent of the cardiac output with an FIO_2 of 0.3 and only 15 percent with an FIO_2 of 0.4. If the clinician reduces PEEP while the patient breathes an FIO_2 of 0.3, venous admixture could increase to 30 percent, indicating a deterioration in pulmonary function. Further reductions in PEEP are contraindicated. However, if PEEP is decreased and the FIO_2 is simultaneously increased to 0.4, venous admixture could be 20 percent. The clinician might erroneously conclude that the reduction of PEEP is well tolerated when, in fact, the patient's pulmonary status has greatly deteriorated. Thus one must always evaluate pulmonary function while FIO_2 is constant and low.

In order to evaluate pulmonary mechanics accurately, the clinician must be sure that respiratory resistance is minimal and that spontaneous respiration is adequate. Respiratory resistance is best minimized with a continuous flow of gas or a sensitive demand valve in the inspiratory circuit of the ventilator; either will prevent inspiratory airway pressure from decreasing significantly during spontaneous inspiration. Decreased inspiratory airway pressure requires a greatly decreased intrapleural pressure.(23) Thus retractions can occur and may erroneously suggest a deterioration in pulmonary function. Therefore, to insure that spontaneous respiration is sufficient to allow accurate evaluation of pulmonary mechanics, the clinician should begin to wean the patient from PEEP only when the mechanical ventilator rate is low enough to insure that there is a pronounced respiratory effort. In most instances, weaning should not be attempted until the respiratory rate includes fewer than 2 or 3 mechanical breaths per minute.

As Robert Kirby recognized in 1971, IMV allows patients to be weaned from PEEP independent of their requirement for mechanical ventilatory support, oxygen therapy, or both.(19) In addition, applying PEEP to the airway pressure pattern may reduce the amount of oxygen and mechanical ventilatory support needed, so PEEP actually may help to wean the patient from oxygen and mechanical ventilation.

Intermittent Mandatory Ventilation

For many years, mechanical ventilation was reserved for patients unable to breathe spontaneously because of neuromuscular dysfunction. Weaning these patients from the mechanical ventilator is often straight-forward. Once they are able to breathe spontaneously without a deterioration in arterial pH secondary to respiratory acidosis, mechanical ventilation may be discontinued safely; weaning from mechanical ventilation is rarely a problem. However, during the last few decades, clinicians have begun to favor the use of mechanical ventilation for patients with inadequate arterial oxygenation and increased work-of-breathing. Many of these patients have no difficulty eliminating CO_2 while breathing spontaneously. Thus, classic criteria for initiating mechanical ventilation, and later for a trial of spontaneous respiration based on respiratory strength and drive, are not applicable to such patients. Without specific guidelines for patients with acute respiratory failure, the decision to initiate and terminate mechanical ventilatory support is often subjective and, consequently, difficult. However, such difficulty can be avoided if

mechanical ventilation is reserved for patients unable to
sustain adequate spontaneous respiration (i.e., those who
suffer acidemia during spontaneous respiration). Thus, we
supply IMV at a rate that will just prevent acidemia, and
weaning may be achieved by lowering that rate in decrements,
as long as acidemia does not occur. Once mechanical
ventilation has been completely discontinued without
acidemia, the patient is considered weaned. It is important
to emphasize the difference between acidemia and respiratory
acidosis, which can occur with a normal arterial pH when
$PaCO_2$ is chronically increased.

For many years, clinicians believed that compensatory
respiratory acidosis did not occur in conscious persons.
However, we have treated several patients with $PaCO_2$
elevated to maintain a normal arterial pH. Therapy
initiated to correct the metabolic alkalosis results in the
prompt reduction of $PaCO_2$, indicating that some patients are
hypoventilating in order to maintain a more normal arterial
pH and are able to breathe well enough to prevent
respiratory acidosis. For this reason, we do not use $PaCO_2$
as the primary index of the patient's ability to maintain
spontaneous respiration, or as the sole criterion for
reduction of the IMV rate. Rather, we continue to reduce
the rate of IMV as long as arterial pH remains greater than
7.35. In this way, we can wean patients rapidly from
mechanical ventilatory support, even when serious metabolic
alkalosis is present.

By promoting spontaneous respiration and expedient
termination of mechanical ventilation, IMV may avoid several
problems observed in conventional therapy.(15)
Occasionally, during prolonged mechanical ventilatory
support, patients develop a psychological dependence upon
the ventilator that may cause weaning problems. Those
allowed to breathe spontaneously throughout the period of
ventilatory support apparently do not develop such
dependence.(13) In addition, for reasons that are not

clear, a pronounced discoordination of the respiratory muscles may occur in patients who have prolonged mechanical ventilatory support. Some reports have indicated that almost all patients requiring ventilatory support for more than 24 hours develop discoordination of abdominal and accessory muscles of respiration.(6) Such discoordination may be great enough to prevent adequate spontaneous respiration and may prolong dependence on the ventilator. Our impression has long been that this discoordination does not occur in patients who breathe spontaneously throughout their treatment with IMV. Recently, Andersen and associates(1) confirmed the absence of respiratory muscle discoordination in patients who received IMV.

Controversy has arisen about whether IMV will permit weaning more quickly than can conventional weaning techniques. We designed a prospective investigation to determine the efficacy of IMV criteria compared with traditional criteria for weaning patients from mechanical ventilatory support. The study involved 30 patients who required short-term postoperative mechanical ventilatory support.(20) Inspiratory pressure, vital capacity, arterial pH, and $PaCO_2$ were recorded every 15 minutes after mechanical ventilatory support was initiated. The ventilator rate was decreased as long as arterial pH was greater than 7.35. When inspiratory occlusion pressure was less than 20 cm $H2O$ and vital capacity was greater than 15 ml/kg, mechanical ventilation was completely discontinued, and 30 minutes later all measurements were repeated. If respiratory acidosis occurred during the 30 minute trial with a T-piece, results based on traditional criteria were considered false positives. If patients breathed spontaneously and had an arterial pH greater than 7.35 before they could generate the necessary peak inspiratory pressure or vital capacity, IMV criteria were considered to have allowed weaning sooner than did the traditional

criteria. If patients met traditional criteria and were
able to breathe spontaneously while they had an arterial pH
greater than 7.35, there was no difference between the two
criteria in the time needed to wean patients. We found that
traditional criteria falsely predicted the ability to wean 5
patients who subsequently became acidemic after breathing
spontaneously. These patients had received narcotics and
had depressed respiratory drive, but they had adequate
neuromuscular function to generate the required peak
inspiratory pressure and vital capacity. Discontinuation of
mechanical ventilatory support was tolerated by 21 patients
before they were able to generate adequate peak inspiratory
pressure and vital capacity. Therefore, IMV results in
faster and safer weaning for the majority of postoperative
patients who require ventilatory support.

Specific Therapy

Although many of the necessary decisions are made
subjectively, the ventilatory care of patients with
respiratory failure has become rather standard. Initially,
oxygen may be added to the inhaled gas to alleviate arterial
hypoxemia. If a satisfactory arterial oxygen tension is not
achieved, the trachea frequently may be intubated and
mechanical ventilation instituted. If an adequate PaO_2 is
still not obtained, a somewhat arbitrary amount of PEEP may
be added. Classically, weaning from mechanical support
proceeds in reverse fashion. First, PEEP is decreased in
decrements as long as PaO_2 remains satisfactory and inspired
oxygen nontoxic. After successful removal of PEEP, the
patient is encouraged to breathed spontaneously from a
T-piece for increasingly longer periods. Once totally
spontaneous respiration is satisfactory, patients are
extubated and an elevated FIO_2 administered to prevent
arterial hypoxemia from recurring. Eventually, patients are
weaned from oxygen and allowed to breathe room air

spontaneously. Use of IMV for primary ventilatory support has allowed revamping and standardizing of the weaning process in such a way that it proceeds in a more objective and efficient fashion.

In general, patients suffering acute respiratory failure require mechanical ventilatory support, CPAP, and oxygen therapy. After patients are orotracheally intubated, we provide mechanical ventilatory support that will supply nearly 100 percent of the required alveolar minute ventilation. Initially, to treat arterial hypoxemia, an elevated FIO_2 is administered. Pulmonary mechanics and gas exchange are evaluated and CPAP is titrated to minimize abnormalities. Once the optimal CPAP is obtained, mechanical ventilation is reduced as long as arterial blood pH remains greater than 7.35. Simultaneously, the FIO_2 is reduced to a level that will maintain PaO_2 between 60 and 80 torr. Finally, CPAP is reduced in 2 cm H_2O decrements, and when gas exchange and mechanics are considered adequate, the patient is extubated. It is important to note that patients are weaned first from mechanical ventilation and last from CPAP. This order reverses the standard mode of therapy previously discussed. In addition, CPAP is titrated to produce the desired response. Recently, we have found that many patients can be treated with CPAP applied with a mask. In such patients tracheal intubation and mechanical ventilation may be unnecessary. This approach may not apply to all patients. Specific therapy for those who have had a major operation, who have chest trauma, or acute exacerbation of chronic obstructive pulmonary disease (COPD) may require alteration based on physiologic principles.

Many patients who receive mechanical ventilation have undergone major operations. They usually have little or no underlying lung disease, but they may require mechanical ventilation and O_2 therapy for a short time because of the effects of anesthesia and/or the operation. Initially, we provide these patients with 100 ml/kg/min of total minute ventilation.(14) Since they usually have no problem with arterial oxygenation, the initial FIO_2 is 0.3. A PEEP of 5 cm H_2O is added to the expiratory limb of the ventilator circuit. An arterial blood sample is analyzed, gas exchange is evaluated, and the setting of the ventilator is changed accordingly within 10 minutes of the time mechanical support is instituted. The rate of ventilation is adjusted to the point where it prevents acidemia. To calculate the FIO_2 needed to achieve a desirable PaO_2, the fraction FIO_2/PaO_2 is multiplied by the desired PaO_2. This fraction is relatively constant and is independent of the O_2 concentration inspired as long as PaO_2 is greater than 100 torr.(16) As the patient recovers from the sedatives, narcotics, and muscle relaxants used for anesthesia, the ventilator rate is reduced rapidly. When arterial oxygenation is adequate with an FIO_2 of 0.3 and PEEP of 5 cm H_2O, and arterial pH is greater than 7.35 without ventilatory assistance, the patient is considered to be weaned from supplemental oxygen, PEEP, and mechanical ventilation. As mentioned previously, the use of IMV for managing such patients has decreased the period of mechanical ventilatory support slightly and has probably made weaning safer.

Ventilatory management of patients with acute respiratory failure and a sharp decrease in FRC and lung compliance is more difficult. Occasionally, lung compliance may deteriorate so much that patients cannot support adequate respiration and must receive mechanical ventilatory support. Even though mechanical support may be necessary at first, CPAP often lessens this need. CPAP may increase both FRC and lung compliance and reduce the work-of-breathing, so that only a very short period of mechanical ventilatory support is required. Thereafter, spontaneous respiration with CPAP and a slightly increased FIO_2 is usually the only therapy necessary. This approach may be beneficial in several respects. For example, weaning from mechanical

ventilatory support may occur within hours of its'
initiation.(7)

Patients who require CMV with PEEP often need
intravenous infusion of large amounts of fluid to stabilize
cardiovascular function.(21) Such intravascular fluid
loading may increase pulmonary capillary hydrostatic
pressure and cause deterioration in pulmonary function
secondary to an increase in lung water when weaning from
mechanical support is attempted. If spontaneous breathing
is allowed and mechanical ventilatory support is
discontinued as soon as possible, intravascular volume
expansion often is unnecessary and PEEP and oxygen may be
withdrawn more rapidly. In addition, pulmonary barotrauma
may occur less frequently during IMV than during CMV.
Barotrauma probably is caused by increased airway pressure
during mechanically supported inspiration. If patients are
weaned rapidly from mechanical ventilation, exposure to
elevated pressure in the airways and thus barotrauma may be
reduced. Available evidence suggests that barotrauma is
lessened when IMV, rather than CMV, is used.(12)

Since Avery, Morch, and Benson(3) introduced internal
pneumatic stabilization for patients with flail chest
injury, CMV has been the therapeutic mainstay for patients
with lung contusion and flail chest. Recently, however,
some clinicians have questioned the efficacy of such
therapy.(25) We believe that the treatment of patients with
severe chest trauma should be similar to that described for
patients with acute respiratory failure. But if the chest
wall is unstable, mechanical ventilatory support should not
be discontinued as rapidly. Patients with lung injury and
flail chest often cannot breathe spontaneously with ambient
airway pressure because of the sharp reduction in lung
compliance. However, as Burford(5) and Jensen(17)
recognized in 1945 and 1952, respectively, elevation of
airway pressure may increase FRC and lung compliance so that
mechanical ventilatory support is not necessary. In such

cases, stabilization of the chest wall occurs without CMV.
Thus, the appropriate function of mechanical ventilation in
the treatment of chest trauma should be to immobilize the
chest wall, but only until lung compliance improves enough
so that spontaneous respiration can occur without disruption
of unstable chest wall segments. In many instances,
mechanical ventilatory support can be discontinued within a
matter of hours. In some cases, the patient may require
support for three or four days. Only in the rarest cases,
when totally unstable chest wall segments make spontaneous
respiration ineffectual, is mechanical ventilatory support
necessary for more than a week.(10) These patients should
be weaned according to evaluation of gas exchange and
pulmonary mechanics.

Ventilatory support of patients with acute
exacerbation of COPD is difficult. These patients have a
high mortality, and their clinical course is often marked by
extreme fluctuation in blood pressure, barotrauma,
electrolyte balance, and other undesirable side effects of
mechanical ventilatory support.(18) Weaning them from
mechanical support often is hampered by respiratory and
metabolic alkalosis, malnutrition, and sedation. The
situation is further complicated by the fact that prolonged
mechanical ventilatory support decreases the patient's
chance of survival. For that reason, we choose not to let
patients "rest" with mechanical ventilatory support after it
is initiated. Within 24 to 48 hours, most have recovered
sufficiently from the cause of the acute crisis, so that a
rest is not necessary. Furthermore, controlling the
patient's respiration and administering sedatives to provide
such a rest often later leads to serious problems in
weaning. Therefore, clinicians who use IMV to manage the
ventilation of patients with COPD usually recommend that
sedatives and muscle relaxants be avoided. We have developed
the following clinical approach.

A patient with COPD often has a hypoxemic drive to

breathe. Therefore, the initial FIO_2 usually does not exceed 0.3. Spontaneous respiration is encouraged for as long as possible. If mechanical ventilation is required, the initial ventilator rate is low, in most cases no more than 2 or 3 breaths per minute, with a V_T of 10 ml/kg. This amount of support usually results in a low but consistent fall in $PaCO_2$ and an increase in arterial pH. In this manner, rapid reduction in $PaCO_2$ and alkalosis may be avoided.(11) COPD is usually accompanied by a large increase in FRC and lung compliance, so PEEP may not improve the V_A/Q. Once ventilatory support with a low FIO_2 has been instituted, a vigorous regimen of bronchodilation and tracheobronchial toilet can be maintained and, as the patient improves, the mechanical ventilator can be withdrawn rapidly. When the ventilator rate has been reduced to zero, the patient should be extubated quickly in order to restore normal glottic function as soon as possible.

Conclusion

Oxygen, CPAP, and mechanical ventilatory therapy should be administered to patients in varying amounts and should be removed gradually and independently. The method of determining optimal CPAP, oxygen concentration, and ventilation is not unlike that recommended for many other therapies. Fifteen years of prospective evaluation have demonstrated numerous clinical advantages of this technique, and relatively few complications have been associated with it. Reduced FIO_2 may promote resistance to atelectasis and allow rapid discontinuation of mechanical ventilation and CPAP. Similarly, optimal levels of CPAP may improve matching of ventilation and perfusion and assist lung mechanics, so that FIO_2 and mechanical ventilation may be reduced. Minimal mechanical ventilatory support eliminates iatrogenic respiratory alkalosis and weaning from ventilatory support may be initiated early. In turn, such

weaning minimizes the detrimental effects of mechanical
ventilation on acid-base balance and cardiovascular
function, as well as lessening barotrauma. We believe that
this approach has simplified the clinical management of
patients with compromised respiratory function and has
decreased their mortality.

1. Andersen JB, Kann T, Rasmussen JP, et al. Am Rev Respir Dis 117:89, 1978.
2. Ashbaugh DG, Petty TL, Bigelow DG, et al. J Thorac Cardiovasc Surg 57:31, 1969.
3. Avery EE, Morch ET, Benson DW. J Thorac Surg 32:291, 1956.
4. Barach AL, Martin J, Eckman M: Ann Intern Med 12:754, 1938.
5. Burford TH, Burbank B. J Thorac Surg 14:415, 1945.
6. Chiang H, Pontoppidan H, Wilson RS, et al. In Abstracts of the 1973 Annual Meeting of the American Society of Anesthesiologists. San Francisco, California, P 211, 1977.
7. Douglas ME, Downs JB. Chest 71:18, 1977.
8. Douglas ME, Downs JB. Anesth Analg (Cleve) 57:346, 1978.
9. Douglas ME, Downs JB, Dannemiller FJ, et al: Anesth Analg (Cleve) 55:688, 1976.
10. Downs JB. Arch Surg 113:903, 1978.
11. Downs JB, Block AJ, Vennum KB. Anesth Analg (Cleve) 53:437, 1974.
12. Downs JB, Chapman RL Jr. Chest 69:363, 1976.
13. Downs JB, Klein EF Jr. Chest 64:331, 1973.
14. Downs JB, Marston AW. Crit Care Med 5:112, 1977.
15. Downs JB, Perkins HM, Modell JH. Arch Surg 109:519, 1974.
16. Horovitz JH, Carrico CJ, Shires GT. Arch Surg 108:349, 1974.
17. Jensen NK. Dis Chest 22:319, 1952.
18. Kilburn KH. Ann Intern Med 65:977, 1966.
19. Kirby R, Robison E, Schultz J, et al. Anesth Analg (Cleve) 51:871, 1972.
20. Millbern SM, Downs JB, Jumper LC, et al. Arch Surg 113:1441, 1978.
21. Qvist J, Pontoppidan H, Wilson RS, et al. ANESTHESIOLOGY 42:45, 1975.
22. Rose DM, Downs JB, Heenan TJ. Crit Care Med 9:79, 1981.
23. Sturgeon CL Jr, Douglas ME, Downs JB, et al. Anesth Analg (Cleve) 56:633, 1977.
24. Suter PM, Fairley HB, Schlobohm RM. ANESTHESIOLOGY 43:617, 1975.
25. Trinkle JK, Richardson JD, Friends JL, et al. Ann Thorac Surg 19:355, 1975.
26. West JB. Anesth Analg (Cleve) 54:409, 1975.

ECMO: A VIEW FROM THE EAST

WARREN M. ZAPOL, M.D.

Department of Anesthesia, Massachusetts General Hospital, Boston, MA 02114

The membrane lung is an extracorporeal device for directly exchanging respiratory gases in blood (1). By preventing hypoxia and hypercapnea in some patients for days or weeks the membrane lung can sustain life while otherwise intolerable pulmonary damage heals. Lung repair will be made possible since bypass with the artificial lung relieves the patient's lungs of their primary burden of respiratory gas exchange and the handicaps of conventional ventilator therapy, high ventilator pressures and inspired oxygen tensions. Temporary circulatory assistance can also be delivered to assist the heart. In newborns with congenital diaphragmatic hernia after surgical repair or meconium aspiration and an unstable pulmonary circulation (pulmonary vasoconstriction and ductal shunting) partial venoarterial perfusion appears to improve survival rates (Fig.1)

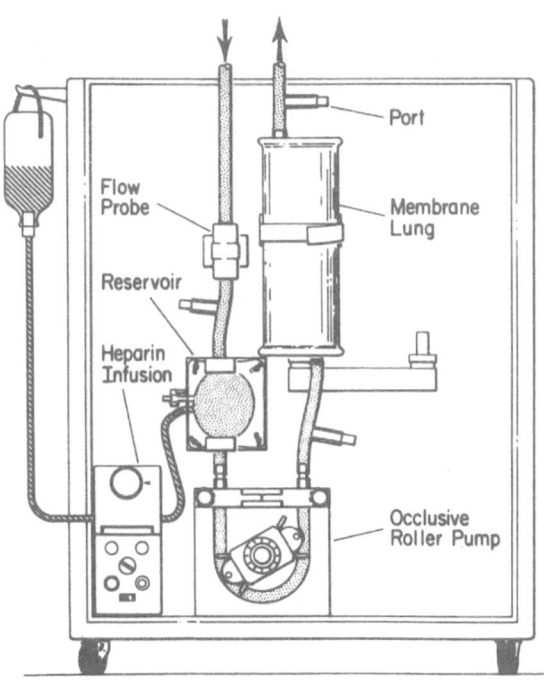

Fig.1 A simple circuit for adult clinical membrane oxygenation. (Reprinted with permission from Zapol WM et al: Anesthesiology 46: 272. 1977).

295

T. H. Stanley and R. J. Sperry (eds.), Anesthesia and the Lung, 295–301.
© 1989 by Kluwer Academic Publishers.

Indications:

    Adults - At present ECMO therapy is only useful for tiding patients over a week-long crisis of insufficient pulmonary gas exchange. The hope that large numbers of patients with respiratory failure due to septicemia or pneumonia would survive with ECMO support has proven fruitless and ECMO should not be used to treat such patients (2). Indeed the best use of ECMO is to tide patients over a brief crisis of insufficient gas exchange, especially when respiratory failure is provoked by reversible circulatory insufficiency. Acute pulmonary embolism is an excellent example of major respiratory embarassment with a reduced cardiac output, amenable to ECMO therapy if surgical embolectomy or thrombolytic therapy is undertaken. Another non-inflammatory cause of respiratory failure, e.g. severe hypoxemic pulmonary alveolar proteinosis unable to be lavaged with a double lumen tube, has been successfully treated with 36 hours of ECMO to support bronchoalveolar lavage. Other transient and reversible causes of cardiorespiratory failure can be successfully treated with ECMO (e.g. iatrogenic venous gas embolism) and such illnesses are now the only appropriate ones for ECMO therapy.

    Before ECMO is instituted for respiratory failure an adequate duration trial of conservative therapy with conventional mechanical ventilation, suctioning, chest physiotherapy, muscle paralysis, positive end-expiratory pressure, cardiotonics and diuretics must be given. However, evaluating the failure of conventional therapy and a decision to institute ECMO must be taken early, before oxygen toxicity, barotrauma and superinfection make attempts at ECMO futile. Most survivors of ECMO have been bypassed early in their course, after receiving a single reversible pulmonary insult. Although determining the reversibility of any pulmonary insult is difficult, several weeks of respiratory illness, extensive pulmonary or multi-organ pathological changes and advanced age make surviving ECMO for respiratory failure unlikely.

    Children - Success has been reported by Bartlett et al. with ECMO venoarterial bypass therapy for neonatal respiratory failure in infants weighing more than 2 Kg (3). These infants had persistent fetal circulation, meconium aspiration syndrome and congenital diaphragmatic hernia (CDH). These children were treated with ECMO after several different criteria were met for acute deterioration (P_aO_2 < 40 mm Hg or pH < 7.15 for 2 hrs), barotrauma, or CDH (P_aO_2 < 80 mm Hg at FIO_2 > 0.8 after honeymoon period) (Fig. 2).

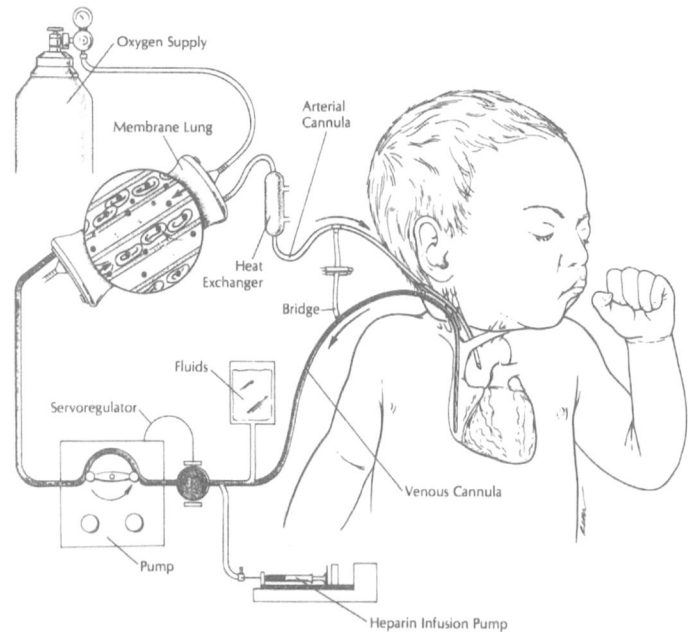

Fig. 2. Extracorporeal membrane oxygenator circuit. Cannulas draw blood from the right atrium and return it to the aorta, thereby functionally bypassing both lungs and heart. (Reprinted with permission from Bartlett RH: Hospital Practice, April 1984, p. 141).

Contraindications:

ECMO causes thrombocytopenia and requires heparin therapy and bleeding is a common complication. Some patients with recent abdominal surgery (< 24 hrs) have been bypassed successfully but patients with recent head trauma can develop intracerebral bleeding. There are reports of thoracic or abdominal surgery during ECMO but hemostasis is difficult to achieve without reducing heparin anticoagulation and clotting the ECMO circuit. Patients often cure their respiratory failure on ECMO but then die after disconnection of multiple organ failure, thus patients with renal or hepatic failure are unsuitable for ECMO. However, several ARDS patients have survived concomitant ECMO and hemodialysis or hemo-ultrafiltration.

In neonates an intracranial hemorrhage, age over 7 days or a concomitant condition incompatible with normal quality life are considered by Bartlett to be contraindications.

Types of ECMO:

Briefly two types of ECMO are in common use. Partial venovenous (VV) bypass and partial venoarterial (VA) bypass; both perfusion routes have advantages and disadvantages which must be weighed in each patient. Both routes can be performed with a single blood pump and a simple extracorporeal circuit (Figs.3 and 4).

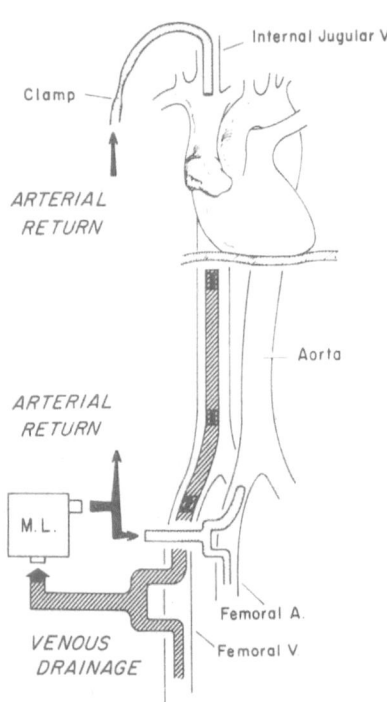

Fig. 3. Venovenous (VV) perfusion route. (Reprinted with permission from Zapol WM et al J Thorac Cardiovasc Surg 69:439, 1975).

VV bypass can be used in children and adults (4). VV or prepulmonary bypass allows the arterial tree to distribute oxygenated blood in a uniform pattern through the left ventricle. Venous blood is drained from the inferior vena cava through the common femoral vein and oxygenated blood returned to the superior vena cava. A double lumen catheter for both venous drainage and arterialized blood return to the thoracic inferior vena cava is available and simplifies VV perfusion to only a single femoral vein cannulation. This simplified cannulation allows blood flows of 2-3 L/min. VV perfusion can be used for infants draining the right atrium via the internal jugular vein and returning via the femoral vein, when possible below the sapheno-femoral junction. VV perfusion is believed best for adult perfusions for respiratory failure without cardiac failure since VV bypass does not reduce the pulmonary blood flow.

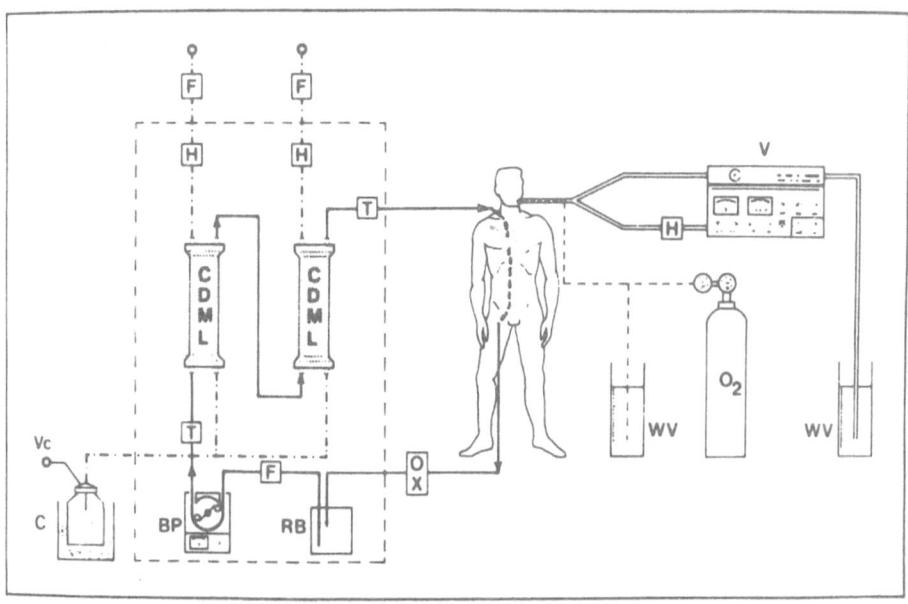

Fig. 4. Low-frequency positive-pressure ventilation with extracorporeal removal of CO_2. (Reprinted with permission from Gattinoni L et al: Lancet, August 9, 1980, p. 292).

VA bypass decreases pulmonary blood flow and requires large bore cannulation of the arterial circulation (Fig. 5). The major flaw of VA bypass is the inappropriate distribution of arterialized blood. Oxygenated blood returned to the distal aorta is distributed to kidneys, mesenteric bed and lower limbs. In severe ARDS we often see a combination of a large cardiac index, intrapulmonary shunt over 50% and a small A-V O_2 content difference. VA perfusion with distal aortic return is then ineffective to increase heart and brain P_aO_2 and proximal aortic cannulation is required. Bartlett et al. cannulates the internal carotid artery of neonates to improve cerebral oxygenation. VA bypass for newborn ECMO has been extensively explored in recent times and this route is recommended for this reason. VA bypass can support the heart by increasing the cardiac output and has been helpful to support adults with reversible right ventricular dysfunction or acute pulmonary embolism.

Results of Bypass:

About 40 adult patients have survived about 300 bypass procedures in my review of known cases (1986). The survivors are listed in Table I. The shock and trauma group provides the largest number of survivors. Although I cannot be certain

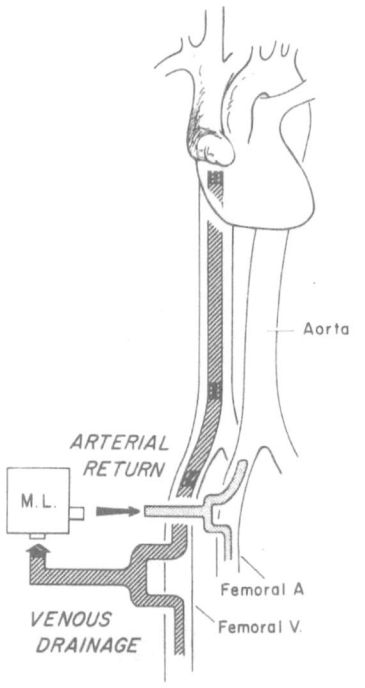

Fig. 5. Venoarterial
(VA) perfusion route
with femoral artery
cannulation and distal
aorta return.
(Reprinted with
permission from Zapol
WM et al: J Thorac
Cardiovasc Surg
69:439, 1975).

if these patients would not have survived with conventional
therapy, I am convinced by a number of my own patients that
hypoxemia and low cardiac output would have killed the patient
without buying time with an ECMO procedure. Clearly membrane
oxygenator perfusion can powerfully support gas exchange and
cardiac output. However each ECMO must be accompanied by
strenuous efforts to improve lung function and remove any
reversible causes of respiratory or cardiac failure (clot,
sepsis, etc.). Only by permanently reversing the natural lung
or heart injury in adults, or relieving the instability of the
pulmonary circulation in neonates can extracorporeal perfusion
with a membrane lung allow the natural organ to heal and the
patient to survive.

Table I

Reported Bypass Survivors with Adult Respiratory Distress
Syndrome to 1986

Disease	Survivors
Shock, trauma, fat embolism	11
Bacterial pneumonia, septicemia	8
Viral pneumonia	5
Cardiac failure after cardiac surgery	4
Goodpasture's syndrome	3
Pulmonary embolism	2
Drowning, inhalation injury	2
Varicella pneumonia	2
Pneumocystis carinii	2
Aspiration pneumonia	1
TOTAL	40

Surviving patients reported over 10 years of age from
approximately 250-300 adult bypass trials.

REFERENCES

1. Zapol WM and Qvist J eds. Artificial Lungs for Acute
    Respiratory Failure: Theory and Practice. New York:
    Academic Press, 1976.

2. Zapol WM, Snider MT, Hill JR, Fallat RJ, Bartlett RH,
    Edmunds LH, Morris AH, Peirce II, PC, Bagniewski A, and
    Miller, Jr, RG. Extracorporeal membrane oxygenation in
    severe acute respiratory failure: A randomized
    prospective study. J Am Med Assoc 1979; 242:2193-2196.

3. Bartlett RH, Roloff DW, Cornell RG, Andrews AF, Dillon PW,
    Zwischenberger JB. Extracorporeal circulation in neonatal
    respiratory failure: A prospective randomized study.
    Pediatrics 76:479-487, 1985.

4. Gattinoni L, Pesenti A, Mascheroni D, Marcolin R, Gumagali
    R, Rossi F, Iapichino G, Romagnoli G, Uziel L, Agostoni A,
    Kolobow T, Damia C. Low-frequency positive-pressure
    ventilation with extracorporeal CO_2 removal in severe
    acute respiratory failure. JAMA 256:881-886, 1986.